60 HIKES
WITHIN 60 MILES
3rd Edition

PHOENIX

Including Scottsdale, Glendale, and Mesa

Dedication

This book is dedicated to the loving memory of my mother, Mary Liu.

60 Hikes Within 60 Miles: Phoenix, Including Scottsdale, Glendale, and Mesa

Published by Menasha Ridge Press
Distributed by Publishers Group West
Third edition, fourth printing 2021

Project editor: Ritchey Halphen
Cover and interior design: Jonathan Norberg
Cover and interior photos: Charles Liu, except where noted
Cartography and elevation profiles: Scott McGrew and Charles Liu
Copy editor: Jackie Doyle

Cover photos: (Front) A stunning view of Battleship Mountain and Weaver's Needle from Boulder Canyon Trail in Superstition Wilderness (see Hike 28, page 151). (Back, top) A hiker explores Bell Pass Trail in Scottsdale's McDowell Sonoran Preserve (see Hike 15, page 90). (Back, bottom left–right) Picketpost Mountain rises steeply above desert plains near the town of Superior (see Hike 25, page 183); Superstition Mountains and the Flatiron loom over Siphon Draw Trail in Lost Dutchman State Park (see Hike 39, page 201); a hiker and companion enjoy Black Mesa Trail in Superstition Wilderness with Weaver's Needle in the distance (see Hike 27, page 146).

Library of Congress Cataloging-in-Publication Data

Names: Liu, Charles, 1968 June 27– author.
Title: 60 hikes within 60 miles, Phoenix : including Scottsdale, Glendale, and Mesa / Charles Liu.
Other titles: Sixty hikes within sixty miles, Phoenix
Description: 3rd edition. | Birmingham, Alabama : Menasha Ridge Press, 2018. | Includes index.
Identifiers: LCCN 2017050209| ISBN 978-163404-074-7 (pbk.) | ISBN 978-163404-075-4 (ebook)
Subjects: LCSH: Hiking—Arizona—Phoenix Region—Guidebooks. | Trails—Arizona—Phoenix Region—
    Guidebooks. | Phoenix Region (Arizona)—Guidebooks.
Classification: LCC GV199.42.A72 P485 2018 | DDC 796.5109791/73—dc23
LC record available at lccn.loc.gov/2017050209

MENASHA RIDGE PRESS
An imprint of AdventureKEEN
2204 First Ave. S, Ste. 102
Birmingham, Alabama 35233

Visit menasharidge.com for a complete listing of our books and for ordering information. Contact us at our website, at facebook.com/menasharidge, or at twitter.com/menasharidge with questions or comments. To find out more about who we are and what we're doing, visit our blog, blog.menasharidge.com.

DISCLAIMER This book is meant only as a guide to select trails in the Phoenix area and does not guarantee hiker safety in any way—you hike at your own risk. Neither Menasha Ridge Press nor Charles Liu is liable for property loss or damage, personal injury, or death that result in any way from accessing or hiking the trails described in the following pages.

Many out-of-town visitors and even seasoned hikers unaware of the dangers of desert hiking have needed to be rescued or even perished. Please be aware that summer temperatures can reach in excess of 115°F, posing serious threat of heatstroke, so stay hydrated, bring ample water, and avoid hiking in extreme temperatures. In addition, be especially cautious when walking on or near boulders, steep inclines, and drop-offs, and do not attempt to explore terrain that may be beyond your abilities.

To help ensure an uneventful hike, please read carefully the introduction to this book, and obtain further safety information and guidance from other sources. Acquaint yourself thoroughly with the areas you intend to visit before venturing out: familiarize yourself with current weather reports, maps of the area you intend to visit, and any relevant park regulations. Ask questions, and prepare for the unforeseen. Though every effort has been made to ensure the accuracy of the information in this book, be aware that prices, phone numbers, websites, and other information may change after publication.

60 HIKES WITHIN 60 MILES
3rd Edition

PHOENIX

Including Scottsdale, Glendale, and Mesa

Charles Liu

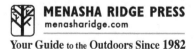

MENASHA RIDGE PRESS
menasharidge.com

Your Guide to the Outdoors Since 1982

60 Hikes Within 60 Miles: Phoenix

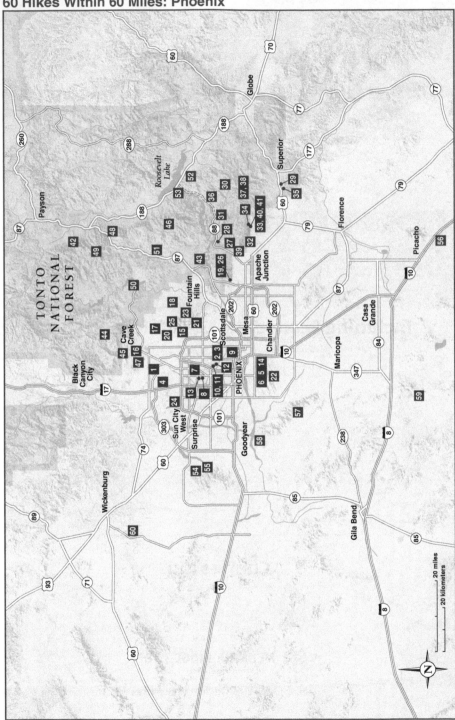

TABLE OF CONTENTS

WEST AND SOUTH
(Including White Tank and Sierra Estrella Mountains)   275

←→ ➡ Directional arrows	▬▬▬▬▬ Featured trail	·················· Alternate trail
═════ Freeway	═══╪═══ Highway with bridge	═════ Minor road
▪▪▪▪▪▪▪▪▪▪ Boardwalk	======= Unpaved road	•–•–•–•– Power line
Park/forest	Water body	River/creek/ intermittent stream

🜲 Amphitheater	✳ Garden	⊼ Picnic area
⛱ Beach	●– Gate	Playground
⊓ Bench	● General point of interest	Δ Primitive campsite
Boat launch	⑦ Information/kiosk	Radio tower
Δ Campground	✕ Mine/quarry	⫪ Restroom
Drinking water	⊥ Monument	Ruins
$ Fee station	▶ One-way (road)	Scenic view
Fishing	Park office/ranger station	○ Spring
¶¶ Food service	℗ Parking	Swimming access
✕ Footbridge	▲ Peak/hill	Trailhead
		// Waterfall/cascades

ACKNOWLEDGMENTS

When I was first presented with the prospect of tackling this project, I felt justifiably elated for such an incredible opportunity and yet equally concerned about the monumental task at hand. Phoenix is the fifth-largest city in the country, and there are hundreds of trails around it. To render adequate coverage and to choose the 60 best trails turned out to be more challenging than I had imagined. Thankfully, over the years I've developed an extensive network of avid hiking friends who are always willing to offer sage advice, trail companionship, and other assistance. Many have contributed to this book in a direct or subtle manner, and some have even done so unknowingly. For their help, I'm sincerely grateful.

The following individuals have contributed in specific ways. I would like to acknowledge them here in alphabetical order; please forgive any accidental omissions.

- **Lisa Cozzetti** provided valuable guidance on South Mountain National Trail and the Boulder Canyon Trail to LaBarge Box and Battleship Mountain.
- **John Daleiden** suggested combining Mormon Trail with the Hidden Valley Loop as an alternative to the popular National–Mormon Loop.
- **Pat Donahue** recommended Fish Creek for its superb scenery.
- **Amy Kemper** assisted with fact-checking and research on the second and third editions.
- **Carrie Behrens McKirchy** suggested the inclusion of Holbert Trail in South Mountain.
- **Skip and Zenda Treaster** brought Circlestone to my attention and gave fascinating insights on this remote archaeological treasure.

The following groups of people also contributed significantly:

A special recognition goes to members of the Take-A-Hike group for tagging along on my often-torturous hiking excursions and for volunteering as photo subjects on these trips.

I also owe a debt of gratitude to Dr. David Pheanis, John Daleiden, and Jim Garvey for writing letters of recommendation.

I'd like to thank Russell Helms, Tim Jackson, Molly Merkle, and the entire AdventureKEEN staff for entrusting me with this book and for providing seasoned advice and guidance.

Many thanks go to webmasters around the Phoenix area for publishing hike information, photos, and other related data. Some notable sources of valuable data include *The Arizona Republic;* HikeArizona.com; the Cities of Phoenix, Tempe, Scottsdale, and Glendale; Maricopa County; Arizona State Parks; the Bureau of Land Management; the U.S. Forest Service; and the National Park Service.

Last but not least, I'd like to acknowledge my family, Kelly Liu, Mary Liu, and Shaung Liu, for offering support in many ways during the writing and rewriting of this book.

—Charles Liu

FOREWORD

Welcome to Menasha Ridge Press's 60 Hikes Within 60 Miles, a series designed to provide hikers with the information they need to find and hike the very best trails surrounding metropolitan areas typically underserved by outdoor guidebooks.

Our strategy was simple: First, find a hiker who knows the area and loves to hike. Second, ask that person to spend a year researching the most popular and very best trails around. And third, have that person describe each trail in terms of difficulty, scenery, condition, elevation change, and all other categories of information that are important to hikers. "Pretend you've just completed a hike and met up with other hikers at the trailhead," we told each author. "Imagine their questions; be clear in your answers."

An experienced hiker and writer, Charles Liu has selected 60 of the best hikes in and around the Phoenix metropolitan area. From city parks and preserves that highlight the diverse Sonoran Desert landscape to rugged Central Arizona mountains and forests, Charles provides hikers (and walkers) with a great variety of hikes—and all within roughly 60 miles of Phoenix.

You'll get more out of this book if you take a moment to read the introduction explaining how to read the trail listings. The "Topographic Maps" section will help you understand how useful topos are on a hike and will also tell you where to get them. And though this is a "where-to," not a "how-to" guide, readers who have not hiked extensively will find the introduction of particular value.

As much for the opportunity to free the spirit as well as to free the body, let these hikes elevate you above the urban hurry.

All the best,
The Editors at Menasha Ridge Press

An acquaintance once questioned my hiking hobby: "So you like to wander around in the desert?" After chuckling at her sardonic observation, I had to explain that my obsession with hiking went far beyond the physical act of walking through the scenery. To me, hiking satisfies many mental, physical, and spiritual needs. This versatile activity is a means to elevate one's intellect as well as heart rate. It forges a bond between man and nature, instills confidence and increases awareness, promotes health and relieves stress, challenges the body, and sharpens the mind. Striking a balance between exercise and travel, hiking can take you to amazing places, where breathtaking vistas, deep canyons, emerald forests, open deserts, tranquil streams, and alpine mountaintops reward those who venture away from the comforts of their air-conditioned homes. Requiring very little up-front investment, hiking is perhaps the perfect hobby, suitable for all ages and any level of physical fitness. It's certainly much more than a walk in the desert!

Of course, I didn't always feel this way about hiking. Indeed, I spent many years living in the Grand Canyon State, oblivious to the wonders that lay in my backyard, before I began exploring the outdoors on foot. I'm embarrassed to admit that what really spurred me into action and kicked off a lifelong pursuit was a fit of hormone-driven teenage angst. Looking to burn off some frustration from "girl problems," I decided on a whim that climbing a mountain would do the trick and make me feel better. I had remembered some friends talking about hiking Piestewa Peak, which was known as Squaw Peak at the time, so I whipped my car around and headed toward the famous Phoenix landmark.

My inaugural hike began on a perfect autumn afternoon. I remembered that it was a cool and breezy day with a clear sky and some lingering clouds—an ideal setting for hiking. I found the trailhead and arrived wearing casual sport sandals, the wrong choice of footwear for the effort, but I didn't care. Charging uphill at full throttle, I quickly felt my chest constricting, my legs burning from lactic acid buildup, and my heart pounding in my throat. Despite the cool breeze, sweat was beading on my forehead and running down my face. That's when I realized that I hadn't brought any water. "What a rookie mistake!" I thought to myself as I labored to catch my breath.

I made it to the summit that day on sheer bravado of youth, and the physical exertion provided a complete catharsis for my woes. By the time I reached the top, I felt winded and spent, yet content. While resting on the rocky summit and admiring a panoramic view of the city some 1,200 feet below me, a perfect Arizona sunset began to play out its colorful drama in the western sky. *Wow!* I caught myself gasping out loud at the beauty of the moment. Some other hikers next to me also echoed their awe. Later that night, as I limped down the mountain in the dark with quivering legs and a parched tongue, I made a mental promise to hike again, and soon.

In general, it takes more than one perfect hike to christen a hiker, and I was no exception to the rule. Over the next few years, I stayed mostly within city limits and occasionally hiked around the islands of mountain preserves. Camelback Mountain became my favorite destination, and for good reason. It was the perfect in-town hike for my tastes. I loved the scenic red rocks, the challenging slope, the friendly fellow hikers, and of course the gorgeous sunsets from the summit. I looked forward to going there after work, to stretch my legs after a day of cubicle imprisonment, and to visit familiar faces on the mountain. Yes, I had slowly but surely begun the metamorphosis into a hiker. Camelback Mountain served as both trainer and proving ground, whipping me into shape and allowing me to test new techniques and gear. I had even developed a custom rating system for hikes, using the Echo Canyon Trail as a standard unit of measure. The transformation was nearly complete.

Then, in the summer of 1995, my experiences on a trip to the Grand Canyon not only validated my self-proclaimed moniker, "Mad Hiker," but accentuated hiking as my defining characteristic. A few friends and I gathered for a trip into the depths of the Grand Canyon, arguably the greatest place on Earth to hike. We ignored all posted warnings and rangers' advice and decided to hike down to the Colorado River and back in one day, a colossal death march of 17 miles with a mile of elevation gain. The challenge was irresistible.

I had visited the Grand Canyon numerous times before but had never stepped foot below the rim. The all-day trek proved more grueling than we could have imagined, but it was also a thrill ride played in slow motion. I realized that day while walking through the Canyon's grandiose splendor, examining its scenery up close and admiring hidden perspectives unseen from rim-side overlooks, that hiking allows me to participate in nature and to witness places that are otherwise unreachable. At the end of a torturous yet exhilarating day, peering back into the Canyon and retracing our steps with my eyes, I felt an overwhelming sense of joy, pride, and wonder. Despite aching muscles and blistered feet, I longed for more. I was addicted, head-over-heels in love with hiking.

Over the next three decades, I sought out increasingly challenging hikes and finally began to explore in earnest the wonders in my backyard. My reach stretched beyond city limits, extended to the rest of Arizona, and eventually broadened to the highest peaks in the western states and around the world. Hiking became a more serious endeavor because I made an extra effort to research each destination, its history, and what I might find along the way. I learned about the intricate ecosystems that make up the Sonoran Desert. I memorized the names of plants and wildflowers, of birds and butterflies, and even of snakes and lizards. I watched in amazement as the most delicate blossoms sprang from the prickliest plants. The more I learned, the more I felt in tune with my surroundings and the more I enjoyed each hike. Every hike became an opportunity to expand my understanding of the world, and I grew eager to share that newfound knowledge. This book is the vessel through which I shall attempt to share the treasures that exist just outside our doors—to help everyone discover what the Phoenix area has to offer.

Visitors from out of town sometimes tell me that before arriving in Arizona, they had imagined it to be a giant sand dune, much like movie scenes of the Sahara Desert. Nothing could be further from the truth. Arizonans are blessed with a wide range of climate zones, supporting rich variations in flora and fauna. If you take the time to study the desert closely, you'll see it teeming with life and buzzing with activity. With ample mountainous terrain nearby and 325 days of sunshine each year, the aptly named Valley of the Sun is ideally suited for outdoor activity.

The City of Phoenix spans a staggering 517 square miles and houses more than 1.5 million people, making it the fifth-largest city in the United States. Within its boundaries, Phoenix has three major mountain preserves where dozens of trails cater to the daily exerciser or the weekend warrior. South Mountain covers the entire southern border of Phoenix, while Piestewa Peak anchors a series of mountains in Phoenix Mountains Preserve. Developed in the late 2000s and early 2010s, Phoenix Sonoran Preserve comprises nearly 22,000 acres of pristine desert foothills. Camelback Mountain stands alone and dominates the central Phoenix skyline. Residents flock to these destinations to take in stunning views, socialize, and exercise.

Phoenix's suburbs also boast their share of parks, greenbelts, and preserves to serve more than 4.5 million residents in the metropolitan area. The City of Scottsdale and the McDowell Sonoran Conservancy in particular have made significant strides in conservation by purchasing state trust land in the McDowell mountain range and turning it into the largest municipal preserve in the country. New trails, trailheads, and access areas entice longtime Valley residents and newbies alike. The third edition of this book explores some new trails in the McDowell and Phoenix Sonoran Preserves. More are on their way in coming years, so check back soon.

Beyond the Valley of the Sun, a ring of rugged mountains awaits exploration. County and state parks provide excellent facilities and convenient access to the foothills trails on the fringes of the city. Tonto and Prescott National Forests encompass several key wilderness areas and hundreds of trails just a short drive from town, transporting hikers into a world that they might not expect to find near Phoenix— one of lush forests, quiet meadows, trickling mountain streams, and thrilling summits. Finally, a series of dams provides the strict water management necessary for desert living. The resultant reservoirs behind these dams also offer scenic settings for hiking and water-related recreation.

Whether you're a complete newbie without a pair of hiking shoes to your name or a seasoned veteran with hundreds of hikes under your belt, you'll likely find something worthwhile between the covers of this book. My hope is that the information provided here will guide you through your own discovery process and help enrich your hiking experience. The possibilities are endless, and this book is merely a beginning.

Happy hiking! —C. L.

60 HIKES BY CATEGORY

REGION / Hike Number/Hike Name	Page #	Mileage/Difficulty	Scenic	Multiuse	Running	Kid-Friendly	Solitude	Best for Dogs	Water Nearby	Fitness (Regular Workouts)	High Altitude (cooler)	Ruins/Petroglyphs	Wildlife	Wildflowers	Scrambling
CITY OF PHOENIX															
1 Apache Vista and Ridgeback Overlook	24	5.6/E–M	✓	✓	✓			✓		✓			✓	✓	
2 Camelback Mountain: Cholla Trail	29	3.8/M–S	✓							✓					
3 Camelback Mountain: Echo Canyon Trail	34	2.6/S	✓							✓					
4 Dixie Mountain Loop	39	5.1/M		✓	✓	✓		✓		✓			✓	✓	
5 Hidden Valley Trail via Mormon Trail	43	3.9/M	✓					✓							
6 Holbert Trail and Dobbins Lookout	47	5.4/M	✓	✓	✓			✓		✓		✓			
7 Lookout Mountain	52	1.1/M						✓		✓					
8 North Mountain National Trail	56	1.6/M	✓			✓		✓		✓					
9 Papago Park	60	2.2/E		✓	✓	✓		✓							
10 Piestewa Peak: Freedom Trail	64	3.8/M			✓					✓					
11 Piestewa Peak: Summit Trail	68	2.4/S	✓							✓					
12 Quartz Ridge Trail	72	4.7/M		✓	✓	✓		✓						✓	
13 Shaw Butte Trail	77	4.2/M						✓		✓					
14 South Mountain: National Trail	82	15.5/M	✓	✓								✓			
PHOENIX SUBURBS (Ahwatukee, Cave Creek, Glendale, Mesa, Scottsdale)															
15 Bell Pass and Windgate Pass Loop	90	9.5/M–S	✓	✓				✓		✓			✓		
16 Black Mountain	96	2.4/S						✓		✓					
17 Brown's Mountain Loop	100	4.1/E		✓	✓	✓		✓						✓	
18 McDowell Mountain Regional Park: Scenic Trail	104	4.5/E	✓	✓	✓	✓	✓	✓							
19 Pass Mountain Trail	108	7.5/E	✓	✓	✓			✓		✓			✓	✓	
20 Pinnacle Peak Trail	112	3.5/M		✓		✓									
21 Sunrise Trail	116	5/M	✓	✓		✓		✓							
22 Telegraph Pass Trail and Kiwanis Trail	121	2.4/E–M			✓	✓		✓		✓		✓		✓	
23 Thompson Peak via Dixie Mine Trail	126	9.4/S	✓				✓						✓		
24 Thunderbird Park: Cholla Loop	130	3.6/E–M		✓				✓		✓				✓	
25 Tom's Thumb	134	4.4/S						✓		✓					
26 Wind Cave Trail	139	3.2/M				✓		✓							
EAST (Including Superstition Wilderness)															
27 Black Mesa Loop	146	9.1/M	✓	✓	✓			✓					✓	✓	
28 Boulder Canyon Trail to LaBarge Box and Battleship Mountain	151	10.5/S	✓				✓		✓				✓	✓	✓
29 Boyce Thompson Arboretum: Main Trail	157	1.5/E				✓		✓							
30 Circlestone from Reavis Ranch	161	6.7/M	✓					✓	✓	✓		✓	✓	✓	
31 Fish Creek	165	3/M	✓					✓	✓				✓		✓
32 Hieroglyphic Trail	169	3/E				✓		✓	✓			✓			
33 Lost Goldmine Trail	174	6/E		✓	✓			✓	✓						
34 Peralta Trail	179	4.6/M	✓			✓		✓							
35 Picketpost Mountain	183	4.3/S	✓				✓							✓	✓
36 Reavis Falls	188	13.3/S	✓	✓			✓		✓				✓	✓	✓
37 Reavis Ranch via Rogers Trough Trailhead	192	15/M–S		✓				✓	✓	✓		✓	✓	✓	

#	REGION / Hike Number/Hike Name	Page #	Mileage/Difficulty	Scenic	Multiuse	Running	Kid-Friendly	Solitude	Best for Dogs	Water Nearby	Fitness (Regular workouts)	High Altitude (cooler)	Ruins/Petroglyphs	Wildlife	Wildflowers	Scrambling
EAST (Including Superstition Wilderness, *continued*)																
38	Rogers Canyon Trail	196	9/M	✓				✓	✓				✓	✓		
39	Siphon Draw Trail	201	6/S	✓							✓				✓	✓
40	Superstition Ridgeline	206	12.2/S	✓				✓						✓	✓	✓
41	Wave Cave	211	4/M				✓	✓								
NORTHEAST (Including Cave Creek and Mazatzal Mountains)																
42	Barnhardt Trail	218	14/M–S	✓	✓			✓	✓			✓			✓	
43	Butcher Jones Trail	223	5/E	✓		✓	✓	✓	✓							
44	Cave Creek Trail and Skunk Tank Trail	227	10.4/E–M		✓	✓	✓	✓	✓					✓		
45	Elephant Mountain Trail	232	9/M–S		✓			✓					✓	✓		
46	Four Peaks: Brown's Peak	237	5/M–S	✓				✓				✓				✓
47	Go John Trail	241	5.8/E–M		✓	✓			✓		✓					
48	Mount Ord	246	15.1/S		✓			✓				✓				
49	Mount Peeley	251	5/M	✓				✓				✓		✓	✓	
50	Palo Verde Trail	255	8.2/E–M	✓		✓	✓		✓	✓						
51	Pine Creek Loop and Ballantine Trail	259	8.8/M		✓			✓	✓					✓	✓	
52	Tonto National Monument: Upper Cliff Dwelling	264	2.4/E	✓									✓			
53	Vineyard Trail	268	6.1/M	✓	✓			✓						✓	✓	
WEST AND SOUTH (Including White Tank and Sierra Estrella Mountains)																
54	Ford Canyon Trail and Mesquite Canyon Trail	276	10.3/M			✓								✓	✓	
55	Goat Camp Trail and Willow Canyon Trail	280	11.5/S			✓								✓	✓	
56	Picacho Peak: Hunter Trail	285	3/S	✓										✓		✓
57	Quartz Peak Trail	289	6/S	✓				✓						✓		
58	Rainbow Valley Trail and Butterfield Trail	294	8.8/M		✓	✓		✓								
59	Table Top Trail	298	7.8/S	✓				✓					✓	✓	✓	
60	Vulture Peak Trail	302	4.2/M	✓				✓						✓		

DIFFICULTY RATINGS		
E = Easy	M = Moderate	S = Strenuous

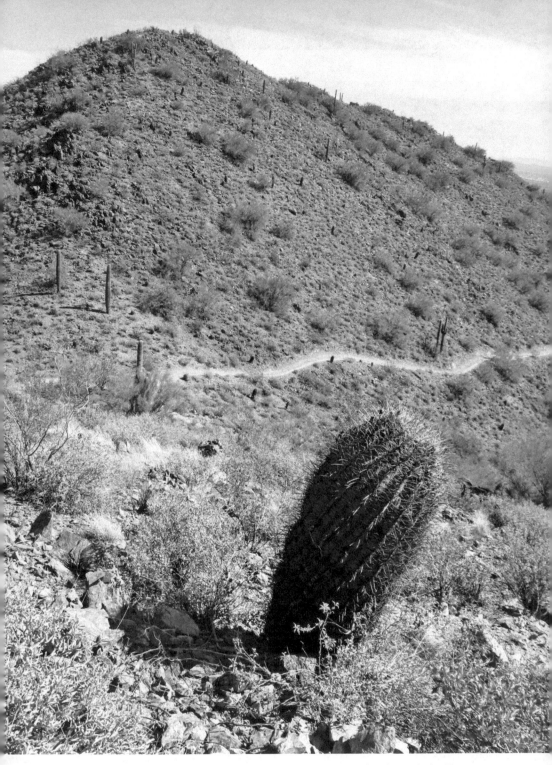

A barrel cactus often points south, earning its nickname "compass cactus." *Photo: Charles Liu*

INTRODUCTION

Welcome to *60 Hikes Within 60 Miles: Phoenix*. If you're new to hiking or even if you're a seasoned trekker, take a few minutes to read the following introduction. We explain how this book is organized and how to use it.

About This Book

Now in its third edition, this book strives to improve on prior releases. Its overall content and organization have been enhanced to make it the best guidebook for Phoenix-area hikes. Since the original publication and the second edition, new preserves have been created, new trails constructed, and some trails rerouted.

Also, in addition to updating information on existing hikes, many readers have provided valuable feedback on their experiences with these 60 hikes and the overall format of the book. Based on these suggestions, *60 Hikes Within 60 Miles: Phoenix* is now organized into five major geographic regions.

Phoenix is the only major city in the United States that contains several mountain ranges within its borders, as well as more than 100 hiking trails. For that reason, the first region is dedicated solely to the City of Phoenix—more specifically, the three mountain preserves within its borders and their scenic trails.

The next region focuses on the Phoenix suburbs, many of which have their own city parks and nature preserves. Scottsdale is especially noteworthy since it operates the McDowell Sonoran Preserve, the largest municipal preserve in the United States.

Surrounding the Valley of the Sun lies a ring of mountainous terrain. The remaining three regions of this book are dedicated to mountains in the East, including those in the expansive Superstition Wilderness; the Northeast, including the Cave Creek Mountains and Mazatzal Wilderness; and finally the West and South, including the Sierra Estrella and White Tank Mountains.

The 60 hikes in this book were carefully chosen for their overall appeal, covering a wide range of locations, hike profiles, terrain, and scenery. There are easy hikes, moderate loops, and long jaunts through the wilderness, along with some very challenging scrambles to thrilling summits. Look through the 60 Hikes by Category table (pages xiv–xv) to pick an adventure that suits your abilities and interests.

How to Use This Guidebook

The following section walks you through this guidebook's organization, making it easy and convenient for you to plan great hikes.

OVERVIEW MAP AND MAP LEGEND

Use the overview map on page iv, opposite the Table of Contents, to assess the general location of each hike's primary trailhead. Each hike's number appears on the overview map, in the table of contents, and on the regional maps (see below). As you flip through the book, a hike's full profile is easy to locate by watching for the hike number at the top of each left-hand profile page.

A map legend that details the symbols on trail maps is found on page viii.

REGIONAL MAPS

Prefacing each regional chapter is an overview map of that region. These maps provide more detail than the overview map at the beginning of the book, bringing you closer to the hikes.

TRAIL MAPS

A detailed map of each hike's route appears with its profile. On each of these maps, symbols indicate the trailhead; the complete route; significant features and facilities; and topographic landmarks such as creeks, overlooks, and peaks.

To produce these maps, I used a handheld GPS unit to gather data while hiking each route and then sent that data to Menasha Ridge's expert cartographers. Note, however, your GPS is no substitute for sound, sensible navigation that takes into account the conditions that you observe while hiking.

Further, despite the high quality of the maps in this guidebook, the publisher and I strongly recommend that you always carry an additional map, such as the ones noted in each entry's listing for "Maps."

ELEVATION PROFILE

Corresponding to the trail map, this graphical element depicts the rises and falls of the trail from the side, over the complete distance (in miles) of that trail. On the diagram's vertical axis, or height scale, the number of feet indicated between each tick mark lets you visualize the climb. To avoid making flat hikes look steep and steep hikes appear flat, varying height scales provide an accurate image of each hike's climbing challenge.

THE HIKE PROFILE

Each hike contains a brief overview of the trail, a description of the route from start to finish, key at-a-glance information—from the trail's distance and configuration to contacts for local information—GPS trailhead coordinates, and driving directions to the trailhead area. Each profile also includes a map (see "Trail Maps," above) and elevation profile. Many hike profiles also include notes on nearby activities.

IN BRIEF

Think of this section as a taste of the trail: a snapshot focused on the historical landmarks, beautiful vistas, and other sights you may encounter on the hike.

KEY INFORMATION

The information in this box gives you a quick rundown of the specifics of each hike.

DISTANCE & CONFIGURATION *Distance* notes the length of the hike round-trip, from start to finish. If the hike description includes options to shorten or extend the hike, those round-trip distances will also be factored here. *Configuration* defines the type of route—for example, a loop, an out-and-back (taking you in and out the same way), a point-to-point (or one-way route), a figure eight, or a balloon.

DIFFICULTY The degree of effort that the typical hiker should expect on a given route. For simplicity, the trails are rated as *easy, moderate,* or *strenuous.* Some trails straddle the line between difficulty ratings (*easy to moderate,* for instance).

SCENERY A short summary of the attractions offered by the hike and what to expect in terms of plant life, wildlife, natural wonders, and historical features.

EXPOSURE A quick check of how much sun you can expect on your shoulders during the hike.

TRAIL TRAFFIC Indicates how busy the trail might be on an average day. Trail traffic, of course, varies from day to day and season to season. Weekend days typically see the most visitors. Other trail users who may be encountered on the trail are also noted here.

TRAIL SURFACE Indicates whether the trail surface is paved, rocky, gravel, dirt, boardwalk, or a mixture of these.

HIKING TIME How long it takes to hike the trail. A slow but steady hiker will average 2–3 miles an hour, depending on the terrain.

WATER REQUIREMENT The minimum recommended amount of water to bring—don't count on finding drinkable water along the trail.

DRIVING DISTANCE The mileage from a familiar place—in this case, Phoenix Sky Harbor Airport. Not that you'd necessarily start from here, but the mileages should give you a good estimate of the travel time from where you live.

ELEVATION GAIN Lists the elevation in feet at the trailhead, plus the elevation of the high point on the trail (or a notation that there is no significant elevation change).

ACCESS Permits or fees required to hike the trail are detailed here—and noted if there are none. Trail-access hours are also listed here (access is daily unless otherwise specified).

MAPS Lists which supplementary maps are best for a particular hike. These generally consist of U.S. Geological Survey (USGS) and/or U.S. Forest Service (USFS) maps, along with maps provided by a particular park or preserve online or on-site.

FACILITIES Lists restrooms, water, picnic tables, and other basics available at or near the trailhead.

WHEELCHAIR ACCESS Lets you know if there are paved sections or other areas where persons with disabilities can safely use a wheelchair.

CONTACT Listed here are phone numbers and website addresses for checking trail conditions and gleaning other day-to-day information.

COMMENTS Here you'll find assorted nuggets of information, such as whether or not dogs are allowed on the trails.

DESCRIPTION

The heart of each hike. Here, the author provides a summary of the trail's essence and highlights any special traits the hike has to offer. The route is clearly outlined, including landmarks, side trips, and possible alternate routes along the way. Ultimately, the hike description will help you choose which hikes are best for you.

NEARBY ACTIVITIES

Look here for information on things to do or points of interest: nearby parks, museums, restaurants, and the like. Note that not every hike has a listing.

DIRECTIONS

Used in conjunction with the GPS coordinates, the driving directions will help you locate each trailhead. Once at the trailhead, park only in designated areas.

GPS TRAILHEAD COORDINATES

As noted in "Trail Maps," on page 2, I used a handheld GPS unit to obtain geographic data and sent the information to the publisher's cartographers. The trailhead coordinates—the intersection of latitude (north) and longitude (west)—will orient you from the trailhead. In some cases, you can drive within viewing distance of a trailhead. Other hiking routes require a short walk to the trailhead from a parking area.

This book lists GPS coordinates as latitude and longitude, in degree–decimal minute format. The latitude–longitude grid system is likely quite familiar to you, but here's a refresher:

Imaginary lines of latitude—called *parallels* and situated about 69 miles apart from each other—run horizontally around the globe. The equator is established to be 0°, and each parallel is indicated by degrees from the equator: up to 90°N at the North Pole, and down to 90°S at the South Pole.

Imaginary lines of longitude—called *meridians*—run perpendicular to latitude lines. Longitude lines are likewise indicated by degrees. Starting from 0° at the Prime Meridian in Greenwich, England, they continue to the east and west until they meet 180° later at the International Date Line in the Pacific Ocean. At the equator, longitude lines also lie approximately 69 miles apart, but that distance narrows as the meridians converge toward the North and South Poles.

As an example, the GPS coordinates for Hike 1, Apache Vista and Ridgeback Overlook (page 24), are as follows:

N33° 46.104' W112° 02.651'

To convert GPS coordinates given in degrees, minutes, and seconds to degrees and decimal minutes, as shown above, divide the seconds by 60. For more on GPS technology, visit usgs.gov.

TOPOGRAPHIC MAPS

The maps in this book have been produced with great care and, together with the hike text, will direct you to the trail and help you stay on course. You'll find superior detail and valuable information, however, in the USGS's 7.5-minute-series topographic maps (or topo maps for short). At mytopo.com and nationalmap.gov, for example, you can view and print free USGS topos of the entire United States. Online services such as Trails.com charge annual fees for additional features such as shaded relief, which makes the topography stand out more. If you expect to print out many topo maps each year, it might be worth paying for such extras.

The downside to USGS maps is that most are outdated, having been created 20–30 years ago; nevertheless, they provide excellent topographic detail. Of course, Google Earth (earth.google.com) does away with topo maps and their inaccuracies . . . replacing them with satellite imagery and its inaccuracies. Regardless, what one lacks, the other augments. Google Earth is an excellent tool whether you have difficulty with topos or not.

If you're new to hiking, you might be wondering, "What's a topo map?" In short, it indicates not only linear distance but elevation as well, using contour lines. These lines spread across the map like myriad intricate spiderwebs. Each line represents a particular elevation, and at the base of each topo a contour's interval designation is given. If, for example, the contour interval is 20 feet, then the distance between each contour line is 20 feet. Follow five contour lines up on the same map, and the elevation has increased by 100 feet.

In addition to the sources listed previously and in Appendix B, you'll find topos at major universities, outdoors shops, and some public libraries, as well as online at nationalmap.gov and store.usgs.gov.

WEATHER

Phoenix is notorious for its blistering summer heat. With the mercury routinely exceeding 110°F, Phoenicians often joke that they live next door to the devil. Peak temperatures occur from late June to mid-July before seasonal monsoons—annual weather disturbances that cause regular thunderstorms—bring some measure of relief. The scorching Arizona sun and oppressive heat can make being outside miserable and often downright dangerous.

Seasoned Phoenix residents have developed strategies to cope with their extreme climate, though. The relatively low humidity causes temperatures to drop significantly at night; therefore, veteran desert hikers take full advantage of cool early mornings and late evenings. They religiously apply sunblock and hydrate well before a hike. Many seek outings to higher elevations and near streams on the hottest days.

In contrast to its merciless summers, Phoenix boasts especially mild and pleasant weather in winter. Measurable snow occurs only once every 20 years in Phoenix. As a matter of fact, locals have coined the term "snowbirds" for the seasonal influx of winter visitors attempting to escape frigid conditions elsewhere in the country. Perpetually low humidity blesses Arizona with ample sunshine and accounts for its magnificent sunsets.

Phoenix receives an average of just 7 inches of rain per year, making it one of the driest regions in the country. That said, desert storms can be sudden and violent: flash floods, blinding dust storms (also known as *haboobs*), and rapidly changing temperatures can wreak havoc on anyone unprepared for monsoon conditions, which typically invade the Valley of the Sun from mid-July through mid-September. Winter rains are somewhat milder and occur between December and March, bringing life and color to desert plants that are poised to respond. Early spring is the most colorful time of year, when wildflowers blanket hillsides with splashes of gold, and fragrant citrus blossoms perfume the air.

The Sonoran Desert can be exquisitely beautiful but also unforgiving to those who are unprepared for its harsh realities. To hike safely in a desert environment requires knowledge and preparation; common sense doesn't hurt either. Bring plenty of water, apply ample sunblock, and always tell someone where you're going. Wilderness areas near Phoenix feature rugged and remote mountains that reach elevations in excess of 7,000 feet. Temperature extremes, sudden storms, and intense solar radiation are common at these altitudes. Whether visiting desert foothills in town or exploring remote mountain trails, hikers need to be aware of their environment and its risks, and come prepared with proper clothing and gear.

The chart at the top of the next page lists average temperatures and precipitation by month for the Phoenix metropolitan region. For each month, "Hi Temp" is the average daytime high (in degrees Fahrenheit), "Lo Temp" is the average nighttime low, and "Rain" is the average precipitation (in inches).

	January	February	March	April	May	June
HI TEMP	67°F	71°F	77°F	85°F	95°F	104°F
LO TEMP	46°F	49°F	53°F	60°F	69°F	78°F
RAIN	0.91"	0.91"	0.98"	0.28"	0.12"	0.04"
	July	August	September	October	November	December
HI TEMP	106°F	104°F	100°F	89°F	76 F	66°F
LO TEMP	83°F	83°F	77°F	65°F	53°F	45°F
RAIN	1.06"	0.98"	0.63"	0.59"	0.67"	0.87"

Source: USClimateData.com

WATER

How much is enough? Well, one simple physiological fact should persuade you to err on the side of excess when deciding how much water to pack: a hiker walking steadily in 90° heat needs about 10 quarts of fluid per day—that's 2.5 gallons.

A good rule of thumb is to hydrate before your hike, carry (and drink) 6 ounces of water for every mile you plan to hike, and hydrate again after the hike. For most people, the pleasures of hiking make carrying water a relatively minor price to pay to remain safe and healthy. So pack more water than you anticipate needing even for short hikes, especially during summer.

Around Phoenix, water sources are scarce at best, so hikers must be prepared to take along all the water they need. Look in the Key Information box for each hike to find the minimum recommended amount of water to bring with you; also, keep in mind that high ambient temperatures and physiological differences among individuals may require you to drink more than this recommended amount.

If you find yourself tempted to drink "found" water, do so with extreme caution. Many ponds and lakes encountered by hikers are fairly stagnant, and the water tastes terrible. Drinking such water presents inherent risks for thirsty trekkers. Giardia and cryptosporidium contaminate many water sources; these parasites cause unpleasant intestinal disturbances that can last for weeks after ingestion. For more information, visit the Centers for Disease Control and Prevention online: cdc.gov/parasites/giardia and cdc.gov/parasites/crypto.

In any case, effective treatment is essential before you drink from any water source found along the trail. Boiling water for 2–3 minutes is always a safe measure for camping, but day hikers can consider iodine tablets, approved chemical mixes, filtration units rated for giardia and cryptosporidium, and UV filtration. Some of these methods (for example, filtration with an added carbon filter) remove bad tastes typical in stagnant water, while others add their own taste. As a precaution, carry a means of water purification if you realize that you've underestimated your consumption needs.

CLOTHING

Weather, unexpected trail conditions, fatigue, extended hiking duration, and wrong turns can individually or collectively turn a great outing into a very uncomfortable one at best—and a life-threatening one at worst. Thus, proper attire plays a key role in staying comfortable and, sometimes, in staying alive. Here are some helpful guidelines:

➤ **Choose silk, wool, or synthetics** for maximum comfort in all of your hiking attire—from hats to socks and in between. Cotton tends to retain moisture, which can be used to your advantage during hot summer days as a means to achieve evaporative cooling.

➤ **Always wear a hat,** or at least tuck one into your day pack or hitch it to your belt. Wide-brim hats offer all-weather sun and wind protection, as well as warmth if it turns cold.

➤ **Be ready to layer up or down** as the day progresses and the mercury rises or falls. Today's outdoor wear makes layering easy, with such designs as jackets that convert to vests and zip-off or button-up legs.

➤ **Wear hiking boots** or sturdy hiking sandals with toe protection. Flip-flopping along a paved urban greenway is one thing, but never hike a trail in open sandals or casual sneakers. Your bones and arches need support, and your skin needs protection.

➤ **Pair that footwear with good socks.** If you prefer not to sheathe your feet when wearing hiking sandals, tuck the socks into your day pack; you may need them if the weather plummets or if you hit rocky turf and pebbles begin to irritate your feet. Plus, in an emergency, you can adapt the socks into mittens if you've lost your gloves.

➤ **Don't leave rainwear behind,** even if the day dawns clear and sunny. Tuck into your day pack, or tie around your waist, a jacket that is breathable and either water-resistant or waterproof. Investigate different choices at your local outdoors retailer. If you hike frequently, you'll ideally have more than one rainwear weight, material, and style in your closet to protect you in all seasons in your regional climate and hiking microclimates.

ESSENTIAL GEAR

Today you can buy outdoor vests that have up to 20 pockets shaped and sized to carry everything from toothpicks to binoculars. If you don't aspire to feel like a burro, however, you can neatly stow all of these items in your day pack or backpack. The following list showcases never-hike-without-them items, in alphabetical order, as all are important:

➤ **Extra clothes:** rain gear, wide-brim hat, gloves, and a change of socks and shirt.

➤ **Extra food:** trail mix, granola bars, or other high-energy foods.

➤ **Flashlight or headlamp** with extra bulb and batteries.

➤ **Insect repellent.** For some areas and seasons, this is vital.

➤ **Maps and a high-quality compass.** Even if you know the terrain from previous hikes, don't leave home without these tools. As previously recommended, bring maps in addition to those in this guidebook, and consult those maps before you hike. If you're GPS-savvy, bring that device too, but don't rely on it as your sole navigational tool—battery life is limited, after all—and be sure to compare its guidance with that of your maps.

➤ **Mirror.** This may come in handy for signaling passing aircraft in remote areas.

➤ **Pocketknife and/or multitool.** Choose one with sturdy tweezers for removing painful cactus needles.

➤ **Sunblock** is an essential layer of protection when hiking in the desert. Regular use protects your exposed skin against UV radiation, sunburn, and potential skin cancer. Use a product with an SPF of 15 or above for day hikes, and reapply often.

➤ **Water.** As emphasized more than once in this book, you should bring more than you think you'll drink. Depending on your destination, you may want to bring an extra container and iodine or a filter for purifying water in case you run out.

➤ **Whistle.** This little gadget will be your best friend in an emergency.

➤ **Windproof matches and/or a lighter,** as well as a fire starter.

FIRST AID KIT

In addition to the aforementioned, the items below may appear overwhelming for a day hike. But any paramedic will tell you that these products—in alphabetical order, because all are important—are just the basics. The reality of hiking is that you can be out for a week of backpacking and acquire only a mosquito bite. Or you can hike for an hour, slip, and suffer a cut, scrape, or broken bone. Fortunately, these listed items will collapse into a very small space. Convenient prepackaged kits are also available at your pharmacy or online.

➤ Adhesive bandages

➤ Antibiotic ointment (Neosporin or the generic equivalent)

➤ Athletic tape

➤ Blister kit (such as Moleskin or Spenco 2nd Skin)

➤ Butterfly-closure bandages

➤ Diphenhydramine (Benadryl or generic), in case of allergic reactions

➤ Elastic bandages or joint wraps

➤ Epinephrine in a prefilled syringe (EpiPen), typically by prescription only, for people known to have severe allergic reactions to hiking mishaps such as bee stings

➤ Gauze (one roll and a half-dozen 4-by-4-inch pads)

- Hydrogen peroxide or iodine
- Ibuprofen (Advil) or acetaminophen (Tylenol)
- Snakebite kit

Note: Consider your intended terrain and the number of hikers in your party before you exclude any article cited above. A botanical garden stroll may not inspire you to carry a complete kit, but anything beyond that warrants precaution. When hiking alone, you should always be prepared for a medical need. And if you are a twosome or with a group, one or more people in your party should be equipped with first aid material.

GENERAL SAFETY

The following tips may have the familiar ring of Mom's voice as you take note of them.

- **Let someone know where you'll be hiking and how long you expect to be gone.** Give that person a copy of your route, particularly if you're headed into an isolated area. Let him or her know when you return.

- **Sign in and out of any trail registers provided.** Don't hesitate to comment on the trail condition if space is provided; that's your opportunity to alert others to any problems you encounter.

- **Don't count on a cell phone for your safety.** Reception may be spotty or nonexistent on the trail, even on an urban walk—especially one embraced by towering trees.

- **Always carry food and water, even for a short hike.** And bring more water than you think you will need. (We can't emphasize this enough.)

- **Ask questions.** State forest and park employees are on hand to help.

- **Stay on designated trails.** Even on the most clearly marked trails, you usually reach a point where you have to stop and consider in which direction to head. If you become disoriented, don't panic. As soon as you think you may be off-track, stop, assess your current direction, and then retrace your steps to the point where you went astray. Using a map, a compass, and this book, and keeping in mind what you have passed thus far, reorient yourself and trust your judgment on which way to continue. If you become absolutely unsure of how to continue, return to your vehicle the way you came in. Should you become completely lost and have no idea how to find the trailhead, remaining in place along the trail and waiting for help is most often the best option for adults and always the best option for children.

- **Always carry a whistle,** another precaution that we can't overemphasize. It may be a lifesaver if you get lost or hurt.

- **Be especially careful when crossing streams,** especially after monsoon rains. Whether you're fording the stream or crossing on a log, make every step count. If you're unsure that you can maintain your balance on a log, ford the stream instead: use a trekking pole or stout stick for balance, and *face upstream as you cross*. If a stream seems too deep to ford, don't chance it—whatever is on the other side isn't worth the risk.

➤ **Be careful at overlooks.** While these areas may provide spectacular views, they're potentially hazardous. Stay back from the edge of outcrops, and make absolutely sure of your footing; a misstep could mean a nasty or possibly fatal fall.

➤ **Standing dead trees** and storm-damaged living trees pose a significant hazard to hikers. These trees may have loose or broken limbs that could fall at any time. While walking beneath trees, and when choosing a spot to rest or enjoy your snack, *look up.*

➤ **Be sun-savvy.** The Valley of the Sun lives up to its name: sunburn is a serious threat to hikers around Phoenix, and Arizona unfortunately leads the nation in skin cancer occurrences. High-altitude hikes exacerbate your risk of overexposure. Aside from the obvious pain, suffering, and unsightly peeling associated with prolonged sun exposure, sunburn can be extremely harmful to the skin. To avoid looking like a lobster at the end of your hike, apply sunblock with an SPF rating of 15 or higher before you set out. Reapply it every few hours to all exposed areas of your body, including your ears, your nose, and the back of your neck. Wear a wide-brim hat and long shirts and pants for ultimate protection.

➤ **Know the symptoms of heat-related illness, or hyperthermia.** Here's how to recognize and handle three types of heat emergencies:

> *Heat cramps are painful spasms in the legs and abdomen, accompanied by heavy sweating and feeling faint. Caused by excessive salt loss, heat cramps must be treated by getting to a cool place and sipping water or an electrolyte solution (such as Gatorade).*

> *Dizziness, headache, irregular pulse, disorientation, and nausea are all symptoms of heat exhaustion, which occurs as blood vessels dilate and attempt to move heat from the inner body to the skin. Find a cool place, drink cool water, and get a friend to fan you, which can help cool you off more quickly.*

> *Dilated pupils, dry, hot, flushed skin, a rapid pulse, high fever, and abnormal breathing are all symptoms of heatstroke, a life-threatening condition that can cause convulsions, unconsciousness, or even death. If you should be sweating and you're not, that's the signature warning sign. If you or a hiking partner is experiencing heatstroke, do whatever you can to cool down and find help.*

➤ **Likewise, know the symptoms of subnormal body temperature, or hypothermia.** Shivering and forgetfulness are the two most common indicators of this stealthy killer. Hypothermia can occur at any elevation, even in the summer, especially when the hiker is wearing lightweight cotton clothing. If symptoms present themselves, seek shelter, hot liquids, and dry clothes as soon as possible.

In summary: Plan ahead. Watch your step. Avoid accidents before they happen.

WATCHWORDS FOR FLORA AND FAUNA

Hikers should be aware of the following concerns regarding plant life and wildlife, described in alphabetical order.

AFRICANIZED BEES

The American Southwest has seen an increase in these bees in recent decades. Though encounters with them are rare, they can be serious and even deadly. Africanized bees are an aggressive strain of honeybee that has migrated north from South and Central America. Though their stings are no more venomous than those of a regular honeybee, Africanized bees are much more reactive to perceived threats: they've been known to chase people for as much as quarter of a mile and are 10 times as likely to swarm and sting humans as non-Africanized bees.

As you would in the case of any other type of wild-animal encounter, be aware of your surroundings, and distance yourself from any area where you see a swarm or hear the buzzing of bees. If you're allergic to bee stings, be sure to carry an epinephrine syringe.

BLACK BEARS

Though attacks by black bears are uncommon, the sight or approach of a bear can give anyone a start. If you encounter a bear while hiking, remain calm and avoid running. Make loud noises, and back away from the bear slowly. In primitive and remote areas, assume that bears are present; in more-developed sites, check on the current bear situation before your hike.

Most bear encounters are food-related, as bears have an exceptional sense of smell and not particularly discriminating tastes. While this is of greater concern to backpackers and campers, on a day hike you may plan a lunchtime picnic or munch on an energy bar or other snack from time to time. So remain aware and alert.

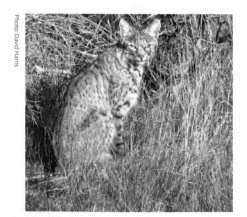

Photo: David Harris

BOBCATS

Resembling large house cats, with tufted ears, large paws, and a short tail, bobcats can be found in nearly any type of terrain in central Arizona and can weigh up to 30 pounds when they are fully mature. Though generally timid, bobcats have been known to encroach on neighborhoods, golf courses, backyards, and tree-lined parks. Like all wild cats, they're efficient and ferocious hunters, generally subsisting on small prey like mice and rabbits but capable of taking down animals as large as a deer.

Bobcats are nocturnal hunters and rarely come out during the day. (Like domestic cats, they prefer to sleep the day away.) If you happen to see a bobcat in the wild, leave it alone. The cats' sharp claws and teeth can do some serious damage, although attacks on humans are extremely rare.

COYOTES

Coyotes freely roam the desert and surrounding mountains, especially in the early morning and during dusk. They can even be seen in city neighborhoods that border parks and preserves. Though coyotes present little danger to hikers, be mindful that they often prey on small pets. A distant relative of the wolf, coyotes are agile and nimble. They can hop fences and chase down small rabbits, cats, and small dogs effortlessly. If you're hiking with a pet, be sure to keep it on a short leash.

GILA MONSTERS

Gila monsters are the largest lizards in the country and one of only two venomous lizard species in the world. They are native to the Southwest and make their home in the mountains near Phoenix. Bulky and awkward-looking, they grow to 2 feet in length and have bright and distinctive brown, pink, yellow, and black markings.

Staying out of sight for most of their lives, Gila monsters rarely make public appearances. They move relatively slowly and pose little threat to hikers, but those who molest these reptiles may receive a very painful and tenacious bite from which it may be nearly impossible to free themselves. Unlike snakes, Gila monsters don't have fangs. Rather, they deliver venom by gripping their prey with steel-like jaws and letting poison seep into the wound. If you happen upon a Gila monster on a hike, count yourself lucky and take some pictures, but don't attempt to touch or otherwise pester it.

JAVELINAS

Also known as collared peccaries, javelinas are tusked animals that resemble pigs, weighing 30–60 pounds; travel in packs and live close to desert washes and dense vegetation; and can be spotted along the outskirts of town and in mountain preserves.

Encounters with javelinas are rare. They will likely run away if approached, but if cornered, they can fight back with their hooves and tusks. Hikers should consider them potentially dangerous and leave them alone.

MOSQUITOES

While it happens only rarely, individuals can become infected with West Nile virus from the bite of an infected mosquito. Culex mosquitoes, the primary species that transmit West Nile virus to humans, thrive in urban rather than wilderness areas. They lay eggs in stagnant water and can breed in any standing water that remains for more than five days. Most people infected with West Nile virus have no symptoms of illness, but some may become ill, usually 3–15 days after being bitten.

The Phoenix area has proved to be one of the riskiest for West Nile virus due to an abundance of stagnant swimming pools. Most at risk are the elderly and those with weakened immune systems. Though the risk of infection is relatively low, hikers should consider taking measures to prevent mosquito bites. Precautions include using insect repellent and wearing clothes that completely cover the arms and legs.

MOUNTAIN LIONS

Also known as cougars, these solitary and elusive cats populate central Arizona in abundance. They live in forests, rocky hills, and mountain preserves but can move down into the desert, golf courses, and suburbs if attracted there. They hunt small game like javelina, deer, and rabbits, mostly in steep mountainous terrain where they can ambush their prey.

Mountain lions dislike company, so they stay out of sight. If you see one of them, count yourself lucky, because they very rarely show themselves to humans. I have been hiking in Arizona for more than 30 years but have seen only one cougar as it was running away.

In the extremely unlikely event of a mountain lion encounter, don't run or crouch. Maintain eye contact, make yourself appear bigger by raising your arms, and make loud noises. Persuade the cat that you aren't an easy meal, and then back away slowly. If attacked, fight back with everything you have: sticks, trekking poles, rocks, and even backpacks. Protect your head and neck with your arms if necessary. Keep pets and small children close, and make sure that they don't run—running will trigger the mountain lion's instinct to give chase.

POISON IVY, OAK, AND SUMAC

Thankfully, these itch-causing plants aren't as common around Phoenix as they are elsewhere, although they do grow locally near perennial streams and ponds. Recognizing and avoiding poison ivy, oak, and sumac are the most effective ways to prevent the painful, itchy rashes associated with these plants.

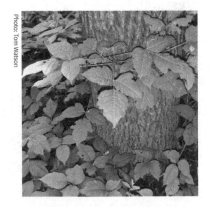
Photo: Tom Watson

Poison ivy (*right*) occurs as a vine or ground cover, 3 leaflets to a leaf; poison oak (*next page, top left*) occurs as either a vine or shrub, also with 3 leaflets; and poison sumac

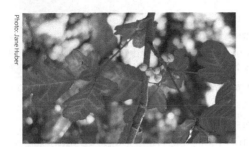

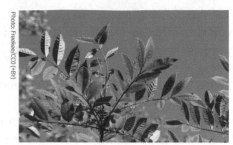

(*above right*) flourishes in swampland, each leaf having 7–13 leaflets. Urushiol, the oil in the sap of these plants, is responsible for the rash. Within 14 hours of exposure, raised lines and/or blisters will appear on the affected area, accompanied by a terrible itch. Refrain from scratching because bacteria under your fingernails can cause an infection. Wash and dry the affected area thoroughly, applying calamine lotion to help dry out the rash. If itching or blistering is severe, seek medical attention.

If you knowingly touch the plant, you have a window of about 15–20 minutes to remove the oil before it causes a reaction. Rinsing it off with cool water is impractical on the trail, but commercial products such as Tecnu are effective at removing urushiol from your skin. To keep from spreading the misery to someone else, wash not only any exposed parts of your body but also any oil-contaminated clothes, hiking gear, or pets.

PRICKLY PLANTS

Cacti grow in abundance in desert environments and can present significant risks to hikers and their pets. When hiking, stay on established trails whenever possible, look before you reach out for balance, and keep pets on a leash at all times. There are dozens of varieties of cacti around Phoenix; noteworthy species include giant saguaros, fishhook barrels, chollas, and prickly pears.

Cactus needles can inflict painful stings if accidentally touched. Two particular varieties, the **teddy bear cholla** (*below*) and **chain fruit cholla,** have earned the dubious nickname "jumping cholla" because of their penchant for quickly attaching themselves to passersby. They don't really jump, of course, but a strong breeze can send them flying onto your clothing or skin.

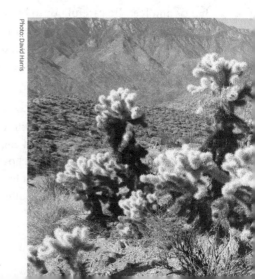

Prickly pear cactus has very fine needles that embed themselves like splinters in your skin if you unknowingly brush against them or accidentally fall onto one. Saguaro and barrel cactus needles don't break off but can still inflict a nasty puncture wound.

Arm yourself with tape, a comb, and tweezers when hiking near Phoenix. If you're unfortunate enough to get into cactus, remove large clusters with a comb rather than trying to pull them off with your hands. Pluck out large needles with strong tweezers. Cholla needles have tiny barbs on them and can be painful when pulled. Fine needles can sometimes be removed using athletic or duct tape, though often not completely.

Besides cacti, there are other prickly plants worth knowing about. Recognizing and avoiding them will save you much aggravation—and perhaps some bloodshed.

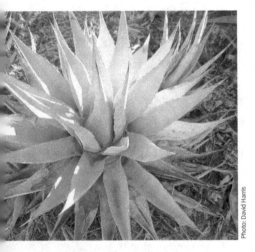

Photo: David Harris

Agave (*left*), or century plant, is a succulent that grows in desert areas. It has very sharp and stiff needles at the tips and along the edges of its fleshy leaves. Careless hikers can accidentally puncture their arms or legs to the bone if they don't pay careful attention to these plants. (On the other hand, these plants give us tequila, so they aren't all bad!)

Catclaw acacia is another particularly annoying plant that grows in abundance next to trails. Its leaves resemble mesquite and ironwood, but they have tiny curved barbs that look like a cat's claw (hence the name). If you brush against this plant, it will likely want to hold onto your clothing, often tearing tiny holes before dislodging itself.

Ocotillos look like spiny dead sticks that grow from the desert during most of the year. Only in spring do they sprout leaves along their stems, and then a bright raceme of delicate trumpetlike flowers during April.

In general, be aware of your surroundings, and pay attention to where you put hands and feet. Be careful not to brush up against any plant, if possible—most flora in the desert have some kind of self-defense adaptation that make them unpleasant to eat or touch. On the brighter side, desert plants bloom with some of the brightest and most delicate flowers during spring.

SNAKES

Hike enough in the desert, and you're bound to meet a snake—it's the price desert dwellers pay for a relative dearth of nagging insects, ticks, and poison ivy. Snakes pose less risk than most people imagine, however, and they certainly need not dissuade you from enjoying a hike. Knowing their habitat, understanding their behavior, and respecting their territory are the keys to minimizing risks associated with a snake encounter.

Rattlesnakes are the most common snakes found in deserts and mountains near Phoenix. They belong to a group of venomous snakes called pit vipers—*pit* because they have concave, pitlike heat-sensing glands on the sides of their faces, and *viper* because they have venom-conducting fangs.

Arizona is home to more than a dozen species of rattlesnakes, many of which are protected by law. The **Western diamondback** (*below*) is the largest and most common, and the nearly identical **Mojave rattler** is the most dangerous. You'd do well to avoid both. True to their name, diamondbacks are usually brown in color, with speckled dark-brown diamond-shaped blotches on their backs. Alternating black and white stripes line the tail just below the rattle. Mojave rattlers share the diamondbacks' blotchy pattern and black-and-white tail stripes, but their white stripes are notably wider than black ones. Mojave rattlers, which sometimes also bear a greenish tint, carry a potent neurotoxin that is 10 times as powerful as the hemotoxins of other rattlesnakes. Because the Mojave rattler is so close in appearance to a diamondback, it can be very difficult to tell them apart, especially during a stressful snake encounter.

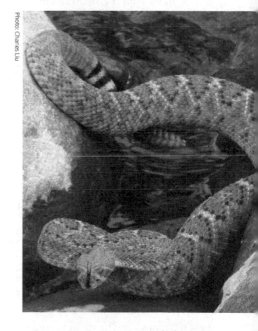

Photo: Charles Liu

Armed with deadly venom, heat-sensing glands, and effective camouflage, rattlesnakes are efficient predators that thrive on small rodents. Fortunately, they aren't aggressive by nature, rarely attacking humans unless sufficiently provoked. Most snakebites occur when an inattentive hiker steps on a snake or when a foolish person bothers one out of curiosity. Always give rattlesnakes plenty of space, and never approach one on purpose.

Rattlesnakes prefer warmth but not searing heat. Most active during spring and around dusk, they like to hang out among rock crevices, in tall brush, and under shady branches. Vigilantly watch your step while hiking, and peer over any rock outcroppings before using them as handholds.

Rattlesnakes do not like company. When you get too close for comfort, they'll let you know by coiling into a defensive posture and emitting a loud rattle that will likely make you jump. Heed their warning: back up slowly, and give them ample space. More often than not, the snake will back down and seek shelter under a nearby rock. If a snake obstinately obstructs the trail, find a way around it. Never provoke snakes by poking them or throwing rocks at them. If you often hike with a dog, keep it on a close leash—dogs often chase snakes, and that can lead to trouble.

Some nonvenomous snakes encountered around Phoenix include gopher snakes, king snakes, and garter snakes. Gopher snakes may be intimidating, with coloring that often resembles a diamondback's and measuring up to 5 feet in length, but they lack a rattle and have a rounded head. King snakes display brightly colored rings and may resemble venomous coral snakes. Remember this little jingle: "Red on yellow kills a fellow; red on black, venom lack."

SPIDERS AND SCORPIONS

Desert areas are home to infamous arachnids such as black widow spiders, scorpions, and tarantulas. Their reputations are far more fearsome, though, than the actual risks of encountering them in the wilderness. In fact, the black widow spider and the scorpion are more often seen near your homes than during a hike. Be careful where you put your hands while hiking in order to avoid contact with these creatures. It may seem like obvious advice, but don't reach into dark areas where these animals like to hide. And if you do see them while hiking, simply avoid them.

Tarantulas are often seen on hiking trails at dusk. Their large, hairy bodies and legs can be startling when you first encounter one. In reality, tarantulas are typically very docile and pose little threat to humans. Even though all spiders are venomous to a degree, tarantulas will not bite unless absolutely cornered. The moral of this story is not to pick them up or otherwise molest them—just take a picture and move on.

TICKS

Thankfully, these arachnids are seldom found in the deserts around Phoenix, though they do exist in higher elevations, around streams, and in lush forested areas. Among local varieties of ticks, brown dog ticks and Rocky Mountain wood ticks are the most common, and they can carry Lyme disease. Adult ticks are most active April–May and again October–November.

Wear light-colored clothing to make it easier for you to spot ticks before they migrate to your skin. At the end of the hike, visually check your hair, the back of your neck, your armpits, and your socks. During your posthike shower, take a moment to do a more complete body check. Use tweezers to remove ticks that are already embedded: grasp the tick close to your skin, and remove it by pulling straight out firmly. Do your best to remove the head, but don't twist. Apply disinfectant solution to the wound.

HUNTING

Various regulations and licenses govern different hunting types and seasons. Though you generally won't run into problems, you may wish to forgo venturing out during big-game season, when the woods suddenly fill with orange and camouflage. For more information, visit azgfd.gov and click "Hunting" at the top of the page.

REGULATIONS

Hikers should familiarize themselves with the rules of each park, preserve, or wilderness area they enter. This book lists such basic information as entrance fees and operating hours in each hike description; a few additional rules are noted below.

- In 2017, the City of Phoenix enacted legislation that prohibits taking dogs on a hike when ambient temperatures exceed 100°F. Though this law affects only trails within Phoenix city limits, it's a good rule to follow regardless of where you hike—dogs have no sweat glands and can be easily overcome by heat. The Arizona sun is unforgiving to humans, and it can be deadly to pets.

- Also introduced in 2017, a state law protects good Samaritans from civil liability for breaking car windows to rescue animals or infants who have been left unattended inside vehicles. Potential rescuers must first perceive that the pet or child is in imminent danger; they must also verify that the vehicle is actually locked and have contacted appropriate authorities before breaking windows and entering a vehicle. In any case, you should *never* leave children or pets inside a locked vehicle, even on a short hike or errand—temperatures inside a vehicle can exceed 150°F within minutes in Phoenix.

- In wilderness areas such as those within Tonto National Forest, there may be group-size limits to be aware of. Hike leaders should know and respect such limits when planning group hikes or when taking large families on an outing. Typically, a group of fewer than 15 people should be fine, but if your group is larger, separate them into smaller groups and depart at least 15 minutes apart.

TRAIL ETIQUETTE

Always treat the trail, wildlife, and fellow hikers with respect. Here are some reminders.

- **Plan ahead in order to be self-sufficient at all times.** For example, carry all necessary supplies for changes in weather or other conditions. A well-planned trip is satisfying.

- **Hike on open trails only.**

- **In seasons or places** where road or trail closures may be a possibility, use the websites or phone numbers in the "Contacts" line for each of this guidebook's hikes to check conditions prior to heading out for your hike. And don't try to circumvent such closures.

- **Avoid trespassing on private land,** and obtain all permits and authorization as required. Also, leave gates as you found them or as directed by signage.

- **Be courteous to other hikers,** bikers, equestrians, and others you encounter on the trails.

- **Never spook wild animals or pets.** An unannounced approach, a sudden movement, or a loud noise startles most critters, and a surprised animal can be dangerous to you, to others, and to itself. Give animals plenty of space.

➤ Observe the YIELD signs around the region's trailheads and backcountry. Typically they advise hikers to yield to horses and bikers to both horses and hikers. Per common courtesy on hills, hikers and bikers yield to any uphill traffic. When they encounter mounted riders or horsepackers, hikers may courteously step off the trail, on the downhill side if possible. So that the horse can see and

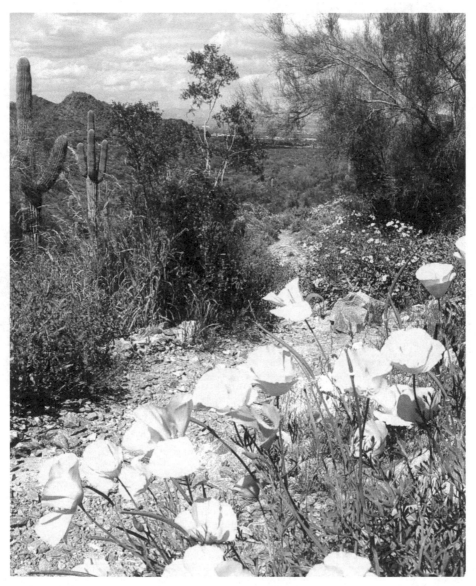

Mexican gold poppies bloom brightly during spring along Phoenix-area trails.   *Photo: Charles Liu*

hear you, calmly greet the rider before he or she reaches you, and don't dart behind trees. Also, don't pet horses unless invited to do so.

➤ **Stay on the existing trail,** and don't blaze any new trails.

➤ **Pack out what you pack in,** leaving only your footprints. Nobody likes to see the trash someone else has left behind.

TIPS ON ENJOYING HIKING IN PHOENIX

Because of Phoenix's mild winter climate, thousands of visitors descend upon the Valley of the Sun to escape frigid conditions elsewhere. Family reunions, weddings, and holiday vacations seem to happen more often here between November and April than other times of the year. Many people spend nearly half the year living in Phoenix and the rest of the time in their respective hometowns.

While the rest of the country shivers under a blanket of snow and ice, Phoenicians enjoy their best hiking weather. Instead of writhing in discomfort after overindulging in Thanksgiving turkey, try burning it off with a family outing to Pinnacle Peak. A Christmas vacation to Phoenix just wouldn't be complete without a hike up Camelback Mountain in shorts and a Santa hat. You can even call your snowbound Midwestern friends from the summit to brag about the weather.

Before winter ice begins to thaw elsewhere, early spring in Phoenix is the best time to attempt longer hikes in the wilderness areas near town. When conditions are ripe, wildflower displays can be absolutely stunning in the Superstition Mountains.

Phoenix also hosts a plethora of large corporations, welcoming thousands of business travelers. These 60 hikes offer perfect getaways from the busy demands of commerce. Some of the largest and best urban parks and mountain preserves in the United States are located here. Instead of eating out, you can pack a lunch and head out to picnic along the Indian Bend Wash Greenbelt or on Tempe Town Lake. Jumpstart your day with a power hike up Piestewa Peak, or wind down from a stress-filled meeting by watching the sunset from atop Camelback Mountain. You can also plan ahead and take a small group of your business comrades on a nearby hike in South Mountain or to the Wind Cave in Usery Park.

No matter how you end up in Phoenix, be sure to take advantage of its superb hiking opportunities.

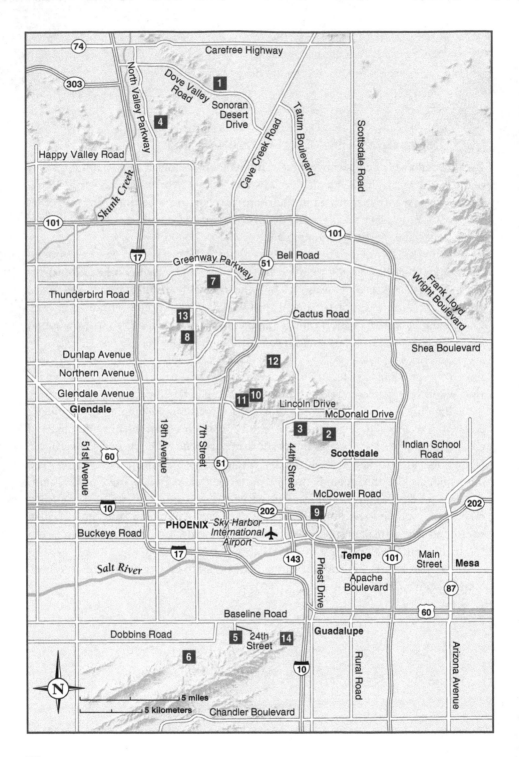

CITY OF PHOENIX

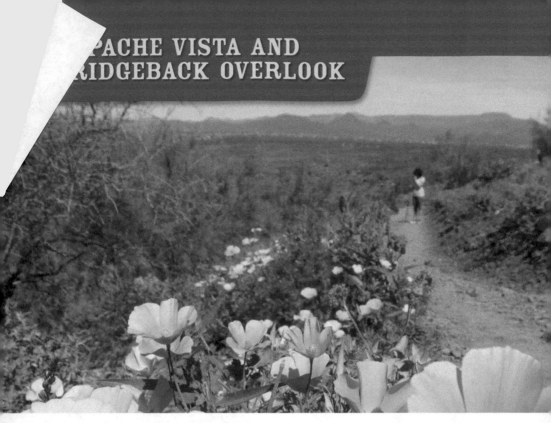

A hiker pauses to admire wildflowers while hiking to Apache Vista.

SEARCHING FOR NEW hiking destinations within the City of Phoenix? Look no further than Phoenix Sonoran Preserve. This enjoyable loop connects six trails in the preserve's northern section and visits two superb vista points overlooking the surrounding desert plains.

DESCRIPTION

The City of Phoenix operates three large open-space areas for preservation and recreation: South Mountain along its southern border, Phoenix Mountains Preserve in central Phoenix, and Phoenix Sonoran Preserve in the north. The newest and largest of the three is Phoenix Sonoran Preserve, focusing on preserving the natural beauty of the Sonoran Desert in which we live. Unlike South Mountain and Phoenix Mountains Preserve, Sonoran Preserve lacks sizable peaks. However, there are several vista points where hikers can enjoy a good workout while climbing to panoramic views. This hike strings together six trails to visit both Apache Vista and Ridgeback Overlook in the northern section of Phoenix Sonoran Preserve.

Begin your hike behind the well-appointed Apache Wash Trailhead building area. Look for trail signage and follow Sidewinder Trail straight, heading northeast. This trail starts on level terrain amid grassy fields, triangle-leaf bursage, creosote, and teddy bear cholla; mountain bikers love to ride these multiuse trails, so watch for cyclists as

DISTANCE & CONFIGURATION: 5.6-mile loop

DIFFICULTY: Easy–moderate

SCENERY: Phoenix Sonoran Preserve, wildflowers, two prominent summits

EXPOSURE: Mostly exposed

TRAIL TRAFFIC: Moderate

TRAIL SURFACE: Packed dirt, rock

HIKING TIME: 3 hours

WATER REQUIREMENT: 2.5 quarts

DRIVING DISTANCE: 28 miles from Phoenix Sky Harbor Airport

ELEVATION GAIN: 1,725' at trailhead, 2,010' at Apache Vista, 2,180' at Ridgeback Overlook

ACCESS: Gates open 5 a.m.–7 p.m.; trails open until 11 p.m.; no permits or fees required

MAP: USGS *New River SE;* park maps available at website below

FACILITIES: Restrooms, horse trailer parking, but no water

WHEELCHAIR ACCESS: Short section near trailhead

CONTACT: 602-495-6939, phoenix.gov/parks /trails/locations/sonoran-preserve

COMMENTS: Dogs on leash permitted except when temperature exceeds 100°F

you hike. Thompson Peak (see Hike 23, page 126), Pinnacle Peak (see Hike 20, page 112), and the rest of the McDowell Mountains grace the horizon to your right. If you happen to hike Sidewinder Trail during spring, especially after a wet winter, you'll see fields of bladderpod and fiddleneck wildflowers blanketing the foothills.

Cross a dry wash 0.25 mile from the trailhead as the trail rounds the side of a hill with Black Mountain (see Hike 16, page 96) to your right. The trail ascends gently, while smooth, packed dirt gives way to slightly rockier terrain. If you catch the peak of wildflower season, you will see poppies and lupines here. Each section of this hike seems to highlight a particular species of wildflower, where minute differences in elevation, temperature, moisture level, and sun exposure cater to their ideal growing conditions.

Continue counterclockwise around the hill. As you pass 0.6 mile from the trailhead, travel along the east edge of the hill, with sandy Apache Wash below you. You'll see Apache Wash Loop snaking its way through the green oasis created by the seasonal creek. Sidewinder Trail soon straightens, dips a bit, and then quickly regains elevation.

At the signed trail junction with Apache Vista Trail, 0.9 mile from the trailhead, turn left to visit Apache Vista. This spur trail is moderately steep and rocky but remains wide and well marked. At 1.1 miles from the trailhead, you'll reach a fork in the trail. Taking either route is fine since this is the beginning of a small loop on the summit ridge.

Apache Vista stands at 2,010 feet, high enough to offer a sweeping view of mountains all around the Valley of the Sun, expansive desert plains below, trails winding their way through the preserve, and distant housing developments. Sonoran Desert Drive threads through the gap between southern hills of the preserve and those of the north. To the west lies Ridgeback Overlook, our next hilltop destination. Take a

Apache Vista and Ridgeback Overlook

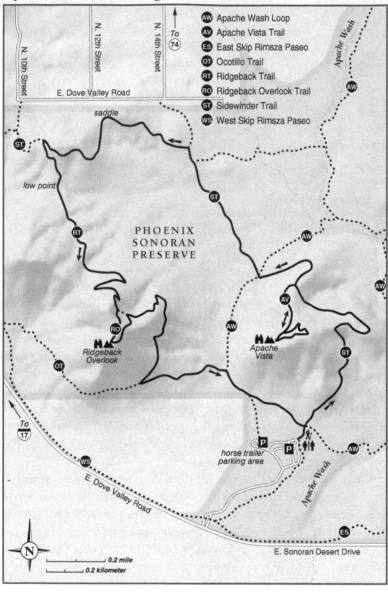

AW Apache Wash Loop
AV Apache Vista Trail
ES East Skip Rimsza Paseo
OT Ocotillo Trail
RT Ridgeback Trail
RO Ridgeback Overlook Trail
ST Sidewinder Trail
WS West Skip Rimsza Paseo

N. 10th Street
N. 12th Street
N. 14th Street
To 74
E. Dove Valley Road

saddle
low point

PHOENIX
SONORAN
PRESERVE

Apache Wash

To 17

Ridgeback
Overlook

Apache
Vista

horse trailer
parking area

E. Dove Valley Road

Apache Wash

N

0.2 mile
0.2 kilometer

E. Sonoran Desert Drive

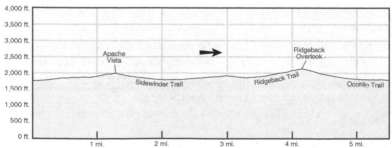

4,000 ft.
3,500 ft.
3,000 ft.
2,500 ft.
2,000 ft.
1,500 ft.
1,000 ft.
500 ft.
0 ft.

Apache
Vista

Ridgeback
Overlook

Sidewinder Trail
Ridgeback Trail
Ocotillo Trail

1 mi.   2 mi.   3 mi.   4 mi.   5 mi.

quick breather here to enjoy the view, and then continue downhill to complete the small summit loop. Follow Apache Vista Trail back to Sidewinder Trail.

When back at the Sidewinder Trail junction, a total of 1.6 miles from the trailhead now, turn left to resume the hike. Sidewinder continues north-northeast, with Black Mountain on the horizon and Cave Creek Road below. The trail soon drops to 1,800 feet in elevation as it heads west through palo verde trees.

Just shy of 2 miles from the trailhead, the trail reaches a slightly confusing junction with Apache Wash Loop. Veer right at the first signpost, onto Apache Wash Loop; then take a left at the second signpost to continue along Sidewinder Trail. You'll cross a dry wash shortly as you hike through a grass-covered plain and a creosote forest sparsely dotted with buckhorn chollas. After yet another dry wash, at 2.3 miles from the trailhead, there are two successive trail junctions at 2.4 and 2.5 miles—stay left at both junctions to remain on Sidewinder Trail, which begins to wind and zigzag through the foothills.

At 2.8 miles is a small saddle point where Mexican gold poppies and desert hyacinth bloom in great numbers during the spring. The Bradshaw Mountains form a backdrop to the housing developments of North Phoenix. The trail then curves south and climbs to the top of a hillock with a few teddy bear chollas adorning the landscape. Sidewinder Trail lives up to its name, twisting through the preserve. You'll see a few hillside homes in the distance on the gradual descent.

When you reach Ridgeback Trail at 3.2 miles, turn left onto it to complete the loop hike. Sidewinder continues another 3.5 miles before terminating at the Desert Hills Trailhead on Carefree Highway. Ridgeback Trail is another well-marked and well-groomed trail. Start hiking the gradual descent south in the direction of Ridgeback Overlook, the highest hill ahead. The White Tank Mountains (see Hike 55, page 280) are to your right, while you can see Four Peaks (see Hike 46, page 237) above some saguaros to your left.

At 1,833 feet elevation, you'll have passed the valley's low point, after which you begin a gradual climb as the trail bends. The slope increases to a moderate grade at 3.6 miles from the trailhead, with Black Mountain ahead. The next section will get your heart rate up as you make the steep climb. Turn right at 4.1 miles, onto Ridgeback Overlook Trail, to visit the summit.

Ridgeback Overlook (2,180') is slightly higher than Apache Vista and other hills in the area. Again, panoramic views reward those who make it to the top. One can see nearly all major peaks around Phoenix from this fantastic vantage point. Take a moment to enjoy the view; then continue following Ridgeback Overlook Trail as it wraps around the hill and dives down the other side. Descend along the hillside until you reach Ridgeback Trail again at 4.4 miles.

Turn right, onto Ridgeback Trail; then continue downhill along the ridge. One advantage of ridge hiking is that it affords open panoramic views. This trail section, with Black Mountain in the foreground, is lined with poppies and brittlebush in spring. Navigate a hairpin turn around a hillside drainage, where you can now see the trailhead parking area on your left. Continue your descent southeast.

At 4.9 miles, you'll reach the junction with Ocotillo Trail. Turn left here to finish the loop. Ocotillo is yet another wide, smooth trail affording a view of many saguaros and teddy bear chollas on the southern slopes as it gently descends. Ocotillo Trail meets Apache Wash Loop at 5.25 miles. Continue straight along the shared section of Apache Wash Loop Trail to reach the original trailhead, completing the 5.6-mile hike.

NEARBY ACTIVITIES

Among the other trails within Phoenix Sonoran Preserve that are worth a visit is **Dixie Mountain Loop** (see Hike 4, page 39), another great loop hike in the south-

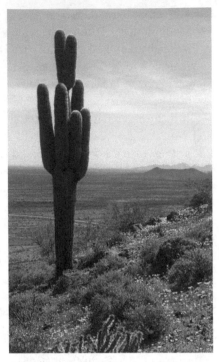

A giant saguaro and Mexican gold poppies adorn the hills near Apache Vista.

ern portion of the preserve. **Black Mountain** (see Hike 16, page 96) lies directly to the east, in the town of Cave Creek. **Cave Creek Regional Park** is traversed by still more outstanding trails (see Go John Trail, Hike 47, page 241).

• •

GPS TRAILHEAD COORDINATES N33° 46.104' W112° 02.651'

DIRECTIONS From Loop 101, take Exit 28 at Cave Creek Road and drive north 4.5 miles to Sonoran Desert Drive. Turn west (left) onto Sonoran Desert Drive; then continue 4 miles to the signed Apache Wash Trailhead entrance.

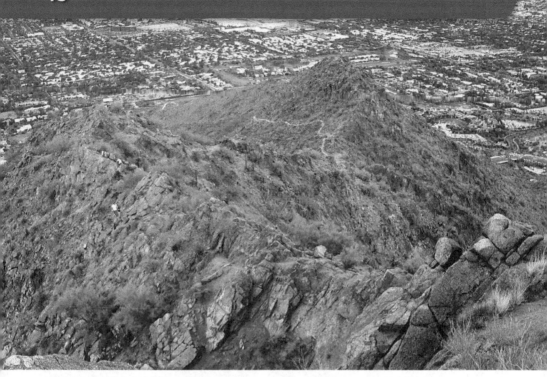

Cholla Trail ascends the east ridge of Camelback Mountain in central Phoenix.

THE SUMMIT OF Camelback Mountain is the highest point in the City of Phoenix. The 2,704-foot summit affords hikers an impressive panoramic view of the city and the surrounding mountain ranges. Cholla Trail offers hikers an easier, albeit longer, way to reach the top of Camelback Mountain than does the popular Echo Canyon Trail (page 34). Fans of cityscape can appreciate Cholla Trail for its open views along the way.

DESCRIPTION

When people say, "I'm hiking Camelback Mountain," they usually mean they're climbing the Echo Canyon Trail on the northwestern side of the mountain, which gets its name from the fact that it looks like a sleeping camel. Echo Canyon Trail (see next hike), which traverses the camel's "head," with its cliffs of red sandstone and huge boulders, does offer a very scenic hike up Camelback Mountain, but it's also steep and sometimes crowded.

A slightly less trafficked and somewhat easier way to summit Camelback Mountain is to hike up the gentler Cholla Trail, on the mountain's eastern side. Nearly 2 miles long, Cholla Trail meanders up the "spine" of the sleeping camel and gives those not endowed with legs of steel a more pleasant route to experience the

DISTANCE & CONFIGURATION: 3.8-mile out-and-back

DIFFICULTY: Moderate–strenuous

SCENERY: Highest point in Phoenix, city views, cliffs

EXPOSURE: Late-afternoon shade, otherwise mostly exposed

TRAIL TRAFFIC: Heavy

TRAIL SURFACE: Packed dirt, gravel, rock, a little easy scrambling

HIKING TIME: 2 hours

WATER REQUIREMENT: 1–1.5 quarts

DRIVING DISTANCE: 9 miles from Phoenix Sky Harbor Airport

ELEVATION GAIN: 1,375' at trailhead, 2,704' on summit of Camelback Mountain

ACCESS: Sunrise–sunset; limited parking; no permits or fees required

MAP: USGS *Paradise Valley*

FACILITIES: None

WHEELCHAIR ACCESS: None

CONTACT: 602-261-8318, phoenix.gov/parks /trails/locations/camelback-mountain

COMMENTS: No parking along Cholla Lane— park along Invergordon Road instead; no dogs allowed

wonders of this mountain. Fans of city views will also appreciate Cholla's ample, wide-open vistas.

Hiking Cholla Trail is not without its own challenges, though, the first of which is to find desirable parking. In the late 1990s, residents near the original Cholla Trailhead petitioned the city to reroute the trail because of noise and vandalism. As a result, you may no longer park near the trailhead on Cholla Lane, for which the trail was named. Instead, you must park in designated spots along the western side of Invergordon Road. The first half mile of your hike, therefore, is spent reaching the trailhead by walking along Invergordon Road and turning west on Cholla Lane. Stay on the south side of Cholla Lane, where a gravel trail ascends gently. Take this opportunity to warm up your leg muscles and gawk at the opulent mansions along the way.

At the end of a white fence along the golf course at The Phoenician resort, about 0.5 mile from your car, a conspicuous plaque marks the official Cholla Trailhead. Your journey up Camelback Mountain begins here. The first section of trail rounds the edge of the golf course. Watch out for low-flying golf balls! As you climb, the trail bends back to the southeast and then levels out. From this flat stretch, you can survey the scenery. To your left lies a palm-lined putting green flanked by white sand traps. Looking toward the northeastern horizon you'll see the McDowell Mountains. Straight ahead, you will recognize the unmistakable shape of Four Peaks in the distance.

At the end of the straightaway, Cholla Trail makes a switchback ascent. Now skirting the eastern flank of the mountain, the trail climbs to the ridge along the sleeping camel's spine. It then becomes a bit more difficult to negotiate as smooth gravel and neat steps give way to rougher terrain. At 0.25 mile and 0.5 mile from the trailhead (0.75 mile and 1 mile, respectively, from your car), wide overlooks provide open views of the East Valley and The Phoenician resort.

The trail alternates between winding switchbacks and gentle straightaways for a while as it ascends, passing creosote bushes, palo verde trees, various cacti, and

Camelback Mountain: Cholla Trail

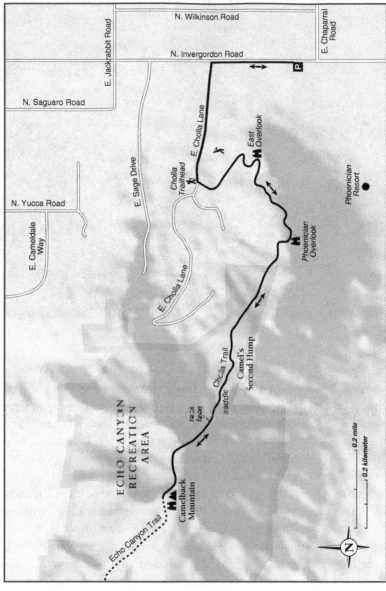

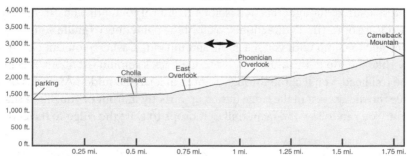

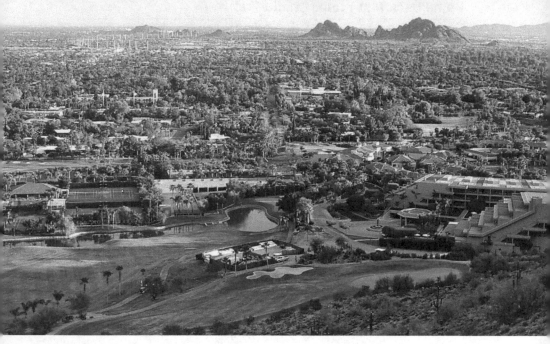

Cholla Trail overlooks The Phoenician Resort, with Papago Buttes in the distance.

ocotillo plants. The trail then bends northwest to take you up along the northern side of the camel's lower hump. At about 0.7 mile from the trailhead, you'll come to a small metal railing along the side of the trail, where a sign reads AREA CLOSED. This is where the original Cholla Trail meets the current one. If you look carefully, you can just see the faint remnants of the old trail snaking downhill toward an empty cul-de-sac, the original parking area for Cholla Trail.

Continue climbing until you reach a prominent saddle point at 1 mile from the trailhead. Take a breather here to enjoy the views on either side. You will need your strength because the remainder of Cholla Trail presents more of a challenge than what you've encountered so far. From here the trail climbs steeply up the ridge, over boulders and slippery gravel-covered slopes. In some spots, such as at the small rock face at 1.1 miles from the trailhead, you may have to use your hands to scramble uphill. Rest assured, though: this trail is not a technical route. Just be careful. If you become unsure of the trail's direction, look for blue paint dots to guide you.

Continue to climb until you reach the summit ridge, where you can clearly see the top. Hike the top of this ridge toward Camelback's summit. At about 1.25 miles from the trailhead, you'll climb through a notch in a large boulder. After this point, you'll see the rocky crest of the ridge jutting up directly in front of you, like a shark's dorsal fin. You can follow the main trail as it drops to skirt the ridge to its left or, if you feel a bit adventurous, tackle the ridge straight on. Look for a lone tree directly in front of the rocky ridgecrest, and use a conveniently extended branch to hoist yourself up and to the right. This seemingly unlikely turn is actually a split in the trail. If you follow it to the right side of the ridgecrest, you'll have 10 feet of exposed traverse to get your adrenaline flowing. The two routes rejoin about 100 feet farther along the trail, and the rest of the climb is obvious.

The 2,704-foot summit of Camelback Mountain is one of my favorite places in Phoenix. From this central vista point, you can see for miles in all directions. As your lungs recover from the climb, take a moment to explore the wide summit. Beautifully landscaped resorts, golf courses, and mansions dot the base of Camelback. A ring of mountains surrounds the sprawling metropolis of the fifth-largest city in the United States. If you aren't afraid of heights, go to the northeastern side of the summit to peer over the sheer cliff. You might find some brave souls rappelling down or parasailing off the cliff. If you are lucky, a beautiful desert sunset will reward your travails, and there's no better place in Phoenix from which to watch it than here.

Return the same way you came, for a 3.8-mile round-trip hike. Alternatively, shorten your hike by 0.7 mile by descending on the more scenic Echo Canyon Trail. Of course, this option requires that you have a ride waiting in Echo Canyon Recreation Area. Biking or jogging around the mountain are other enjoyable possibilities.

NEARBY ACTIVITIES

Enjoy one of the many upscale resorts and spas, such as **The Phoenician** or **Camelback Inn,** that surround Camelback Mountain. The **Indian Bend Wash Greenbelt,** a system of parks, golf courses, bike paths, and lakes, lies 4 miles to the east along Hayden Road. **Piestewa Peak** (see Hikes 10 and 11, pages 64 and 68), another popular urban hiking destination, lies just 4 miles to the northwest. The smaller **Mummy Mountain** is directly north of Camelback Mountain.

• •

GPS TRAILHEAD COORDINATES N33° 30.813' W111° 56.907'

DIRECTIONS *From Loop 202:* Exit onto 44th Street and drive 3.5 miles north to Camelback Road. Turn east (right) on Camelback Road and continue 2.7 miles to Invergordon Road. Turn north (left) onto Invergordon Road, drive 0.7 mile, and park in marked spots on the west side of the street.

From Loop 101: Exit onto Chaparral Road and drive west 3.2 miles until you reach a T-intersection at Invergordon Road. Turn north (right) on Invergordon and park on the west side of the street.

3 CAMELBACK MOUNTAIN:
Echo Canyon Trail

The Praying Monk kneels in awe of Camelback Mountain against a colorful desert sunset.

PERHAPS THE BEST in-town hike in Phoenix, Camelback Mountain is centrally located, offers a rigorous climb of 1,264 feet to its summit, and features rugged sandstone cliffs, a panoramic view from the top, and the chance to see a perfect sunset. Whether you're a resident or a visitor, this hike is a must-do.

DESCRIPTION

Named for its double-hump silhouette, Camelback Mountain, in the middle of metropolitan Phoenix, resembles a giant sleeping camel. Like an oasis of wilderness in a sea of housing developments and shopping centers, Camelback is a welcome respite from the hustle and bustle of urban life.

There are two trails to the summit of Camelback Mountain. The popular Echo Canyon Trail runs up the western side, while the slightly easier Cholla Trail (see previous hike) scales Camelback Mountain's gentler eastern ridge.

Echo Canyon Trail starts at the end of a small parking lot inside Echo Canyon Recreation Area. A drinking fountain, shaded benches, and restrooms give hikers one last chance to prepare for the challenge ahead. The 1,264-foot climb to its summit is just over a mile in length but can humble all but the most accomplished athletes, so remember to take the hike at your own pace to avoid exhaustion.

DISTANCE & CONFIGURATION: 2.6-mile out-and-back

DIFFICULTY: Strenuous

SCENERY: Highest point in Phoenix; sandstone cliffs; Praying Monk

EXPOSURE: Partial early-morning and late-afternoon shade; otherwise exposed

TRAIL TRAFFIC: Heavy

TRAIL SURFACE: Packed dirt, gravel, stairs, boulders, handrail-assisted steep sections

HIKING TIME: 1.5 hours

WATER REQUIREMENT: 1–1.5 quarts

DRIVING DISTANCE: 8 miles from Phoenix Sky Harbor Airport

ELEVATION GAIN: 1,440' at trailhead, 2,704' on summit of Camelback Mountain

ACCESS: Sunrise–sunset; limited parking at Echo Canyon; no permits or fees required

MAPS: USGS *Paradise Valley;* trailhead plaque

FACILITIES: Restrooms, water, picnic areas

WHEELCHAIR ACCESS: None

CONTACT: 602-261-8318, phoenix.gov/parks /trails/locations/camelback-mountain

COMMENTS: No dogs allowed

Every year, many ill-prepared hikers experience dehydration and heat exhaustion and must be rescued from Camelback. *Do not underestimate the difficulty or potential perils of this trail.* During summer, when the temperature soars above 100°F, consider splashing water on your clothing before starting the hike to keep cool. You'll be completely dry again before you reach the summit.

Begin your hike by crossing a dry wash to reach the packed-dirt trail that ascends Echo Canyon. In February and March wildflowers dot the landscape along this section. Purple lupines, yellow brittlebush, and Mexican gold poppies stand in stark contrast to green grasses and red rocks. At about 0.15 mile, the trail begins a series of steep switchbacks. As you huff and puff up the trail, the city fades and the beauty of Echo Canyon engulfs you. Sheer cliffs and red sandstone formations reminiscent of Sedona frame your field of view. These rocks form the sleeping camel's head, which is relatively young compared with the metamorphic rock that composes the rest of Camelback Mountain. At 0.3 mile, you will arrive at the first of several saddle points on this hike. Take a quick breather here to enjoy the view. The town of Paradise Valley lies straight ahead, and you can turn around to see the parking lot, already 250 feet below. Above and to the right looms a famous rock formation known as the Praying Monk. It doesn't look like it from this vantage point, but when seen from the East Valley, this formation resembles a person kneeling in prayer at the base of Camelback Mountain.

Continue your hike by following the obvious trail to the right, sandwiched between formidable cliffs and a chain-link fence shielding houses below from falling rocks and wandering hikers. After you ascend the stairs, approach a handrail-assisted scramble up a steep slope in the shadows of a towering precipice. Don't worry— this part looks scarier than it really is. When you eventually descend this section, however, remember that it may be easier to lower yourself down backward (facing uphill). One more handrail-assisted climb up some boulders, and you're done with the camel's head at about 0.6 mile. From here, you're on your own—there are no more steps or rails to guide you.

Camelback Mountain: Echo Canyon Trail

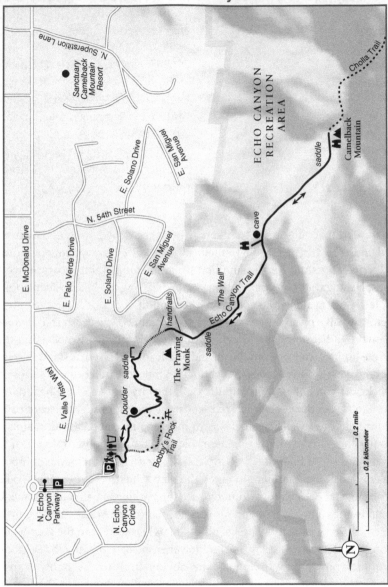

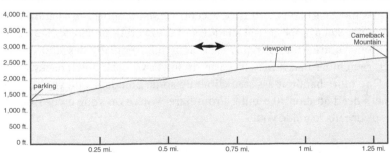

Traverse a small flat stretch in the trail; then, just before it climbs again, the trail forks. The left fork takes you up a smooth rock face some locals call "The Wall," while the right fork runs up a boulder-strewn gulley. Bear right here and brave the boulders unless you're sure-footed enough to tackle a 45-degree incline with a steep drop-off.

At the top of the gulley, admire your first open view toward the south. The trail bends left and climbs relatively gently to another small saddle. If you are adventurous, leave the trail here and turn left to visit the best-kept secret on Camelback Mountain. Skirt the right edge of the hill on your left and be careful with your footing. About 100 feet farther, you will find a small shallow cave. At the cave opening, you can rest while enjoying a secluded view of Paradise Valley's many mansions and golf courses. Remember to duck when leaving the cave to avoid hitting your head; then return to the trail.

What comes next is a long, steep section of boulder-hopping. Just keep your head down and work your way slowly up this beast. If you need to take a break, do so at about 1.1 miles, where you have a view of a castlelike home to your right, nestled in the mountainside. Right about here, the trail makes a nearly 90-degree bend to the left. On the way down, however, this little bend is not obvious, so make a mental note of where the trail is.

By now your lungs and legs are probably burning, and you might be wondering when you're ever going to reach the top. Be aware that you can't see the summit from here. The top of this steep section is a false peak, though it isn't far from the true summit. The trail bends one last time to the left and ascends the final 0.1 mile to the 2,704-foot peak of Camelback Mountain.

The wide summit of Camelback can easily accommodate a large crowd, and it usually has one. Everyone from sweaty trail-runners to camera-toting tourists is enjoying this view from the highest point in Phoenix. And who can blame them? From here, you command a sweeping 360-degree view of metropolitan Phoenix. Take a well-deserved rest and see if you can find the following landmarks in a clockwise survey of the landscape: the Phoenician Resort at the base of the mountain to the southeast, South Mountain, Sky Harbor International Airport, downtown Phoenix and Chase Field, Piestewa Peak, McDowell Mountains, Four Peaks, Superstition Mountains, and Cholla Trail running down the eastern ridge of Camelback (see previous hike). If you're lucky enough to hike Camelback at the right time on a partly cloudy day, you might also experience an amazing display of color. Nothing beats the silhouette of a saguaro cactus or an ocotillo plant against a brilliant Arizona sunset. *Warning:* Avoid dawdling, because hiking down in near-darkness can be treacherous, and you risk getting a parking ticket if you stay too long.

After you soak up the scenery, return the way you came. Alternatively, descend the 1.4-mile Cholla Trail down the eastern ridge of Camelback Mountain. This option requires a car shuttle to Invergordon Road, the parking area for Cholla Trail.

The truly ambitious day-hiker can attempt a "double crossing," descending Cholla Trail and then coming back up. Insane as it may seem, many fit locals make this double crossing a daily routine. Cross-trainers sometimes jog the additional 3 miles from the Cholla Trailhead back to Echo Canyon Park.

NEARBY ACTIVITIES

Many upscale resorts and spas, such as **The Phoenician** and **Camelback Inn,** surround Camelback Mountain. The **Indian Bend Wash Greenbelt,** a system of parks, golf courses, bike paths, and lakes, lies 4 miles to the east along Hayden Road. **Piestewa Peak** (see Hikes 10 and 11, pages 64 and 68), another popular urban hiking destination, is 4 miles to the northwest. The smaller **Mummy Mountain** is directly north of Camelback Mountain.

• •

GPS TRAILHEAD COORDINATES N33° 31.283' W111° 58.410'

DIRECTIONS *From Loop 202:* Exit onto 44th Street and drive north 4.5 miles. Follow 44th Street as it bends east into McDonald Drive. As McDonald Drive curves north into Tatum Boulevard, turn east (right) onto McDonald Drive, and then take the second right turn at the roundabout to enter Echo Canyon Park.

From Loop 101: Exit onto McDonald Drive and drive west for 5 miles to Echo Canyon Park.

A secluded cave near Echo Canyon Trail offers an intimate view of Paradise Valley.

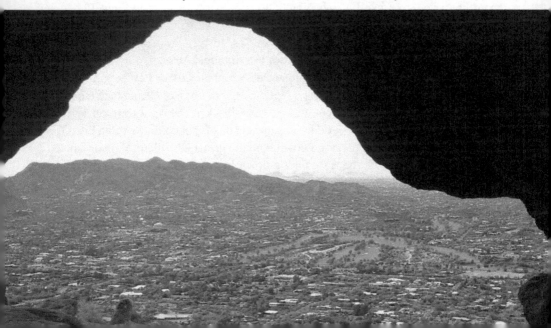

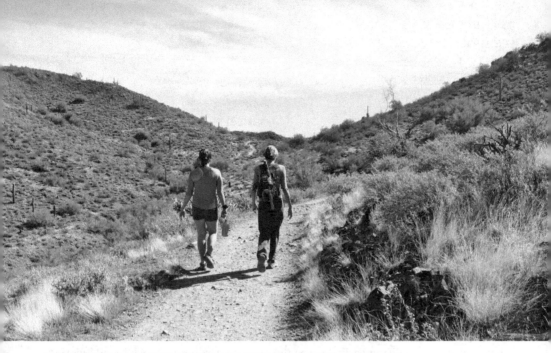

Mild winters beckon hikers to enjoy the great outdoors in Phoenix Sonoran Preserve.

A SCENIC LOOP takes hikers around Dixie Mountain, and a detour along Dixie Summit Trail affords a bird's-eye view from the top.

DESCRIPTION

North Phoenix residents have ample opportunities to explore trails within Phoenix Sonoran Preserve, the newest addition to the City of Phoenix's nature preserve system. The state trust land is still in the process of being acquired and developed; the resulting preserve's master plan calls for the conservation of more than 20,000 acres of pristine northern-Phoenix desert. Many miles of trails are already open; the hike described here traverses one popular loop in the southern section of the preserve.

From the marked Desert Vista Trailhead, hike north along Hawk's Nest Trail, a wide, packed-dirt path. Cross a dry wash about 500 feet into your hike as the trail begins to leave the housing development behind. The desert holds many surprises for the observant hiker. You may not find a hawk's nest along this short trail, but often there are owls perched in the arms of tall saguaros, especially at dawn or dusk.

The trail turns east to begin a moderate climb. Stay left to pass the signed junction for Hawktail Trail and Desert Tortoise Trail. Continue hiking along a hillside where the desert blooms in vibrant colors during spring. Hawk's Nest Trail meets

DISTANCE & CONFIGURATION:
5.1-mile balloon

DIFFICULTY: Moderate

SCENERY: Dixie Mountain, Phoenix Sonoran Preserve, city views, wildlife

EXPOSURE: Mostly exposed

TRAIL TRAFFIC: Moderate

TRAIL SURFACE: Rock, gravel, packed dirt

HIKING TIME: 2.5 hours

WATER REQUIREMENT: 2 quarts

DRIVING DISTANCE: 28 miles from Phoenix Sky Harbor Airport

ELEVATION GAIN: 1,600' at trailhead, 2,285' on summit of Dixie Mountain

ACCESS: Sunrise–sunset; no fees or permits required

MAPS: USGS *Union Hills* and *New River SE;* trailhead map kiosk

FACILITIES: Restrooms but no water; horse-trailer parking

WHEELCHAIR ACCESS: None

CONTACT: 602-495-6939, phoenix.gov/parks /trails/locations/sonoran-preserve

COMMENTS: Dogs permitted on leash except when temperature exceeds 100°F

Dixie Mountain Loop at a saddle point 0.4 mile from the trailhead; turn right to head counterclockwise on Dixie Mountain Loop Trail.

The trail levels off as you hike toward a gap between two hills. Notice the contrast between the tranquil desert basin and the sea of tile roofs behind you. The trail begins another gentle ascent and soon crests a small hill where eastern views open up. In the distance, Red Mountain, Four Peaks (see Hike 46, page 237), Pinnacle Peak (see Hike 20, page 112), and Thompson Peak (see Hike 23, page 126) line the horizon. The trail levels off again, making it easier to scan the scenery. You'll soon reach a trail junction for Valle Verde Trail—stay left here to continue hiking Dixie Mountain Loop.

Past the trail junction, rockier terrain requires you pay a bit more attention to your footing, but the trail remains easily navigable. The eastern section of this loop showcases vibrant desert flora such as the ocotillo, whose delicate, bright-red flowers bloom in April. Palo verde trees and creosote bushes are also common sights. However, not as many chollas or saguaro cacti live here compared with the warmer western foothills. At 1 mile from the trailhead, reach a saddle point with an unmarked spur trail to the left, which leads to a viewpoint overlooking north Phoenix. Head around the hill to soon reach the junction with Dixie Summit Trail.

Turn left to visit the summit of Dixie Mountain. The summit trail switchbacks up the steep hill in a field of palo verde trees and creosote bushes. You'll reach the top of Dixie Mountain at 1.6 miles from the trailhead and 2,285 feet elevation. Several hilltops within the preserve are visible from the wide and rocky summit, as is the sprawling city beyond. The panoramic view encompasses the White Tank Mountains to the west, plateaus to the east, and the other Phoenix mountain preserves to the southeast. Retrace your steps down Dixie Summit Trail; then turn left onto Dixie Mountain Loop to continue the hike.

At 2 miles from the trailhead, you arrive at the easternmost point of the loop, a saddle dotted with teddy bear chollas, barrel cacti, and a saguaro. Follow the trail as it turns sharply northwest. Even fewer cacti live on the cooler northern slopes, but

Dixie Mountain Loop

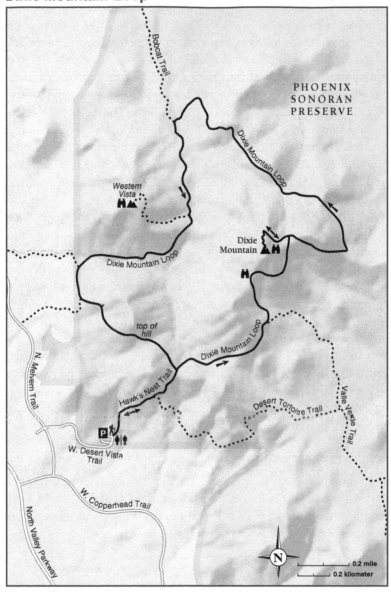

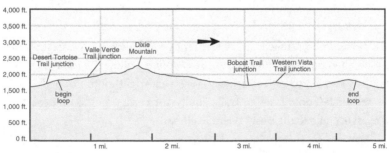

the ubiquitous creosote bushes cover the landscape. The wide, rocky trail undulates but generally descends from Dixie Mountain, with the massive Bradshaw Mountains in the distance. Cross a significant drainage at 2.5 miles; then pass a field of teddy bear chollas—stay clear of them, and keep your pets from a prickly encounter, too. Follow Dixie Mountain Loop north-northwest until it sweeps around to face south.

Pass a dry wash to reach the junction with Bobcat Trail. Again, stay left to remain on Dixie Mountain Loop, hiking south. The wide gravel trail begins another climb through the Sonoran Desert landscape, with Dixie Mountain in full view. Cross the same dry wash again several times within the next 0.25 mile, and continue climbing as you begin the final stretch of the loop. At 3.5 miles from the trailhead, you'll arrive at the Western Vista Trail junction, where you'll see a dense forest of teddy bear chollas. If you'd like to add another summit excursion to your loop, the Western Vista Trail climbs to an unnamed peak (2,040' elevation) within 0.33 mile. Otherwise, stay left and continue along Dixie Mountain Loop. Soon after the trail junction, you'll hike parallel to a deep ravine on your left before crossing a dry creek bed.

Notice the rusty carcass of an old SUV at 4 miles from the trailhead. Someone must have tried to drive this narrow mountain path but took an unfortunate slide into the ditch. Now hiking on the western edge of Dixie Mountain Loop, you pass two unmarked trail junctions; keep left each time to stay on the main trail. Then climb a steep hill on the edge of some housing developments to complete the loop.

Cresting the steep hill at 4.5 miles from the trailhead, take a quick breather here before completing the final ascent on Dixie Mountain Loop. The trail levels off and then returns to the Hawk's Nest Trail junction. Turn right, onto Hawk's Nest Trail, and hike 0.4 mile to return to the Desert Vista Trailhead.

NEARBY ACTIVITIES

More than 50 miles of trails crisscross Phoenix Sonoran Preserve. The nearby **Apache Wash** and **Desert Hills Trailheads** lead to many of these trails. **Cave Creek Regional Park** (see Hike 47, page 241) and **Black Mountain** (see Hike 16, page 96) are both a short drive northeast of Phoenix Sonoran Preserve.

• •

GPS TRAILHEAD COORDINATES N33° 44.472' W112° 05.833'

DIRECTIONS From I-17, take Exit 218 for Happy Valley Road. Drive east on Happy Valley 0.5 mile; then turn north (left) onto 19th Avenue. Follow the road 1.8 miles as 19th Avenue turns into North Valley Parkway. Turn east (right) onto Copperhead Trail, and take the second left onto Malvern Trail. Finally, turn east (right) onto Desert Vista Trail, and follow it 0.3 mile to the Desert Vista Trailhead.

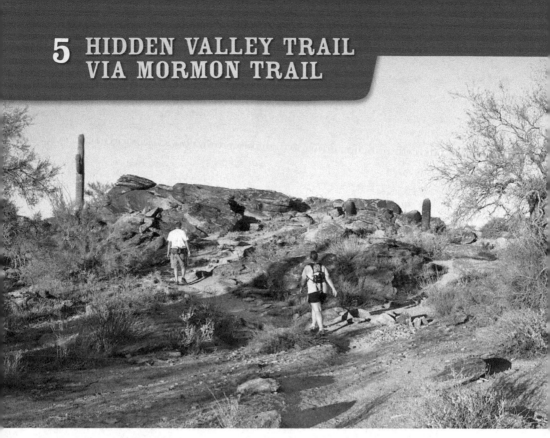

A setting sun paints the rugged landscape along South Mountain's Mormon Trail.

HIDDEN VALLEY TRAIL, traversing an enclave of wilderness where all signs of the city disappear, is South Mountain's hidden gem. High atop the Guadalupe Range, this quiet half-mile trail boasts some of the most picturesque rock formations in the region, including a natural rock tunnel and Fat Man's Pass.

DESCRIPTION

Covering more than 16,000 acres, South Mountain Park/Preserve spans almost the entire southern boundary of Phoenix. Since 1924, visitors have enjoyed its desert and mountain lands for their rustic beauty. The Civilian Conservation Corps built numerous trails, roads, picnic facilities, and lookouts in the park. Today, more than 3 million visitors come here annually to enjoy splendid hiking, mountain biking, and other recreational activities. Though both the population of Phoenix and the number of visitors to South Mountain have skyrocketed in recent decades, one part of the park remains relatively untouched by the influx of people: Hidden Valley.

Atop the Guadalupe Range, the half-mile Hidden Valley Trail takes hikers through a stretch of charming wilderness that holds the most scenic rock formations in the entire park. Two such formations, a natural rock tunnel and Fat Man's Pass, act as sentinels, one at either end of the trail, guarding entrances into Hidden Valley. Once

DISTANCE & CONFIGURATION: 3.9-mile balloon

DIFFICULTY: Moderate

SCENERY: Desert, city views, Hidden Valley, Fat Man's Pass, unique rock formations

EXPOSURE: Mostly exposed

TRAIL TRAFFIC: Moderate

TRAIL SURFACE: Gravel, packed dirt, smooth bedrock, a little easy scrambling

HIKING TIME: 2 hours

WATER REQUIREMENT: 2 quarts

DRIVING DISTANCE: 6 miles from Phoenix Sky Harbor Airport

ELEVATION GAIN: 1,325' at trailhead, 2,100' at highest point

ACCESS: Gates open 5 a.m.–7 p.m.; trails open until 11 p.m.; no permits or fees required

MAPS: USGS *Lone Butte;* trailhead plaque

FACILITIES: Water and shaded ramada, but no restrooms

WHEELCHAIR ACCESS: None

CONTACT: 602-262-7393, phoenix.gov/parks /trails/locations/south-mountain

COMMENTS: Shortest route to reach Hidden Valley and Fat Man's Pass; dogs permitted on leash except when temperature exceeds 100°F

you're inside, all signs of the city vanish, along with most traffic and noise from the busy National Trail (see Hike 14, page 82). This tranquil valley further entices you with sandy wash beds and beautiful granite boulders and rocks unlike any found elsewhere on South Mountain.

Hidden Valley Trail is really just a detour along National Trail, forming a small loop beginning at 2.6 miles on National's 15-mile course. The easiest way to reach Hidden Valley is to hike up Mormon Trail, which intersects this loop on the National Trail side. The resulting Mormon–National–Hidden Valley balloon, one of the most enjoyable short hikes on South Mountain, is a desirable alternative to the often over-crowded National–Mormon Loop, accessible from the east end of South Mountain.

Park in a small lot on 24th Street and Valley View Drive, and begin by ascending a hill at the western end of the parking area up to the ridge, where a trailhead plaque displays park information and a map. Mormon Trail heads southeast atop the ridge and begins a moderate climb up South Mountain. Along the trail, you'll find familiar desert plants, such as creosote bushes, palo verde trees, and saguaro cacti. At 0.3 mile, top out on a small saddle, where you can turn and survey the parking lot below and the housing developments encroaching on the base of the mountain. From here, you can also see downtown Phoenix, Piestewa Peak, Camelback Mountain, the McDowell Mountains, and the red sandstone buttes in Papago Park.

Continue on Mormon Trail as it snakes uphill. The trail gets progressively more difficult, and at 0.6 mile it switchbacks up a steep hillside. Power through this sec-tion—it's the only moderately difficult ascent on this hike. The slope soon gives way to a high, flat basin at 0.9 mile and 1,900 feet elevation. Mormon Loop Trail, which joins from the left at 1.1 miles, parallels National Trail and takes you to Pima Canyon Park at the eastern end of South Mountain. Continue straight on Mormon Trail until it ends and makes a T with National Trail at a signed junction 1.4 miles into the hike.

At this point you can go either way; I prefer to ascend first and hike the loop counterclockwise, because route-finding in Hidden Valley is slightly easier from

Hidden Valley Trail via Mormon Trail

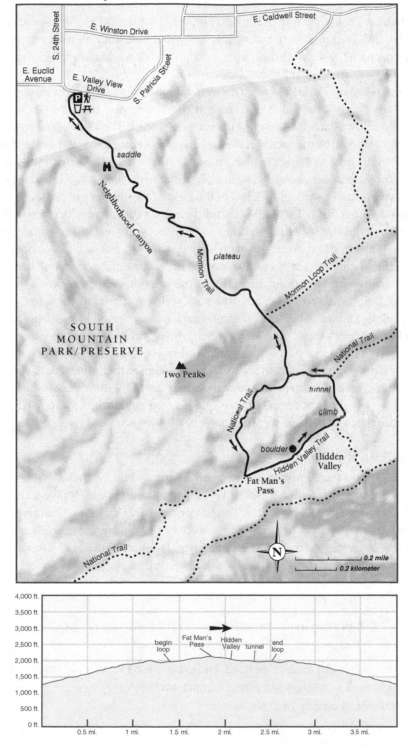

west to east. Turn right, onto National Trail, watching out for speedy mountain bikers. National Trail meanders and climbs gently 0.4 mile until it crests at 2,100 feet before dropping slightly. At this point, look for a trail marker at the Hidden Valley Trail junction. Turn left and leave National Trail here.

You'll soon see Fat Man's Pass. This misnamed wonder is one of the most popular features on South Mountain. A thin crack nearly 25 feet long and only 9 inches wide at one point, Fat Man's Pass tempts kids and adults alike. The walls of the crack have been worn smooth by thousands of sweaty torsos squeezing through it over the years. Take off your pack and cram yourself through sideways (suck in that gut!), or just scoot over the boulders instead of sliding through the crack. Kids will also enjoy sliding down a naturally smooth rock just to the right of the entrance to Fat Man's Pass.

On the other side of Fat Man's Pass, follow a dry wash dotted with riparian brush. At 2 miles from the trailhead, a cluster of large boulders blocks the path. You can squeeze under or climb over them, then jump down a few feet into a large open bowl and continue along the sandy creekbed. At 2.2 miles, a natural granite wall challenges you to climb down 5 feet or so. Be careful on the smooth, slippery rock.

The trail turns north soon after the rock wall and arrives at the other striking feature along Hidden Valley Trail, a natural rock tunnel formed by overlapping boulders. Look through the 30-foot-long tunnel, whose worn walls shimmer in the light coming from the other side. Watch your head as you walk through. Once through, look for petroglyphs etched into the rock by Hohokam natives hundreds of years ago.

Hidden Valley Trail rejoins National Trail at 2.4 miles from the Mormon Trailhead. Turn left onto National Trail here, and hike 0.2 mile to the Mormon Trail junction. Turn right and descend via Mormon Trail with the skyline of Phoenix before you.

NEARBY ACTIVITIES

South Mountain Park/Preserve boasts many hiking and biking trails, including **Holbert** (see next hike), **National** (see Hike 14, page 82), **Pyramid, Ranger,** and **Telegraph Pass** (see Hike 22, page 121). The **Environmental Education Center,** near the Central Avenue entrance, has a superb visitor center, complete with historical exhibits and a three-dimensional model of the entire park. **Dobbins Lookout** and **Buena Vista,** both accessible by car, offer superb views of Phoenix by day and its city lights by night.

• •

GPS TRAILHEAD COORDINATES N33° 21.983' W112° 1.862'

DIRECTIONS Exit I-10 at Baseline Road, and drive west 3.7 miles to 24th Street. Turn south (left) onto 24th Street and follow it until it ends at Valley View Drive. Turn left to find the trailhead parking lot.

Holbert Trail offers splendid views of the Valley of the Sun.

THIS SHORT HIKE offers visual variety to visitors seeking an alternative to South Mountain's main corridor trails. Along the hike, visit Hohokam petroglyphs, which were carved into the boulders; gaze on a perfectly framed view of the Phoenix skyline; and enjoy the steady moderate incline for a great workout.

DESCRIPTION

Three of the five largest municipal parks and preserves in the country are right here in the Phoenix area. Valley of the Sun residents are truly lucky to have access to so many hiking destinations. Situated on Phoenix's southern border, South Mountain Park/Preserve provides a natural setting for outdoor activities and exploration on foot, mountain bike, or horseback.

The dozens of trails within the park's boundaries span three mountain ranges and their foothills. These trails vary greatly in length, difficulty, popularity, and accessibility. From the main park entrance, however, perhaps no other trail is as convenient and as visually appealing as Holbert Trail. Rising from the desert floor, Holbert leads hikers on a scenic approach via Box Canyon, continues steadily up a picturesque mountainside to Dobbins Lookout, and then culminates at a junction with National Trail (see Hike 14, page 82) along the spine of South Mountain.

DISTANCE & CONFIGURATION: 5.4-mile out-and-back

DIFFICULTY: Moderate

SCENERY: City views from Dobbins Lookout, South Mountain Park/Preserve, Hohokam petroglyphs, Box Canyon

EXPOSURE: Mostly exposed

TRAIL TRAFFIC: Moderate

TRAIL SURFACE: Packed dirt, sand, uneven rock, pavement

HIKING TIME: 2.5 hours

WATER REQUIREMENT: 2 quarts

DRIVING DISTANCE: 9 miles from Phoenix Sky Harbor Airport

ELEVATION GAIN: 1,345' at trailhead, 2,400' at end of trail where it meets National Trail

ACCESS: Gates open 5 a.m.–7 p.m.; trails open until 11 p.m.; no permits or fees required

MAPS: USGS *Lone Butte*; park maps available from website below

FACILITIES: Restrooms, water, picnic tables

WHEELCHAIR ACCESS: None

CONTACT: 602-262-7393, phoenix.gov/parks /trails/locations/south-mountain

COMMENTS: Ample parking; dogs permitted on leash except when temperature exceeds 100°F

Make your way from the almost ridiculously large parking area between the Activity Complex and Environmental Education Center to the Holbert Trailhead, which is near the restrooms and picnic area. Hike south on a level trail toward Box Canyon and the rugged mountains. You'll travel over sandy packed dirt and rocky steps as you hike around a large rock outcrop on your left. The trail soon curves east. You might hear some gunfire in the distance as you hike, but relax: those shots are likely from a nearby shooting range. Pass through a large open area with fire rings used for guided walks and other events; then pass a series of dry-wash crossings. To your left is a sea of tiled roofs, downtown Phoenix's tall buildings, and, on the distant horizon, numerous mountains north of town.

A quarter mile from the trailhead, you'll arrive at some wooden guardrails and large boulders covered with petroglyphs. These primitive drawings, made by etching into the dark, topmost patina of the rock, offer a glimpse into desert life some 600–800 years ago. The color of the etchings indicates whether they are original designs left by the Hohokam or scribbles made by modern "artists."

After the petroglyph area, continue hiking through relatively level terrain to cross a large dry wash at 0.4 mile from the trailhead. To your left, look for a deep-cut canyon formed by powerful desert flash floods. Even an arid area such as Phoenix can experience violent storms, the runoff from which can cut a deep swath through the desert floor. Holbert Trail soon meets a paved service road leading to a large water tank. Hike along the road about 100 yards; then veer away from it at a signpost near the water tank.

The trail begins its steady ascent from this point, 0.6 mile from the trailhead. The initial uphill slope is steep enough to raise your heart rate in a hurry, but it soon eases into a gentle climb. Uneven rocky landscape covers most of this trail, so be sure to watch your footing to avoid ankle injuries.

Holbert Trail and Dobbins Lookout

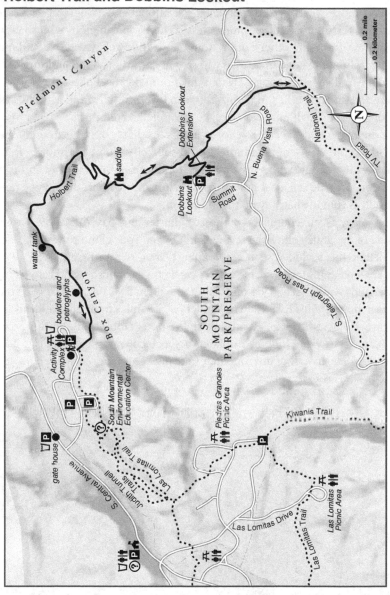

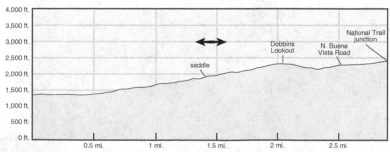

Unlike more-well-traveled trails such as National and Telegraph Pass (see Hike 22, page 121), Holbert Trail sees much less traffic. You can enjoy superb city views rivaling those from any other South Mountain trail in relative peace and quiet. At 0.75 mile, follow the edge of a ridge where you can still see the parking lot behind you and the trail ahead wrapping around the mountainside. Follow the trail as it contours around the next hill, alternating between level stretches and a gradual ascent.

Along the next half mile, you'll make a couple hairpin turns as you cross major hillside drainages and traverse a set of switchbacks that lessen the strain of the steep climb. Along the way, stop to admire picturesque city views charmingly framed by the hills. A small saddle with a vista point, 1.4 miles from the trailhead and 1,880 feet in elevation, provides an ideal setting to take a longer breather, should you need one. This saddle is roughly halfway up the mountain.

The steady ascent continues southeast a quarter mile past the saddle. Cross to the right side of the gulley at a large ravine, and resume your climb toward the ridgetop. Hills encircle this secluded section of Holbert Trail, obscuring any sight of the city below. Seasonal rains feed a sparse crop of catclaw acacia bushes and canyon ragweed near the sandy wash. Ascend via another set of switchbacks next to a striking rock wall to arrive at the Dobbins Extension trail junction, 1.8 miles from the trailhead.

Leave Holbert Trail here, turning right, onto Dobbins Extension. Continue uphill 0.2 mile to visit Dobbins Lookout, a spectacular vantage point at 2,330 feet that overlooks nearly all of metropolitan Phoenix. This site was named for James C.

Petroglyphs along Holbert Trail and other sites in South Mountain offer a glimpse into the past.

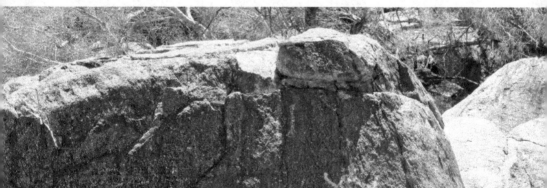

Dobbins, the chairman of the committee responsible for creating what would become South Mountain Park/Preserve. You'll find a parking area and restrooms here. Be sure to visit the circular observation platform, which has a compass map of the valley's landmarks. Next, walk through the stone ramada, which provides shade during the warmer months and allows a cool breeze through its large windows.

Leaving Dobbins Lookout, retrace your steps to reach Holbert Trail.

At this point, you can choose to turn back or continue following Holbert Trail another 0.6 mile to its end. If you choose the latter, turn right and climb to a hillock overlooking the large basin atop South Mountain. Descend about 30 feet and cross the sandy wash that feeds the ravine you just ascended.

The landscape and scenery atop South Mountain are quite different from what you saw on your ascent. A wide basin stretches in all directions. Needlelike saguaros rise from the landscape in the same way that cactus needles might jut out from their trunks. A forest of antennas reaches skyward from the summit of Mount Suppoa, seemingly mimicking the saguaros below. At night, the flashing lights on these antennas can be seen from anywhere in Phoenix.

After crossing the sandy wash, follow the trail gently uphill until it reaches Buena Vista Road. Cross here and hike up a small ridge with open views of the winding road to either side. The Sierra Estrella Mountains loom behind the antenna farm. Holbert Trail ends when it meets National Trail at a paved service road. There is no trail access to the highest point on South Mountain, so you'll return from here via Holbert Trail.

NEARBY ACTIVITIES

South Mountain is one of the largest city parks in the United States. There are many miles of interconnected South Mountain trails, with **National Trail** (see Hike 14, page 82) anchoring them. Other notable hikes within South Mountain Park/Preserve include **Telegraph Pass Trail** (see Hike 22, page 121), **Mormon Trail** (see previous hike), **Alta Trail,** and **Pyramid Trail.** The South Mountain area also offers other activities, such as horseback riding, target shooting, and go-kart racing.

• •

GPS TRAILHEAD COORDINATES N33° 21.098' W112° 04.203'

DIRECTIONS From Central Avenue and Baseline Road, drive south on Central for 2 miles; then follow the road as it curves west. Just past the South Mountain Park/Preserve entrance gate, turn left, toward the Environmental Education Center. Follow this road to the Holbert Trailhead, which is near the Activity Complex.

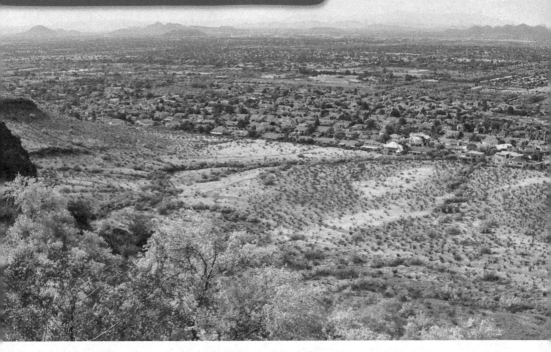

Blooming palo verde trees add a splash of color to the view from Lookout Mountain.

LOOKOUT MOUNTAIN OFFERS hikers a short but challenging climb to a panoramic view from its summit. The longer and easier Circumference Trail winds around Lookout Mountain's base for a more leisurely hike.

DESCRIPTION

At 2,054 feet, Lookout Mountain's summit ranks among the highest peaks in Phoenix and provides choice views of the city below. The crowds that swarm more-popular trails such as Piestewa Peak Summit Trail (Hike 11, page 68) largely stay away from this rocky outpost on Phoenix Mountains Preserve's northern edge. Lookout Mountain Summit Trail 150 extends only 0.6 mile, but it presents a respectable 500-foot elevation gain along a rocky path to the top. Milder and longer, Circumference Trail 308 offers a gentler hike sans steep ascents. Both trails are short enough that you can easily hike both of them within a few hours.

The main trailhead for both Summit Trail and Circumference Trail is on 16th Street, south of Bell Road. Lookout Mountain Park, on the southeastern corner of the mountain, has an alternate trailhead and additional amenities, such as a larger parking lot, a restroom, and shaded picnic areas. A short connecting trail links the park with Circumference Trail, but access to Summit Trail from the park requires a hike to the main trailhead.

DISTANCE & CONFIGURATION: 1.1-mile out-and-back; add 2.6 miles for optional Circumference Trail loop

DIFFICULTY: Moderate for main hike; easy for optional loop

SCENERY: Lookout Mountain, city panorama, desert views

EXPOSURE: completely exposed

TRAIL TRAFFIC: Light–moderate

TRAIL SURFACE: Crushed rock, gravel, scree

HIKING TIME: 1 hour for main hike; add 1.5 hours for optional loop

WATER REQUIREMENT: 1 quart for main hike; add 1 quart for optional loop

DRIVING DISTANCE: 18 miles from Phoenix Sky Harbor Airport

ELEVATION GAIN: 1,580' at trailhead, 2,054' on summit of Lookout Mountain

ACCESS: Gates open 5 a.m.–7 p.m.; trails open until 11 p.m.; no permits or fees required

MAPS: USGS *Sunnyslope;* trailhead plaque

FACILITIES: *Main trailhead:* water only; *alternate trailhead:* restrooms, picnic area, tennis courts, and playground

WHEELCHAIR ACCESS: None

CONTACT: 602-262-7901, phoenix.gov/parks /trails/locations/lookout-shadow-mountain

COMMENTS: Dogs permitted on leash except when temperature exceeds 100°F

From the main trailhead, which is next to a large cylindrical water tank, begin by hiking southwest along an obvious trail covered in gravel and crushed rock. Open desert terrain characterizes the foothills here. Only occasional creosote bushes and palo verde trees break the wide expanses. Cacti seem conspicuously absent from the landscape. Many smaller use trails branch out from the main trail, making navigation a hassle; the main trail is fairly easy to follow, however, if you stay left at the first few forks. Brown, rectangular posts mark the correct route. At 0.1 mile, Summit Trail breaks from Circumference Trail and heads uphill at the end of a wide turn.

Gentle turns give way to switchbacks beginning at 0.2 mile from the trailhead. Loose rocks challenge your footing, while steeper slopes demand more effort from your legs. There are some confusing forks along the ascent, but in general, you want to stay with the switchbacks and avoid any spur trails that go straight. Nearly halfway up the mountain, Summit Trail straightens and gets considerably steeper as it heads for a saddle between the main summit and a smaller summit to the west. Climb the scree-covered trail to a prominent saddle point at 0.4 mile from the trailhead. This saddle, at 1,875 feet, already commands a fine view. From here, finish your climb by turning left to ascend the southern side of Lookout Mountain. There are some loose and rocky steps here, and you might have to duck under a palo verde tree. Once on the summit ridge, the going gets considerably easier, and you can make a beeline for the peak.

As one might expect, Lookout Mountain's flat summit overlooks the vast city surrounding the mountain preserve. To the south, major peaks within Phoenix Mountains Preserve, such as Piestewa Peak, North Mountain, and Shaw Butte, frame the distant downtown buildings. Behind them lie the long ridges of South Mountain and the jagged Sierra Estrella peaks. This panoramic view encompasses nearly all of the major

Lookout Mountain

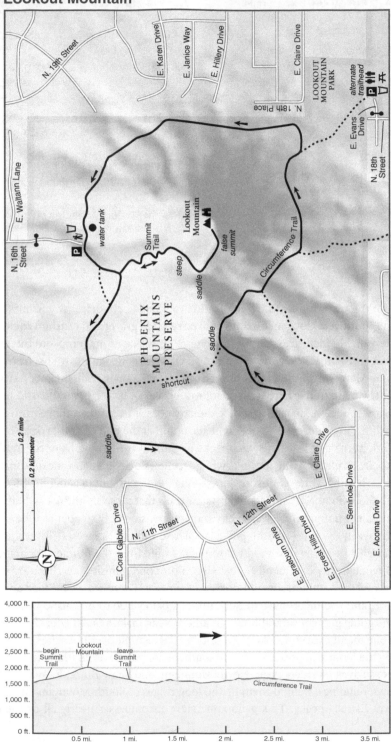

mountain ranges that surround metropolitan Phoenix, so take your time to soak it all in. Return via the same route to the Summit Trail and Circumference Trail junction.

If you have time, consider tacking on the 2.6-mile Circumference Trail 308, which encircles Lookout Mountain and a smaller peak to its west. From the aforementioned trail junction, turn west onto Circumference Trail and descend a gentle slope toward a deep but dry wash. The trail crosses the wash and veers left uphill. At a marked trail fork 0.3 mile from where you left Summit Trail, break right and hike west toward a saddle point. Cross this saddle and then turn left at a fork about 30 yards downhill.

The trail parallels the preserve's western boundary and skirts the backyard fences of some homes. Near the mountain's southwestern edge, make a moderate climb east on loose rock. Roughly 1.4 miles from where you left Summit Trail, you'll reach a boulder-strewn, 1,670-foot-high saddle point between Lookout Mountain and its western sibling; here, turn southeast and skirt the southern side of Lookout Mountain. Many use trails crisscross this area, so look for the brown posts to stay on Circumference Trail.

At 1.9 miles from where you left Summit Trail, a wide path leads toward Lookout Mountain Park and the alternate trailhead. Follow this path southeast, toward the park, but turn left to leave the access trail. Another left turn takes you close to some backyards. Now hiking between Lookout Mountain and backyard fences, continue north along Trail 308. The trail eventually curves around the eastern flank of the mountain to take you back to the water tank and the main trailhead in 2.6 miles.

NEARBY ACTIVITIES

Phoenix Mountains Preserve contains many popular trails, including **Piestewa Peak** (see Hikes 10 and 11, pages 64 and 68), **Shaw Butte** (see Hike 13, page 77), and **North Mountain** (see Hike 8, page 56). **Shadow Mountain,** on the eastern side of Cave Creek Road and Sharon Drive, has a few short trails. On Central Avenue and the Arizona Canal, **Murphy's Bridle Path** offers a pleasantly shaded urban walk.

• •

GPS TRAILHEAD COORDINATES
N33° 37.623' W112° 02.897' (Main Trailhead)
N33° 37.112' W112° 02.578' (Lookout Mountain Park)

DIRECTIONS *Main Trailhead:* Take AZ 51 to Bell Road. Exit onto Bell Road and drive west 2.6 miles to 16th Street. Turn south (left) onto 16th Street and follow it 0.9 mile to a small parking lot next to the water tank.

Lookout Mountain Park: Take AZ 51 to Cactus Road. Exit onto Cactus Road, and drive west 1.6 miles to Cave Creek Road. Follow Cave Creek Road north (right) 1 mile to Sharon Drive. Turn west (left) onto Sharon Drive, and continue 0.5 mile. Then turn north (right) onto 18th Street, and proceed 0.5 mile to Lookout Mountain Park.

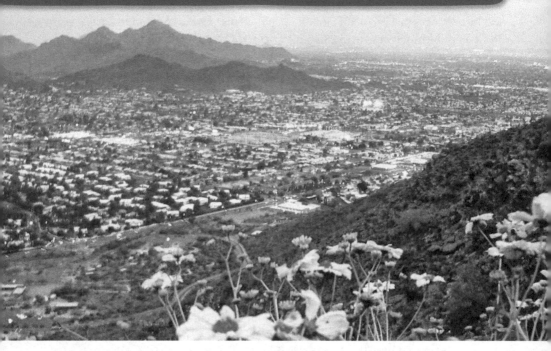

Brittlebush blossoms accentuate a twilight city view from North Mountain National Trail.

SHORT, STEEP, PAVED, and accessible nearly around the clock, the centrally located North Mountain National Trail offers Phoenix residents excellent daily exercise.

DESCRIPTION

North-central Phoenix residents are really fortunate to have the likes of North Mountain in their backyards. North Mountain National Trail 44 is only 1.6 miles round-trip, and most of it is paved. A decent elevation gain of 654 feet induces a cardio workout, and the panoramic scenery from North Mountain's 2,104-foot summit indulges the senses. It's an ideal place for a quick workout any time of the day and well into the night. Imagine how much money you can save on gym memberships by incorporating this trail into your daily routine!

Unlike other popular hikes, such as Camelback Mountain (see Hikes 2 and 3, pages 29 and 34), Piestewa Peak (see Hikes 10 and 11, pages 64 and 68), and Shaw Butte (see Hike 13, page 77), North Mountain seems to have ample parking to handle the crowds. Though the Maricopa Picnic Area, where the trail begins, has only a few spaces, there is a large parking lot in the center of North Mountain Park; other parking areas are sprinkled around the loop drive. There's even an alternate access

DISTANCE & CONFIGURATION: 1.6-mile out-and-back or 1.6-mile loop

DIFFICULTY: Moderate

SCENERY: North Mountain, city panorama, desert views

EXPOSURE: Partial shade in early mornings and late afternoons

TRAIL TRAFFIC: Heavy

TRAIL SURFACE: Rock, gravel, pavement

HIKING TIME: 1 hour

WATER REQUIREMENT: 1 quart

DRIVING DISTANCE: 13 miles from Phoenix Sky Harbor Airport

ELEVATION GAIN: 1,450' at trailhead, 2,104' on summit of North Mountain

ACCESS: Gates open 5 a.m.–7 p.m.; trails open until 11 p.m.; no permits or fees required

MAPS: USGS *Sunnyslope*

FACILITIES: Restrooms, water, picnic areas, playground, ranger station

WHEELCHAIR ACCESS: Yes, at North Mountain Visitor Center

CONTACT: 602-262-7901, phoenix.gov/parks/trails/locations/north-mountain

COMMENTS: Dogs permitted on leash except when temperature exceeds 100°F

point outside the park on Seventh Street. North Mountain Visitor Center, just north of the park, is yet another parking option.

Most people hike to the summit and return along the paved service road, which is a fine route. North Mountain National Trail is actually a loop, however. The unpaved southern half of the trail sees much less traffic and offers fantastic south-facing views. Those who prefer a rugged hiking experience appreciate the unpaved and steeper southern route.

Begin from the Maricopa Picnic Area, at the park's northern end. The trail ascends a steep, rocky slope to a saddle at 0.15 mile, where a spur trail heads right, toward some vista points. Turn left up a flight of stairs to meet the paved service road, which allows access to the mountaintop antennas. You can see the alternate parking area at the base of the service road, on Seventh Street. Looking down the service road, you can also see a gate. Trail 100A lies just beyond that gate and links North Mountain with trails near Shaw Butte and North Mountain Visitor Center.

Follow the steep service road toward the summit. Enjoy a picturesque view at every bend in this road. North-facing turns overlook a wide basin below and Shaw Butte to the northwest. A saddle at 0.4 mile overlooks North Mountain Park and the city to the south. Just below the antenna-studded summit, turn left to find a vista point where a memorial bench beckons you to sit and take a break. From here you actually look down upon Pointe Hilton Tapatio Cliffs Resort and its Different Pointe of View Restaurant, which is poised atop a hill across Seventh Street. Piestewa Peak, Four Peaks, and South Mountain are all within view. On a clear day, you can even see Weaver's Needle, in the Superstition Mountains.

North Mountain's true summit is fenced off, so the bench is a good turnaround point if you wish to stick to the pavement. Consider, however, taking the less-traveled southern route back down to North Mountain Park. Just below the summit, look for

North Mountain National Trail

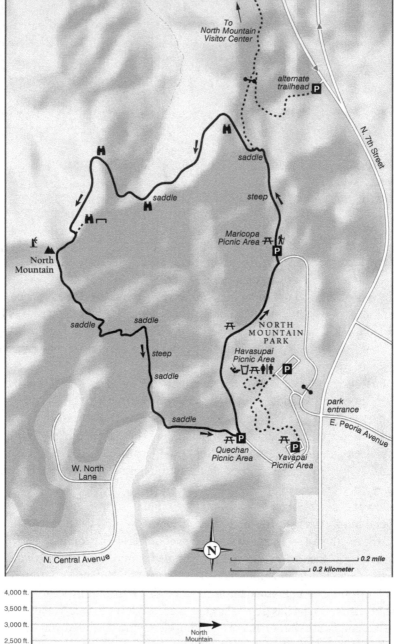

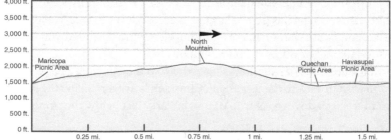

a brown post marking the spot where the trail leaves the road. Hike a short distance up to the ridgeline south of the summit. Walk the ridge heading south on a trail of crushed rock with open views to both sides.

At 0.9 mile from the trailhead, the trail begins to descend from the ridgeline's southern tip. Desert plants such as triangle-leaf bursage and creosote bush line the trail. You might see some colorful flowers here in spring, including yellow brittle-bush, blue phacelia, and purple lupine. Enjoy an impressive view of Phoenix and its downtown skyline from the end of the ridgeline.

The remainder of the hike is a steep but short descent of the southern slope of North Mountain. Along the way, you'll pass several view-studded saddles and numerous switchbacks. The turns are obvious and well marked. The trail eventually emerges at the Quechan Picnic Area, inside North Mountain Park. Complete the 1.6-mile loop by hiking north along the one-way road to return to Maricopa Picnic Area. Hikers who crave thigh-burning steep climbs may choose to tackle this loop in the opposite direction because the southern trailhead is lower and the trail itself is considerably steeper than the paved service road.

NEARBY ACTIVITIES

Phoenix Mountains Preserve encompasses many popular hiking trails, including **Piestewa Peak** (see Hikes 10 and 11, pages 64 and 68), **Shaw Butte** (see Hike 13, page 77), **Lookout Mountain** (see previous hike), and **Perl Charles. Camelback Mountain** (see Hikes 2 and 3, pages 29 and 34), another Valley favorite, is located at the preserve's southeast end.

North Mountain Visitor Center, on Seventh Street, offers educational classes and interpretive displays explaining the richness of the Sonoran Desert landscape.

• •

GPS TRAILHEAD COORDINATES N33° 35.139' W112° 03.973'

DIRECTIONS Exit AZ 51 onto Northern Avenue and drive west 1.8 miles to Seventh Street. Turn north (right) on Seventh Street, and continue 2 miles to Peoria Avenue. Turn west (left) at Peoria Avenue to enter North Mountain Park; then follow the one-way road to the Maricopa Picnic Area. If the parking lot there is full, use any of the other parking areas in the park.

A small alternate parking area is just outside North Mountain Park, on Seventh Street, 0.5 mile north of Peoria. However, this parking lot is accessible only from the southbound lanes of Seventh Street.

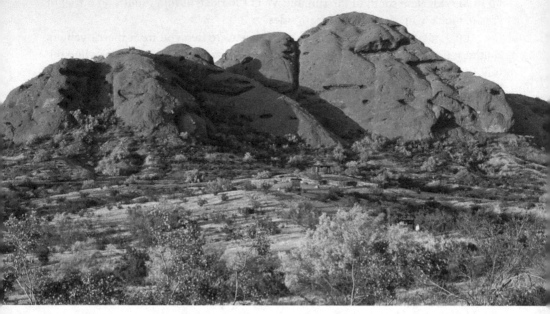

Red sandstone buttes of Papago Park glow in the late-afternoon sun.

A LARGE OASIS amid the sprawling city, Papago Park is to Phoenix what Central Park is to New York. Its distinctive red sandstone buttes and reflective lakes adjacent to the zoo are all trademark features of Papago Park. This backdrop provides the setting for a relaxing and view-studded hike.

DESCRIPTION

Few parks in Phoenix offer as much to enjoy as Papago Park. Home of the Phoenix Zoo and Desert Botanical Garden, a golf course, a fire museum, a sports complex, and many biking, walking, and hiking paths, Papago Park caters to everyone.

Papago Park's colorful history dates to 1879, when it became a reservation for Pima and Maricopa Indians. The park is named for the Papago, a Native American people who inhabited southern Arizona. In the early 1900s, under President Woodrow Wilson's administration, the park was designated Papago Saguaro National Monument, but Congress later rescinded that designation. During World War II, a POW camp erected at the base of Papago Buttes housed more than 400 German prisoners. Today, the Army Reserve Motor Park still occupies the area. The City of Phoenix purchased the park in 1959 and has been operating it ever since.

Oddly eroded by wind and rain, several red sandstone buttes throughout the 1,200-acre park provide the backdrop for many park features. These distinctive

DISTANCE & CONFIGURATION: 2.2-mile figure eight

DIFFICULTY: Easy

SCENERY: Papago Buttes, unique rock formations, desert, city panoramas

EXPOSURE: Completely exposed

TRAIL TRAFFIC: Moderate

TRAIL SURFACE: Gravel, dirt

HIKING TIME: 1 hour

WATER REQUIREMENT: 1 quart

DRIVING DISTANCE: 3 miles from Phoenix Sky Harbor Airport

ELEVATION GAIN: 1,250' at trailhead, with no significant rise

ACCESS: Sunrise–sunset; no fees or permits required

MAPS: USGS *Tempe;* trailhead plaque

FACILITIES: Water, ramada, picnic areas

WHEELCHAIR ACCESS: Yes, to Eliot Ramada

CONTACT: 602-495-5458, phoenix.gov/parks /trails/locations/papago-park

COMMENTS: Dogs permitted on leash except when temperature exceeds 100°F

holey rocks can be seen from nearly anywhere in Phoenix. The largest buttes are in the northern part of the park, straddling McDowell Road. Galvin Parkway bisects the park lengthwise, and the busy eastern half of Papago Park encompasses the much-visited zoo and botanical garden, while the quieter western half appeals more to hikers and mountain bikers.

The route suggested here encircles two prominent buttes in the park's western half and composes part of the West Park Loop Trail. Start from a parking lot west of Galvin Parkway, opposite the main entrance to the Phoenix Zoo. The trailhead is located next to a ramada with drinking water. Begin by hiking north on a gravel path toward the largest butte, which, for lack of imagination, is named Big Butte. Many confusing use trails crisscross the landscape, but don't worry about getting lost: just aim straight for the large mound of rock and the elevated ramada at its base.

Approximately 0.6 mile from the trailhead, arrive at Eliot Ramada, where the Phoenix skyline comes into view on the western horizon. Continue across the paved road and pick up a trail that skirts the left side of the butte. Hike toward the busy McDowell Road, and notice the typical desert flora: triangle-leaf bursage, brittle-bushes, creosotes, palo verdes, and fragrant desert lavender line the trail. North of the butte and adjacent to McDowell Road, an old amphitheater lies unused, undoubtedly because of the incessant road noise.

Continue past the amphitheater to a small mound with a northeastern view. All major mountains on the periphery of the East Valley can be seen here. Camelback Mountain dominates the north, while the McDowell Mountains, Four Peaks (see Hike 46, page 237), Red Mountain, and the Superstitions frame the eastern skyline. On a clear day, one can even see the needlelike Pinnacle Peak (see Hike 20, page 112). Complete your loop around the largest butte, staying close to the red rock at all forks. As you round the hill's eastern flank, you'll glimpse Desert Botanical Garden across Galvin Parkway, Tempe's Hayden Butte, and Hole-in-the-Rock, an eroded red sandstone butte next to the Phoenix Zoo.

Papago Park

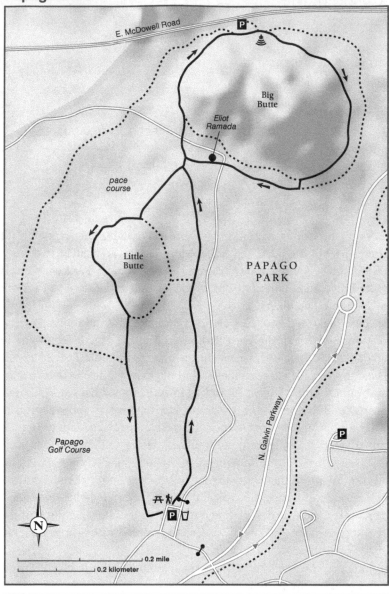

E. McDowell Road

P

Big
Butte

*Eliot
Ramada*

*pace
course*

Little
Butte

PAPAGO
PARK

N. Galvin Parkway

Papago
Golf Course

P

P

N

0.2 mile
0.2 kilometer

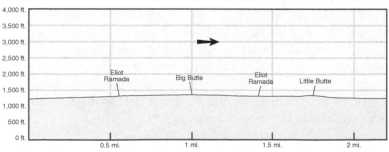

4,000 ft.				
3,500 ft.				
3,000 ft.				
2,500 ft.				
2,000 ft.	Eliot Ramada	Big Butte	Eliot Ramada	Little Butte
1,500 ft.				
1,000 ft.				
500 ft.				
0 ft.	0.5 mi.	1 mi.	1.5 mi.	2 mi.

Approximately 1.3 miles from the trailhead, break away from the large butte and head downhill toward Eliot Ramada again. From there, aim for the right side of a smaller butte, named (you guessed it) Little Butte, where many wooden signs mark the start of an orienteering course and a pace course. As the trail skirts the small butte, enjoy an expansive view toward the southwest. Papago Golf Course lies below the trail, while South Mountain, the Sierra Estrellas (see Hike 57, page 289), and the White Tank Mountains complete a sweep of the western horizon.

At the southwestern corner of the small butte, head south downhill parallel to the golf course fence. Marvel at the striking contrast between the arid landscape and the greens and fairways inside the golf course, proof positive that the grass is indeed greener on the other side of the fence. The trail passes several junctions and eventually meets the parking lot from which you began, completing a 2.2-mile hike. If you have extra time, consider following the trail all the way around the golf course for an additional 2 miles.

Before leaving Papago Park, be sure to visit Hole-in-the-Rock and Hunt's Tomb, two of the park's most popular features. Both are located in the eastern half of the park, so you'll need to drive across Galvin Parkway; make a left after the park gate, and then follow the signs to Ramada 8. A short but steep trail climbs to a natural rock window for a splendid sunset vista overlooking the city and the lakes near the zoo. The ancient Hohokam people used the projection of sunlight through Hole-in-the-Rock as a natural sundial.

Farther south in the park and beyond Ramada 16, a white pyramid entombs Arizona's first governor, George W. P. Hunt, and his family. Though the pyramid itself is worth a visit, its western platform is a must-see, as the view from here is one of the finest in the park. A bench provides the perfect setting for admiring part of Phoenix Zoo as well as the desert sky reflected in several adjacent lakes. With so many attractions, Papago Park is a delightful destination for the entire family.

NEARBY ACTIVITIES

Both the **Phoenix Zoo** and **Desert Botanical Garden** lie within Papago Park. The park also provides a golf course, a sports complex, picnic areas, and even a fish hatchery. **Camelback Mountain** (see Hikes 2 and 3, pages 29 and 34), **Hayden Butte,** and the **Indian Bend Wash Greenbelt** are all within a short distance of Papago Park.

• •

GPS TRAILHEAD COORDINATES N33° 27.316' W111° 57.256'

DIRECTIONS From Loop 202, exit onto Priest Drive. Drive north 1.25 miles on Priest, which becomes Galvin Parkway. At the traffic signal for the Phoenix Zoo, turn left into the trailhead parking lot.

10 PIESTEWA PEAK: Freedom Trail

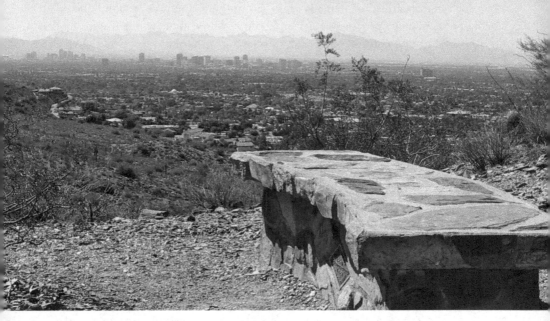

Memorial benches along the Freedom Trail offer resting hikers a view of the Phoenix skyline.

THERE ARE MANY reasons to choose Freedom Trail over the popular Piestewa Peak Summit Trail (see next hike). Some do it to get more scenic variety. Others prefer to get closer to the desert. Some hike it because it's less strenuous than Summit Trail, while others want a longer hike. Whatever your reason for hiking Freedom Trail, you'll enjoy this loop around Piestewa Peak.

DESCRIPTION

Coiled around the base of Piestewa Peak in Phoenix Mountains Preserve, Freedom Trail (formerly Piestewa Peak Circumference Trail) 302 offers a moderate hike and a scenic route through the splendors of Phoenix Mountains Park. In lieu of towering views from the summit, this trail showcases the best desert flora and fauna in the park and takes you on a wide loop around the peak. Freedom Trail is the second-most popular hike in Phoenix Mountains Park. Though it shares 0.5 mile with the often busy Summit Trail 300, most of Freedom Trail is relatively uncrowded.

The trailhead elevation is 1,520 feet. Begin your hike at a well-signed egress from the parking lot at the northern end of Phoenix Mountains Park. Immediately descend to cross a dry creek, and climb up the other side to join the Freedom Trail loop.

I prefer to hike this loop counterclockwise, avoiding the steeper climb on the first part of Summit Trail. To do this, turn right at the T-intersection, and then head

DISTANCE & CONFIGURATION: 3.8-mile loop

DIFFICULTY: Moderate

SCENERY: Desert, Piestewa Peak, Phoenix Mountains Preserve

EXPOSURE: Completely exposed

TRAIL TRAFFIC: Moderate

TRAIL SURFACE: Gravel, crushed rock, stone stairs, sharp and uneven rock

HIKING TIME: 2 hours

WATER REQUIREMENT: 2 quarts

DRIVING DISTANCE: 10 miles from Phoenix Sky Harbor Airport

ELEVATION GAIN: 1,520' at trailhead, 2,090' at highest point on loop

ACCESS: Gates open 5 a.m.–7 p.m.; trails open until 11 p.m.; no permits or fees required

MAPS: USGS *Sunnyslope;* trailhead plaque

FACILITIES: Water, toilets, covered picnic tables, ranger station in Phoenix Mountains Park

WHEELCHAIR ACCESS: None

CONTACT: 602-261-8318, phoenix.gov/parks /trails/locations/piestewa-peak

COMMENTS: Also known as Piestewa Peak Circumference Trail; no dogs allowed on the portion of the hike shared with Piestewa Peak Summit Trail

north along the obvious trail. As you walk along the crushed-rock surface up a gentle incline, admire the abundant variety of desert plants around you. Tall saguaros, prickly chollas, hardy creosotes, and nearly leafless palo verdes line the trail. During spring, Mexican poppies and brittlebush blossoms paint the mountainsides gold.

This part of Freedom Trail overlaps Nature Trail 304, which features many educational plaques detailing various plants and their desert habitat. The basin through which you are hiking hosts the richest variety of desert flora within Phoenix Mountains Preserve. Try to identify all of the following species of cacti as you hike: buckhorn cholla, teddy bear cholla, giant saguaro, strawberry hedgehog, pincushion, prickly pear, and fishhook barrel. Depending on the time of day and time of year, you can also spot many species of birds here. Look for cactus wrens, mockingbirds, quails, owls, and hawks.

At 0.5 mile from the trailhead, an obvious sign directs you to take the left fork at a trail junction—stay on the combined Trail 302/Trail 304. A tenth of a mile farther, you'll pass a plaque detailing the giant saguaro cactus and a memorial bench dedicated to Janet. This is where Perl Charles Memorial Trail 1A merges into Freedom Trail. You've already climbed 200 feet from the trailhead, but a steeper ascent awaits. Look up to see the peaks and saddles directly in front of you. Keep left and follow the trail as it climbs steep switchbacks toward the saddle on the right. At 0.75 mile and an elevation of 1,830 feet, follow the combined Trail 302 and Trail 1A to the left at a well-signed junction.

One mile into the hike, top out on a prominent saddle point at 2,090 feet, Freedom Trail's highest point. Two memorial benches provide convenient resting places to reward your efforts. Take a moment to enjoy the view here before heading down the western side of the saddle. The trail descends steeply via a series of tight switchbacks. As you descend, you can see a trail in the basin below heading for a saddle to the northwest. Resist the temptation to take this unmarked trail, which

Piestewa Peak: Freedom Trail

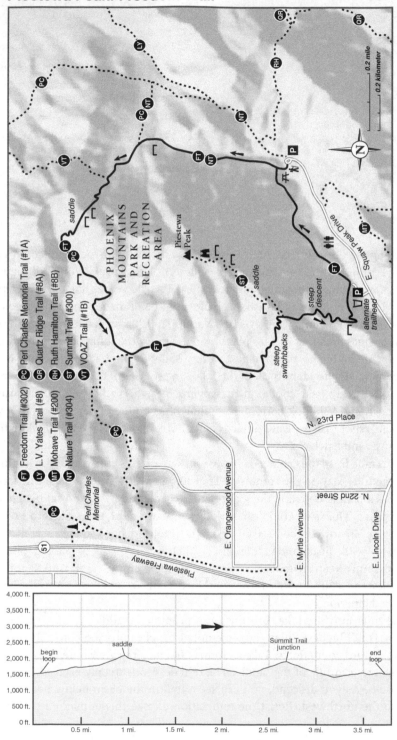

meets Freedom Trail at 1.15 miles at an elevation of 1,890 feet. Instead, follow the main trail south along a fairly flat and long traverse on Piestewa Peak's northwestern slope. Soon, you should see a white triangular sign confirming that you are still on Trail 1A, which coincides with Freedom Trail here.

Hike along the gently sloping traverse to a bench dedicated to Mark Hoff at 1.5 miles. A ring of peaks surrounds you, with only a small window of city views opening to the southwest. Continue hiking gently downhill along the trail as it rounds the western side of Piestewa Peak. At 1.75 miles, reach the halfway point of Freedom Trail and a bench dedicated to Richard Daleiden, where you can rest and admire the view of downtown Phoenix. This spot is also where Trail 1A leaves Freedom Trail and heads downhill toward the west. In the shadow of towering Piestewa Peak, continue south, traversing the hill until you reach a trail junction at 2.25 miles. From here, take the left fork and follow Freedom Trail steeply uphill along tight switchbacks.

Half a mile of hard work later, arrive at a 1,900-foot-high saddle where Freedom Trail meets Piestewa Peak Summit Trail 300. A reminder to those who enjoy hiking with four-legged friends: *dogs are not allowed on Summit Trail.* If you intend to complete the Freedom Trail loop, remember to leave your pets at home. Descend along Summit Trail 0.5 mile until just before you reach the parking lot at the base of the mountain. Freedom Trail breaks away from Summit Trail and turns north, paralleling the paved road inside Phoenix Mountains Park. Hike another 0.6 mile of mild inclines to complete the 3.8-mile loop and then return to the trailhead at the Apache Picnic Area.

NEARBY ACTIVITIES

Phoenix Mountains Preserve offers many other trails, including **Perl Charles Memorial Trail 1A, Piestewa Peak Summit Trail 300** (see next hike), **Shaw Butte Trail 306** (see Hike 13, page 77), and **North Mountain National Trail 44** (see Hike 8, page 56). Some trails are accessible to mountain bikes. Historic **Murphy's Bridle Path** lies along Central Avenue, 2 miles to the west. **Camelback Mountain** (see Hikes 2 and 3, pages 29 and 34), another Valley favorite, is only 4 miles to the southeast.

• •

GPS TRAILHEAD COORDINATES N33° 32.574' W112° 0.929'

DIRECTIONS Exit AZ 51 at Lincoln Drive, and drive east 0.5 mile. Turn north (left) onto Squaw Peak Drive, and continue 0.5 mile to the gated entrance to Phoenix Mountains Park. Go through the gate and follow the road 0.5 mile until it dead-ends at Apache Picnic Area.

11 PIESTEWA PEAK: Summit Trail

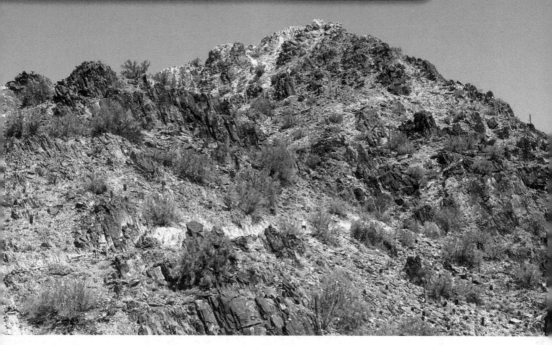

Craggy terrain and a steep ascent challenge Piestewa Peak Summit Trail hikers.

FOR DECADES, Piestewa Peak (formerly Squaw Peak) Summit Trail 300 has carried the title of Phoenix's most popular hiking trail. More people trample this well-trodden path up magnificent Piestewa Peak than any other trail in the Phoenix metropolitan area. This hike has become an institution in Phoenix culture and requires enough oomph to challenge even the fittest athletes. The summit's gorgeous panoramic view justifies its huge popularity.

DESCRIPTION

The 2,608-foot Piestewa Peak towers over Phoenix Mountains Preserve. Its pointy arête is one of the most prominent features on the Phoenix skyline. During mild weather, thousands of people hike Summit Trail 300 every day, making it the second-most popular trail in Arizona. Only Bright Angel Trail in Grand Canyon National Park attracts more visitors.

From the moment skies brighten in the morning until well after nightfall, a seemingly endless stream of hikers dots Summit Trail, making it a people-watching hot spot. If you like to socialize with fellow hikers, there's no better place in Phoenix. On this trail, I've seen everyone from cane-assisted nonagenarians to slumbering infants bouncing along in Mom's backpack. You'll meet weekend warriors trying to shed a few pounds as they labor up steep and rocky stairs, and glistening goddesses

DISTANCE & CONFIGURATION: 2.4-mile out-and-back

DIFFICULTY: Strenuous

SCENERY: City panorama, Piestewa Peak summit, desert, Phoenix Mountains Preserve

EXPOSURE: Completely exposed

TRAIL TRAFFIC: Very heavy

TRAIL SURFACE: Stone stairs, gravel, sharp and uneven rock

HIKING TIME: 1.5 hours

WATER REQUIREMENT: 1–1.5 quarts

DRIVING DISTANCE: 10 miles from Phoenix Sky Harbor Airport

ELEVATION GAIN: 1,400' at trailhead, 2,608' on Piestewa Peak summit

ACCESS: Gates open 5 a.m.–7 p.m.; trails open until 11 p.m.; no permits or fees required

MAPS: USGS *Sunnyslope*; trailhead plaque

FACILITIES: Water, toilets, covered picnic tables, ranger station in Phoenix Mountains Park

WHEELCHAIR ACCESS: None

CONTACT: 602-261-8318, phoenix.gov/parks /trails/locations/piestewa-peak

COMMENTS: Busy trail offers great people-watching; no dogs allowed

in tight sportswear jogging past you on their daily runs. You'll hear the exclamations of camera-wielding tourists and the chitchat of gossiping office workers. Some even come for a chance to flirt with more than Mother Nature.

Summit Trail originated as a pack trail in the 1930s but has seen consistent improvement over the years. Today, it's a veritable staircase of stony steps with some sharp exposed bedrock thrown in to twist your ankles in case of a misstep. Though landscape along the trail appears barren and rocky, rugged Sonoran Desert flora dots the hills around you. Creosote bushes and various species of cacti dominate the area. Occasional palo verde trees provide limited shade. During spring, golden brittlebush flowers add a dash of color to an otherwise gray and rocky terrain.

Hiking 1,190 vertical feet to Piestewa Peak is no small undertaking. Your challenge begins with the search for an open parking spot if you happen to arrive on a nice day. The small trailhead parking area is usually full. Instead, try parking at any of the picnic areas farther up the road. You can hike along Freedom Trail (see previous hike) or along the road to get to the trailhead. Summit Trail starts at a shaded ramada where you can slather on sunblock and fill your water bottle from a drinking fountain. Once you start climbing, consistently steep steps increase your heart rate and adrenaline in a hurry.

As you climb the steep trail, several memorial benches provide ample excuses and convenient places for you to rest and catch your breath. As an interesting diversion from the arduous task of climbing the hill, try to see if you can count the number of benches along Summit Trail. One such bench is dedicated to Robert D. Hill at 0.4 mile from the trailhead; it has a small palo verde tree behind it, yielding some late-afternoon shade. At 0.5 mile, the trail mercifully flattens a bit and heads toward a saddle, where Freedom Trail forks downhill—stay to the right to continue toward the summit.

At two-thirds of a mile from the trailhead and an elevation of 2,030 feet, Summit Trail jumps over a saddle to the western side of the mountain. This saddle overlooks an interior basin below and the AZ 51 freeway in the distance. At about 0.9 mile,

Piestewa Peak: Summit Trail

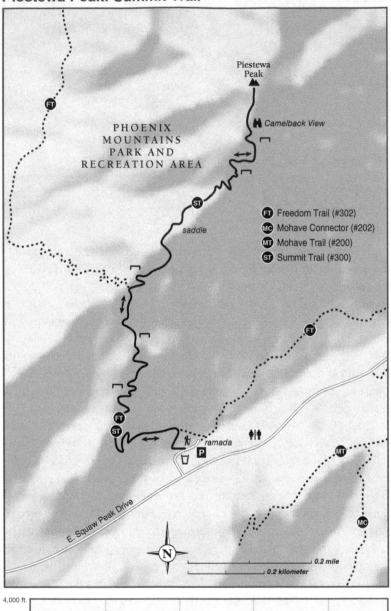

Piestewa
Peak

Camelback View

PHOENIX
MOUNTAINS
PARK AND
RECREATION AREA

saddle

FT Freedom Trail (#302)
MC Mohave Connector (#202)
MT Mohave Trail (#200)
ST Summit Trail (#300)

ramada

E. Squaw Peak Drive

N

0.2 mile
0.2 kilometer

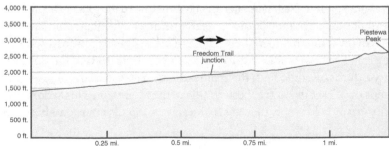

climb a steep hill and head straight toward the trail's most inviting bench, which has a large palo verde draped over it and provides welcome shade even on the hottest days. Take a rest here and enjoy the view of Camelback Mountain to the west, because the rest of the trail gets noticeably steeper and narrower.

While you grind out the last 0.3 mile, pass several old metal hitching posts. Although the days of pack animals on this trail are long gone, these posts are painful reminders that a horse or mule would come in handy right about now. The last few feet of trail near the summit requires a little careful stepping and clambering, especially if you want to get to the absolute highest point on Piestewa Peak, where the USGS survey disk is cemented into the ancient Precambrian granite. Most people settle for a rock outcropping a few feet lower than, and just to the west of, the true summit. From 2,608 feet, enjoy sweeping vistas in all directions. Unlike the wide summit of Camelback Mountain, chiseled Piestewa Peak gives you even better open views. You can see the antenna-covered North Mountain and Shaw Butte to the northwest, downtown Phoenix and Chase Field to the south, Camelback Mountain to the southeast, and the McDowell Mountains to the northeast. The top of the peak is also a great place to catch a beautiful Arizona sunset if you happen to be up here at dusk.

Descend the same route back to the parking lot. For a little variety, especially during hot summer months, try hiking Summit Trail after sundown; just be sure to park outside the entrance gate, which closes at 7 p.m. Flashlights can often be seen dancing up the mountain on a clear night, though under a bright full moon or when low clouds reflect the shimmering city lights, you hardly need artificial lighting at all. Watching the lights of the metropolis from atop Piestewa Peak is also a wonderfully romantic way to spend an evening.

NEARBY ACTIVITIES

Phoenix Mountains Preserve offers many other trails, including **Perl Charles Memorial Trail 1A, Freedom Trail 302** (see previous hike), **Shaw Butte Trail 306** (see Hike 13, page 77), and **North Mountain National Trail 44** (see Hike 8, page 56). Some trails are accessible to mountain bikes. Historic **Murphy's Bridle Path,** along Central Avenue, is 2.5 miles to the west. **Camelback Mountain** (see Hikes 2 and 3, pages 29 and 34), another Valley favorite, is only 2 miles to the southeast.

• •

GPS TRAILHEAD COORDINATES N33° 32.376' W112° 1.391'

DIRECTIONS Exit AZ 51 at Lincoln Drive, and drive east 0.5 mile. Turn north (left) onto Squaw Peak Drive, and continue 0.5 mile to the gated entrance to Phoenix Mountains Park. Take the first left inside the gate to reach the Summit Trailhead. If the small parking lot at the trailhead is full, try any picnic area inside the park.

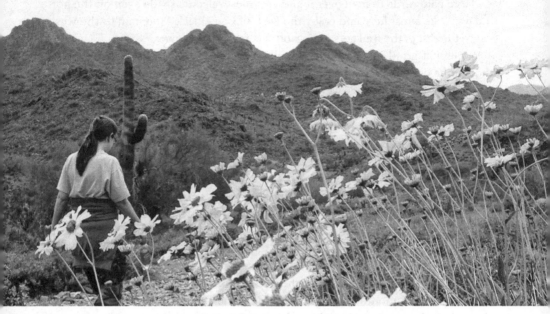

Stacy Herman Lang of Chandler hikes past blooming brittlebush along Quartz Ridge Trail.

DOTTED WITH BREATHTAKING views of Piestewa Peak and Camelback Mountain, Quartz Ridge Trail offers yet another scenic jaunt through Phoenix Mountains Preserve. Though it sits in the middle of the city, this trail visits many secluded desert basins where you experience a real sense of wilderness.

DESCRIPTION

Two prominent trails—L. V. Yates Trail 8 and Quartz Ridge Trail 8A—span the entire eastern border of Phoenix Mountains Preserve. Along with sections of Ruth Hamilton Trail 8B and Nature Trail 304, these trails form an enjoyable loop in the vicinity of Quartz Ridge. Three trailheads serve this network, offering ample opportunities to pick a balloon, loop, or out-and-back route to suit your hiking tastes. Add a shuttle vehicle, and you have several more options for one-way hikes.

Quartz Ridge Trail starts from the northeast corner of 32nd Street and Lincoln Drive, where a rather small trailhead parking area offers easy access to the preserve's interior. This route takes visitors through a striking canyon dotted with white quartz boulders for which the area is named. If parking is unavailable here, consider using alternate parking areas inside Phoenix Mountains Park or the 40th Street Trailhead south of Shea Boulevard.

DISTANCE & CONFIGURATION: 4.7- or 6-mile balloon, plus a variety of other options

DIFFICULTY: Moderate

SCENERY: Desert, Phoenix Mountains Preserve, Piestewa Peak, city views

EXPOSURE: Mostly exposed

TRAIL TRAFFIC: Moderate

TRAIL SURFACE: Gravel, rock

HIKING TIME: 2–3 hours

WATER REQUIREMENT: 2 quarts

DRIVING DISTANCE: 10 miles from Phoenix Sky Harbor Airport

ELEVATION GAIN: 1,400' at trailhead, 1,925' at highest point

ACCESS: Gates open 5 a.m.–7 p.m.; trails open until 11 p.m.; no permits or fees required

MAPS: USGS *Sunnyslope;* trailhead plaque

FACILITIES: Water, restrooms, covered picnic tables, ranger station in Phoenix Mountains Park

WHEELCHAIR ACCESS: None

CONTACT: 602-261-8318, phoenix.gov/parks /trails/locations/piestewa-peak

COMMENTS: Many trailheads serve the Quartz Ridge area, giving you plenty of options to customize the length and difficulty of this hike. Dogs permitted on leash except when temperature exceeds 100°F.

Start this trek from the 32nd Street Trailhead parking lot, which affords a head-on view of Camelback Mountain (see Hikes 2 and 3, pages 29 and 34). Quartz Ridge Trail rounds a hill and then turns north away from the noisy city and into a quiet mile-long basin. At 0.2 mile, you'll pass the junction with Mohave Connector Trail 202 to continue along the wide, crushed-rock path. The trail crosses a large creekbed and follows its eastern bank through rugged hills. You'll begin to ascend a gentle incline, with only the sound of crushed rock underfoot.

At 0.5 mile, the trail passes next to a huge quartz boulder whose white, marble-like surface contrasts against the surrounding desert. A short distance farther, the trail reaches a hilltop that is 130 feet higher than the trailhead before dropping into an upper basin where all signs of the city disappear. A prominent drainage runs through the basin, while a ring of hills surrounds you. At the head of this basin, you'll ascend steeply via a series of switchbacks and straights. The trail bends west halfway up the slope, contouring along a hillside often covered in wildflowers during spring. Along this stretch, you'll also enjoy open views of the valley below and a stunning outline of downtown Phoenix. Then the steep climb resumes, eventually leading to a prominent saddle and the intersection of Quartz Ridge Trail 8A and Ruth Hamilton Trail 8B. At 1.3 miles from the trailhead, this point marks the beginning of a counterclockwise loop.

Continue following Quartz Ridge Trail north over the saddle to descend into a larger basin where the only sign of civilization is a rather conspicuous house perched atop the hill to your right. Ahead, you can see where L. V. Yates Trail 8 approaches the basin from a saddle due north. Hike down a mildly sloped hill on loose crushed rock, taking care with your footing to avoid injury. As the slope tapers, the trail conditions improve. Gravel and packed dirt eventually take the place of loose rock.

At 1.6 miles from the trailhead, the trail enters a dry wash but then immediately veers away from it heading uphill. Strolling through this inner basin is an exercise

Quartz Ridge Trail

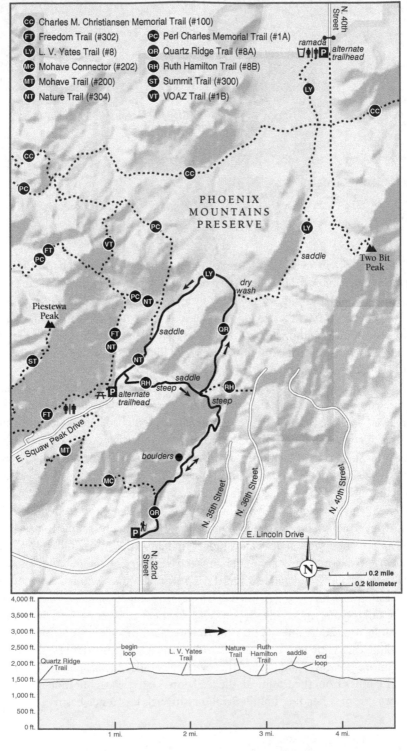

CC Charles M. Christiansen Memorial Trail (#100)
FT Freedom Trail (#302)
LY L. V. Yates Trail (#8)
MC Mohave Connector (#202)
MT Mohave Trail (#200)
NT Nature Trail (#304)
PC Perl Charles Memorial Trail (#1A)
QR Quartz Ridge Trail (#8A)
RH Ruth Hamilton Trail (#8B)
ST Summit Trail (#300)
VT VOAZ Trail (#1B)

N. 40th Street

ramada
alternate trailhead

PHOENIX MOUNTAINS PRESERVE

saddle

Two Bit Peak

dry wash

Piestewa Peak

saddle

saddle
steep

steep

alternate trailhead

E. Squaw Peak Drive

boulders

N. 35th Street
N. 36th Street
N. 40th Street

E. Lincoln Drive

N. 32nd Street

N

0.2 mile
0.2 kilometer

4,000 ft.
3,500 ft.
3,000 ft.
2,500 ft.
2,000 ft.
1,500 ft.
1,000 ft.
500 ft.
0 ft.

Quartz Ridge Trail
begin loop
L. V. Yates Trail
Nature Trail
Ruth Hamilton Trail
saddle
end loop

1 mi.   2 mi.   3 mi.   4 mi.

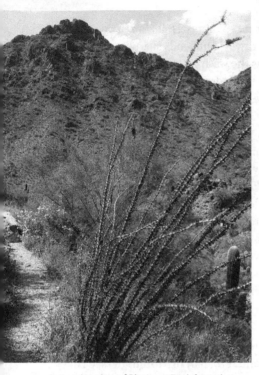

A stunning view of Piestewa Peak from the Quartz Ridge Trail

in serenity, unlike hiking the bustling Piestewa Peak trails nearby. Often the only sound you can hear is an occasional passing airplane. Continue following Quartz Ridge Trail 8A north to its terminus inside a surprisingly large creekbed, 1.9 miles from the trailhead. Here, you'll find the marked junction with L. V. Yates Trail 8. Turn left onto Trail 8 and then wind along the deep, wide creekbed. Some riparian bushes and trees, fed by occasional rainfall and water runoff, can provide limited shade on a warm day. Several trail markers guide you through the twists and turns until you eventually emerge from the dry wash onto a wide thoroughfare.

Follow Trail 8 as it bends southwest, staying left at all of the trail junctions, both marked and unmarked. The jagged summit of Piestewa Peak dominates the view as you begin a gentle ascent toward the 1,800-foot saddle at the head of this inner basin. Trail 8 passes imperceptibly into Phoenix Mountains Park and ends at the prominent saddle where it merges into Nature Trail 304.

Cross the saddle and begin a steep descent along Trail 304. At 2.9 miles, reach the well-marked intersection with Ruth Hamilton Trail 8B, which branches left. If you parked at the Piestewa Peak Trailhead, Trail 304 continues another 500 feet and terminates at the Apache Picnic Area inside Phoenix Mountains Park. Otherwise, turn left onto Trail 8B to embark upon the toughest stretch of trail on the entire circuit.

Trail 8B heads abruptly uphill and follows a ridge east. The path is steep and rocky, and it can quickly elevate your pulse—if you need a breather, turn around for an awesome view of Piestewa Peak. A half mile of hard climbing takes you to a 1,925-foot saddle, the highest point of the entire hike. Camelback Mountain pops into view ahead, and the junction of Trails 8A and 8B from earlier on lies just over the saddle. Descend toward that junction and then turn right onto Quartz Ridge Trail to finish your balloon hike for a total distance of 4.7 miles.

An alternate route for this hike starts from the 40th Street Trailhead, where you'll likely find ample parking. This course originates from the preserve's northern boundary and adds 1.3 miles to the total hike distance, but it offers an easier jaunt through Quartz

Ridge. From the large 40th Street Trailhead, find L. V. Yates Trail 8 on the west end of the parking lot. The trail begins by heading northwest but bends sharply south to cross a dry wash lined with dense brush. The trail exits the wash to the right, meanders southwest for a short distance, and then crosses the same dry wash again. After the second crossing, the trail makes an unmarked 90-degree left turn and heads toward distant hills.

At 0.5 mile from the trailhead, you'll cross Charles M. Christiansen Memorial Trail 100, the most popular mountain-biking trail in the preserve. Look out for speedy bikers! Past this marked trail junction, continue hiking south through a wide valley with the mountains directly ahead. As the trail gently ascends, you'll cross some dry washes typical of desert hillsides. Wildflowers you'll likely see here during spring include purple lupine and Mexican gold poppies. At 1.4 miles, reach a wide saddle with an inviting bench. A giant quartz boulder lies on the hill to your left. Over the saddle, you'll see the wide inner basin described earlier along Quartz Ridge Trail 8A. The trail descends into this basin and then turns sharply west, eventually meeting Trail 8A in the wide creekbed. Turn right to continue on Trail 8 and complete the counterclockwise loop described above before returning to the 40th Street Trailhead.

NEARBY ACTIVITIES

Phoenix Mountains Preserve encompasses many popular hiking trails including **Piestewa Peak** (see Hikes 10 and 11, pages 64 and 68), **North Mountain** (see Hike 8, page 56), **Lookout Mountain** (see Hike 7, page 52), and **Perl Charles. Camelback Mountain** (see Hikes 2 and 3, pages 29 and 34), another Valley favorite, is southeast of the Phoenix Mountains Preserve.

• •

GPS TRAILHEAD COORDINATES
N33° 31.927' W112° 0.740' (32nd Street Trailhead)
N33° 32.574' W112° 0.929' (Piestewa Peak Trailhead)
N33° 34.071' W111° 59.764' (40th Street Trailhead)

DIRECTIONS *32nd Street Trailhead:* Exit AZ 51 onto Lincoln Drive and drive east 2 miles to 32nd Street. The trailhead parking lot is located on the northeastern corner of 32nd Street and Lincoln Drive.

Piestewa Peak Trailhead: Exit AZ 51 onto Lincoln Drive and drive east 0.5 miles. Turn north (left) onto Squaw Peak Drive and continue 0.5 mile to the gated entrance to Phoenix Mountains Park. Once inside the park, follow the road until it ends at Apache Picnic Area. Hike a short distance northeast on Nature Trail 304 to access the loop.

40th Street Trailhead: Exit AZ 51 onto Shea Boulevard and drive east 0.8 miles to 40th Street. Turn south (right) and follow 40th Street 1 mile to the trailhead parking lot.

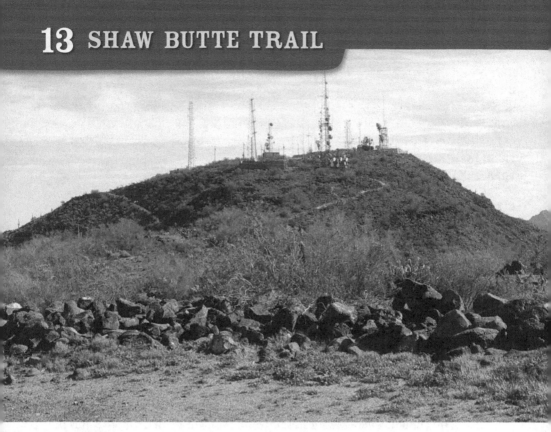

Antenna-studded Shaw Butte sports a coat of green after spring rains.

SHAW BUTTE TRAIL 306 may be the best all-around hike in Phoenix Mountains Preserve. It offers a challenging trek to the summit, a scenic loop through the desert floor, panoramic overlooks around nearly every turn, and fewer crowds than Piestewa Peak or North Mountain.

DESCRIPTION

In the northwestern corner of Phoenix Mountains Preserve, Shaw Butte offers another popular and challenging hike in the heart of Phoenix. Its antenna-studded summit overlooks most of north and central Phoenix. Much like neighboring North Mountain National Trail (see Hike 8, page 56), this well-established trail to the top of Shaw Butte is used by nearby residents for regular exercise. However, the 4-mile Shaw Butte Trail 306 is quite a bit longer than North Mountain and therefore caters to those in search of a longer excursion. It also tends to be less crowded than North Mountain and Piestewa Peak, adding to its appeal.

Panoramic views abound along the Shaw Butte Trail, and a new perspective opens around each bend. This loop hike takes on many personalities. The most popular section climbs a paved road up the northeastern ridge of the mountain. Past the summit, the trail begins a steep and rugged descent. The loop around the base of the mountain

DISTANCE & CONFIGURATION: 4.2-mile loop

DIFFICULTY: Moderate

SCENERY: Shaw Butte, Phoenix Mountains Preserve, city panorama, desert

EXPOSURE: Completely exposed

TRAIL TRAFFIC: Moderate

TRAIL SURFACE: Gravel, pavement, packed dirt, rock

HIKING TIME: 2 hours

WATER REQUIREMENT: 2 quarts

DRIVING DISTANCE: 18 miles from Phoenix Sky Harbor Airport

ELEVATION GAIN: 1,390' at trailhead, 2,149' at highest point

ACCESS: Gates open 5 a.m.–7 p.m.; trails open until 11 p.m.; no permits or fees required

MAPS: USGS *Sunnyslope;* trailhead plaque

FACILITIES: Water but no restrooms

WHEELCHAIR ACCESS: None

CONTACT: 602-262-7901, phoenix.gov/parks /trails/locations/north-mountain

COMMENTS: Dogs permitted on leash except when temperature exceeds 100°F

provides a gentle stroll through a secluded basin. There's something for everyone here, and the total distance is just right for a morning hike. For these reasons, Shaw Butte Trail may be the best all-around hike in Phoenix Mountains Preserve.

On most loop trails, hiking in one direction is easier than the other—for Shaw Butte Trail 306, the easier route is counterclockwise. From the rather small trailhead parking lot, begin by ascending an obvious and wide dirt road on the northeastern side of the mountain. This steep and rocky track passes a gate at 0.25 mile and then bends sharply uphill, where sections of broken pavement remind you that this is a service road for the towers atop Shaw Butte. Attain the ridgeline at 0.4 mile, where you'll have a clear view of North Mountain and Piestewa Peak toward the southeast.

Turn southwest atop the ridge, where you have open views to either side. The towers at the summit still seem quite far. Continue following the wide road as it steadily climbs. The slope levels off as the trail passes a patch of fishhook barrel cacti and reaches a saddle point at 0.8 mile that overlooks the wide basin between Shaw Butte and North Mountain and Pointe Hilton Tapatio Cliffs Resort. To the east, outlines of the Superstition Mountains and Four Peaks form the horizon. The trail resumes its climb toward the summit and reaches another saddle at 1 mile from the trailhead. This vista point provides a clear view down Seventh Avenue toward downtown. South Mountain and the Sierra Estrellas can be seen in the distance.

Finish the ascent on gravel, and pass another gate at 1.25 miles. Just beyond this gate, you'll find an obvious trail junction where the service road continues toward the summit and Trail 306 heads downhill toward the west. Take a short detour along the service road to visit Shaw Butte's 2,149-foot summit. The scenery from the top is impressive, as you might imagine, but the numerous antennas strewn about the wide peak may partly obstruct your view. The constant buzz from transformers also detracts from the experience. Don't worry—plenty of vistas await you farther along the trail, so return quickly to the trail junction just below the summit.

Shaw Butte Trail

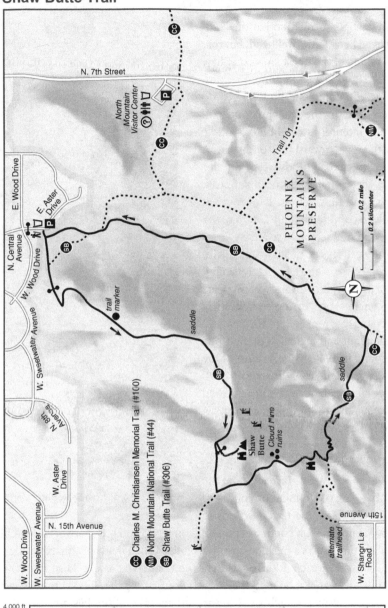

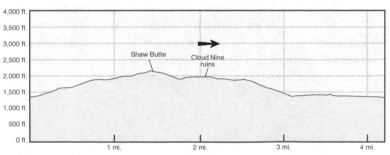

Many people turn around at the summit and head back to the trailhead, but that sacrifices some of the finest views on Shaw Butte Trail. If you have the time, I recommend that you complete the loop. To do that, turn west at the trail junction and descend an intensely steep hill to a saddle point with views toward the southwest. A concrete service road heads west from this saddle to service antennas on a subpeak, involving a half-mile detour. Turn south at the saddle to continue hiking Trail 306.

The next trail section is relatively flat as it hugs the western side of Shaw Butte, with steep drop-offs to the right. At 1.9 miles, you'll reach a trail junction and what appears to be a concrete bunker directly ahead of you. This is all that remains of Cloud Nine, a fancy restaurant and nightclub that burned to the ground in 1964. Though most of the building is covered in graffiti and buried under concrete rubble, the top of Cloud Nine commands an impressive panoramic view and is definitely worth a visit.

The trail is poorly marked here, and it can get confusing. Resist the temptation to descend to the west—instead, take the trail that hugs the old foundations of Cloud Nine. Past the ruins, the trail descends to

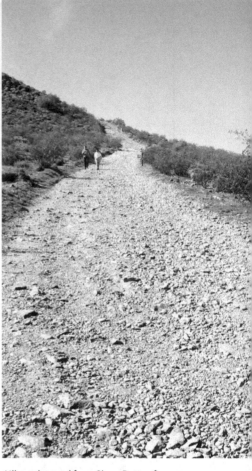

Hikers descend from Shaw Butte after a morning workout.

another vista point, then continues downhill on steep and scree-covered switchbacks where every turn offers a fresh perspective on the valley below. A quarter mile below Cloud Nine, you'll reach a lookout where the trail splits again. Turn left down the smaller trail, and you'll soon see a trail marker confirming that this is the correct route.

Descend the steep switchbacks toward the interior of the basin below. Pass two marked trail junctions in the basin, staying to the left and heading for a narrow gap on the hill flanked by rocky outcrops. Over this small saddle, the trail drops into the main drainage between Shaw Butte and North Mountain. Hikers who seek more of a challenge may choose to go clockwise and climb these steep sections toward the summit.

The remainder of the hike is a cool-down for those hiking counterclockwise. Shaw Butte Trail 306 merges with Christiansen Memorial Trail 100 at the bottom of the basin, just past a dry wash. The combined trail turns left and heads north east. A quarter mile farther, the trail forks at an unsigned junction. Take the left fork to remain on Shaw Butte Trail, which meanders through the picturesque basin and crosses several washes. One mile beyond the fork, Trail 306 skirts a dirt berm and returns to the trailhead on Central Avenue.

NEARBY ACTIVITIES

Phoenix Mountains Preserve encompasses many popular hiking trails, including **Piestewa Peak** (see Hikes 10 and 11, pages 64 and 68), **North Mountain** (see Hike 8, page 56), **Lookout Mountain** (see Hike 7, page 52), and **Perl Charles. Camelback Mountain** (see Hikes 2 and 3, pages 29 and 34), another Valley favorite, is in the southeast corner of Phoenix Mountains Preserve.

• •

GPS TRAILHEAD COORDINATES N33° 36.225' W112° 4.461'

DIRECTIONS *From AZ 51:* Exit onto Cactus Road and follow it west 4 miles to Central Avenue; note that past the Cave Creek Road intersection, Cactus Road becomes Thunderbird Road. Turn south (left) onto Central Avenue, and continue 0.3 mile to the trailhead parking area. If the parking lot is full, wait until a spot becomes available—*please don't park in the nearby residential area.*

From I 17: Exit onto Thunderbird Road and drive east 2.5 miles to Central Avenue. Turn south (right) on Central Avenue, and drive 0.3 mile to the trailhead parking area.

Note: There are alternate access points at Mountain View Park on 7th Avenue, at North Mountain Visitor Center on 7th Street, and at 15th Avenue and Yucca Street. However, they require additional connecting trails.

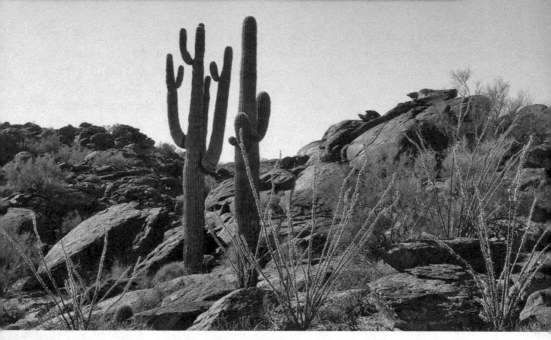

Saguaros and ocotillos thrive in the harsh desert along South Mountain National Trail.

NATIONAL TRAIL IS the longest and grandest of all the trails in South Mountain Park/Preserve. It offers sweeping city vistas, secluded desert valleys, interesting rock formations, ancient Hohokam petroglyphs, historic abandoned mineshafts, and an all-day hike to delight hardy outdoors enthusiasts.

DESCRIPTION

South Mountain Park/Preserve spans more than 16,000 acres of desert and mountain preserves at the southern edge of Phoenix. Ironically, the most recognizable feature in the park is the human-made forest of television, microwave, and radio antennas atop 2,690-foot Mount Suppoa. At night, blinking aircraft warning lights on these antennas can be seen from nearly anywhere in the valley and serve as a welcome beacon for the directionally challenged. Visitors to South Mountain, however, don't care for the antennas. They come to enjoy a wide variety of recreational activities, including hiking, mountain biking, horseback riding, picnicking, and sightseeing.

National Trail, the longest trail in the park, offers day hikers a complete South Mountain experience. It's also a segment of the regional Sun Circle and Maricopa trail systems. In addition to being a superb hike showcasing the best features of the park, National Trail is one of the country's premier mountain-biking destinations. On weekends, dozens of cyclists share the trail with just as many, if not more, hikers.

DISTANCE & CONFIGURATION: 15.5-mile point-to-point with vehicle shuttle

DIFFICULTY: Moderate but long

SCENERY: Desert, city overlooks, mountain vistas, abandoned mineshafts

EXPOSURE: Completely exposed

TRAIL TRAFFIC: Heavy on eastern half, light on western half

TRAIL SURFACE: Gravel, packed dirt, rock

HIKING TIME: 7.5 hours

WATER REQUIREMENT: 4 quarts, 5–6 quarts during summer

DRIVING DISTANCE: 8 miles from Phoenix Sky Harbor Airport

ELEVATION GAIN: 1,300' at trailhead, 2,500' near Mount Suppoa

ACCESS: Gates open 5 a.m.–7 p.m.; trails open until 11 p.m.; no permits or fees required

MAPS: USGS *Guadalupe, Lone Butte, Laveen*; trailhead plaque; available at visitor center

FACILITIES: Picnic areas, visitor center, ranger station, restrooms, water

WHEELCHAIR ACCESS: Yes, at Pima Canyon Trailhead

CONTACT: 602-262-7393, phoenix.gov/parks /trails/locations/south-mountain

COMMENTS: This iconic trail has been designated a segment of the Sun Circle and Maricopa Trails, which run through metropolitan Phoenix and Maricopa County, respectively. Dogs permitted on leash except when temperature exceeds 100°F.

Running east–west along the top of South Mountain's two longest mountain ranges, National Trail intersects almost every other trail in the park. If you plan to hike the whole 15.5 miles along this trail, prepare to spend an entire day enjoying its many wonders. You also need to do a shuttle or arrange a ride from one end of the trail back to the other. *Be aware that the west-end trailhead is reachable by car only during the first full weekend each month.* Lyft or Uber is a good option if you don't feel like driving.

I prefer to hike this trail from east to west, facing the Sierra Estrella mountain range and avoiding an otherwise steep uphill on the western end. Begin your hike from the parking lot at the end of Pima Canyon Park, in the shadows of the Arizona Grand Resort. The first 1.3 miles is a gentle promenade along a wide and level dirt road. On weekend mornings, prepare to share this road with many speedy mountain bikers and slow baby strollers. The road ends in a wide turnaround. You can find petroglyphs left by the ancient Hohokam on the backside of some boulders at the western end of this circular area. At the northwestern end of the turnaround, find obvious trail markers for National Trail, which heads uphill. As you hike, watch out for mountain bikers racing downhill. Although foot traffic has the right of way, sometimes bikers can't see you or stop in time. After a gentle half-mile climb, walk along the top of a ridge and enjoy open views of the Phoenix skyline to the north.

At 2.6 miles National Trail intersects Hidden Valley Trail (see Hike 5, page 43), a particularly attractive and secluded bypass that rejoins National Trail 0.5 mile later. Hidden Valley is a popular detour for National Trail hikers, and its length is similar to the circumnavigated section along National Trail. Hidden Valley Trail, however, is harder to follow and requires a little scrambling over rocky obstacles. If you opt for this half-mile jaunt through Hidden Valley, you'll be treated to a natural rock tunnel,

South Mountain: National Trail

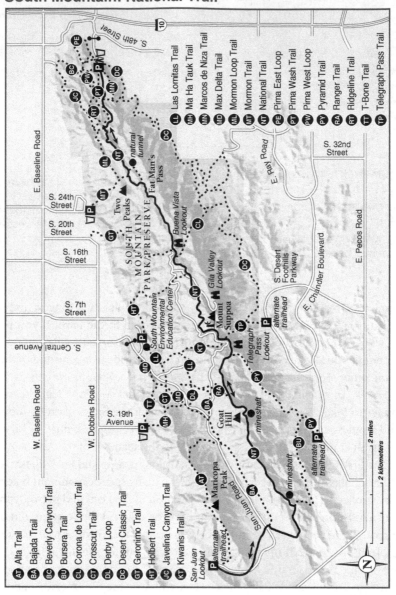

Las Lomitas Trail — LL
Ma Ha Tauk Trail — MH
Marcos de Niza Trail — MN
Max Delta Trail — MD
Mormon Loop Trail — ML
Mormon Trail — MT
National Trail — NT
Pima East Loop — PE
Pima Wash Trail — PT
Pima West Loop — PW
Pyramid Trail — PY
Ranger Trail — RA
Ridgeline Trail — RT
T-Bone Trail — TT
Telegraph Pass Trail — TP

Alta Trail — AT
Bajada Trail — BA
Beverly Canyon Trail — BC
Bursera Trail — BU
Corona de Loma Trail — CL
Crosscut Trail — GT
Derby Loop — DI
Desert Classic Trail — DC
Geronimo Trail — GT
Holbert Trail — HT
Javelina Canyon Trail — JC
Kiwanis Trail — KT

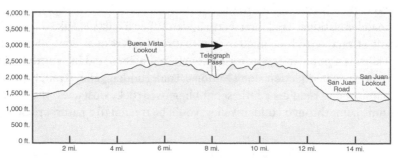

a quiet valley with scenic rocks, and a 9-inch-wide crack through two large boulders, ironically named Fat Man's Pass. Take off your backpack and squeeze through sideways. Try the natural slide on the smooth rock surface immediately after going through Fat Man's Pass. Claustrophobics and heavier hikers need not worry—you can take an easy bypass route over the boulders. Just beyond Fat Man's Pass, Hidden Valley Trail merges back into National Trail at 3.2 miles.

If you choose to stay on the smoother and easier-to-follow National Trail, you can still visit the rock tunnel and Fat Man's Pass, both of which are only a few feet from either end of Hidden Valley Trail. Simply return to National Trail after you check out these formations. An added advantage of staying on National Trail is that the Mormon Trail junction, at 2.75 miles, offers a convenient escape from your commitment in case you are hesitant about finishing this long hike. Mormon Trail leads you to Mormon Loop Trail, which then loops back to the dirt road and Pima Canyon Park.

Continue hiking west along National Trail after Fat Man's Pass, facing the array of antenna towers on Mount Suppoa, the highest point in South Mountain Park/Preserve. At 4.5 miles, look to your left for the Chinese Wall, a dark-colored dike of Tertiary Period granite and diorite. The trail reaches Buena Vista Lookout at 5 miles. Cross the paved parking area to find the trail on the other side of the road. After a small hill, and now at 5.7 miles, the trail joins a paved service road. Walk west along this road 50 yards to rejoin the trail, which then heads straight for the massive antennas on the summit of Mount Suppoa. The trail skirts the fenced-off antenna complex on its northern side. At roughly 2,500 feet, this trail section is the highest accessible point in the park, but don't dawdle too long. Rumor has it that the Federal Communications Commission allows its technicians to work only 2-hour shifts here because of the high-power transmitters.

At 7.5 miles, with the antennas now safely behind you, continue hiking National Trail along a rocky ledge above Summit Road. Here, you may spot strange-looking elephant trees with smooth red bark and fragrant leaves. The trail drops to the road to meet Telegraph Pass Trail (see Hike 22, page 121) at 8 miles from the trailhead. The Army Signal Corps built a telegraph line running from Maricopa Wells, through this mountain pass, to the territorial capital of Prescott back in the late 1800s. From this saddle point, you can see matchboxlike houses in Ahwatukee to the south and tall buildings in downtown Phoenix to the north. Congratulations! You're now halfway through the hike.

The western half of National Trail runs atop the Gila Range and sees much less traffic than the eastern Guadalupe range. Expect to encounter fewer crowds and hardly any mountain bikers. From Summit Road, climb a steep section of trail to Telegraph Pass Lookout, a stone rest house built by the Civilian Conservation Corps. This is a great place to rest and admire the views.

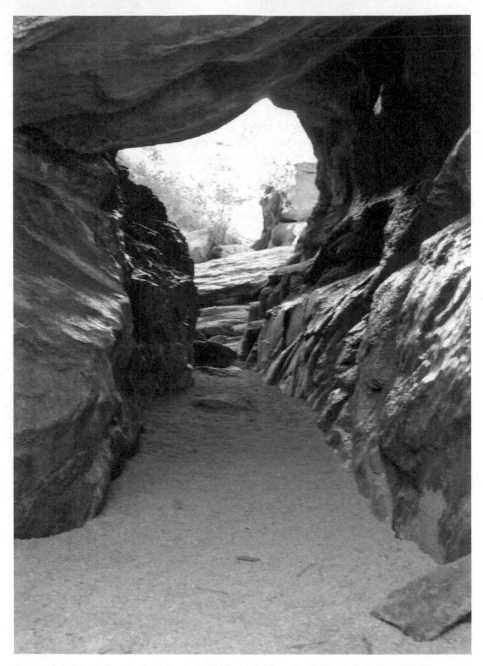

A natural rock tunnel marks the entrance to Hidden Valley from South Mountain National Trail.

National Trail then passes the Pyramid Trail junction and climbs Goat Hill, atop the Gila Range, where it overlooks a small go-kart racing course at the base of the mountain and the Phoenix skyline in the distance. Pass the Ranger Trail junction at 9.6 miles, and continue hiking along a ledge on the southern side of Goat Hill (2,504'). Clusters of furry teddy bear cholla dot the steep hill below you. Enjoy the scenery here in relative isolation, and notice that the trail is obviously less worn here than it was in the first 8 miles. Many abandoned mineshafts lie just off the trail in the next few miles; a particularly large one can be found at 10.8 mile at trail marker 39. Most mineshafts have been sealed, but resist the temptation to climb into any dark and potentially unsafe mineshaft openings.

National Trail finally begins its descent from the Gila Range at 12 miles from the trailhead. Hike steeply downhill as the trail winds through a secluded narrow canyon with colorful rocks to pass the Bursera Trail junction. At 13 miles, cross a dry wash and climb toward a notch where the trail bends into the wide valley between the Gila Range and the Ma Ha Tauk Range to the north. Hike along the valley floor toward San Juan Road. National Trail intersects Bajada Trail at 13.9 miles and crosses San Juan Road shortly thereafter. The elevation in the valley is 1,250 feet, the lowest of the entire hike.

The final 1.5 miles of this long hike are relatively flat and unremarkable as the trail parallels the road, skirting the southern tip of the Ma Ha Tauk Range below Maricopa Peak. The 15.5-mile National Trail ends at San Juan Lookout, where you should have a vehicle or a ride waiting.

• •

GPS TRAILHEAD COORDINATES
N33° 19.820' W112° 08.650' (San Juan Trailhead)
N33° 21.775' W111° 59.157' (Pima Canyon Trailhead)

DIRECTIONS *San Juan Trailhead:* Exit I-10 at Baseline Road, and drive west 6 miles to Central Avenue. Turn south (left) onto Central Avenue, and drive 2 miles to the park entrance. Once inside the park, drive 2.2 miles to the San Juan Road junction. Take San Juan Road west (right) 4 miles until it ends at the San Juan Lookout. *Note:* San Juan Road is open only the first full weekend of each month. Check phoenix.gov/parks/trails /locations/south-mountain for the latest road conditions.

Pima Canyon Trailhead: From the San Juan Trailhead, return east on San Juan Road and, after 4 miles, turn left at the junction to head north on Central Avenue. In 3.8 miles, turn east (right) on Baseline Road. In 5.5 miles, turn south (left) on 48th Street, which becomes Pointe Parkway. Follow this curvy road 1 mile, skirting the Arizona Grand Resort. Just past Guadalupe Road, turn west (right) onto 48th Street, and then make an immediate left to enter Pima Canyon Park. Drive to the parking lot at the west end of the park.

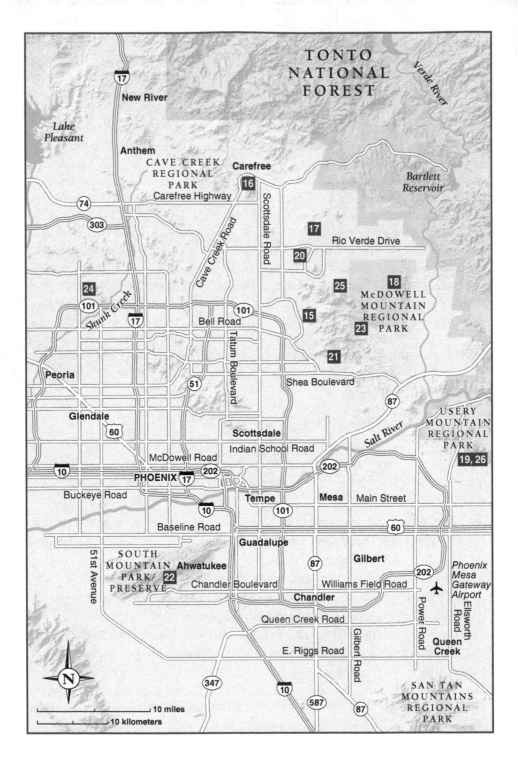

TONTO NATIONAL FOREST

Verde River

New River

Lake Pleasant

Anthem

CAVE CREEK REGIONAL PARK

Carefree

Bartlett Reservoir

Carefree Highway

Scottsdale Road

Rio Verde Drive

Cave Creek Road

McDOWELL MOUNTAIN REGIONAL PARK

Skunk Creek

Bell Road

Tatum Boulevard

Peoria

Shea Boulevard

Glendale

Salt River

USERY MOUNTAIN REGIONAL PARK

Scottsdale

Indian School Road

McDowell Road

PHOENIX

Buckeye Road

Tempe

Mesa

Main Street

Baseline Road

Guadalupe

SOUTH MOUNTAIN PARK/ PRESERVE

Ahwatukee

Chandler Boulevard

Gilbert

Williams Field Road

Phoenix Mesa Gateway Airport

51st Avenue

Chandler

Queen Creek Road

E. Riggs Road

Gilbert Road

Power Road

Ellsworth Road

Queen Creek

N

SAN TAN MOUNTAINS REGIONAL PARK

10 miles

10 kilometers

PHOENIX SUBURBS

(Ahwatukee, Cave Creek, Glendale, Mesa, Scottsdale)

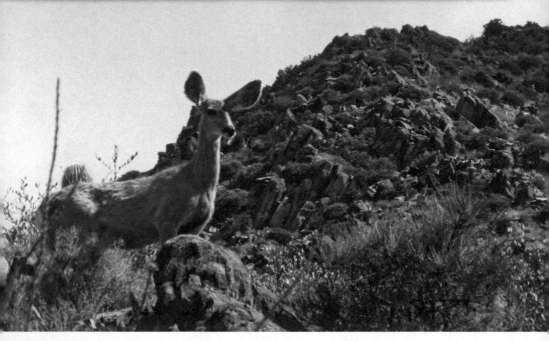

A curious mule deer watches over Windgate Pass Trail during late afternoon.

EASILY ACCESSIBLE AND highly enjoyable, this extensive loop encircles McDowell Peak, one of three prominent peaks within McDowell Sonoran Preserve. Along the way, take in sweeping city views, rugged yet tranquil desert and mountain scenery, and perhaps even some wildlife sightings. You'll get a decent workout, too.

DESCRIPTION

McDowell Sonoran Preserve and the City of Scottsdale operate one of the newest and best trail systems near metropolitan Phoenix. Easy access, ample parking, immaculate facilities, and clear trail signage all contribute to a pleasant hiking experience. Gateway Trailhead is the largest and most visited of all access points into the preserve. On weekends, volunteer trail stewards greet you, answering questions, providing maps, and even leading guided hikes. Handy trail maps are freely available even when the trailhead is unstaffed; just be sure to reuse or recycle the maps when you are done.

Begin this enjoyable loop hike from the back of Gateway Trailhead's building area. First cross a metal bridge spanning a desert wash; then strike out on a level gravel nature trail. In front of you, from right to left, antenna-studded Thompson Peak (see Hike 23, page 126), McDowell Peak, and Tom's Thumb (see Hike 25, page 134)

DISTANCE & CONFIGURATION: 9.5-mile balloon

DIFFICULTY: Moderate–strenuous

SCENERY: McDowell Sonoran Preserve, Tom's Thumb, Fountain Hills, Scottsdale

EXPOSURE: Completely exposed

TRAIL TRAFFIC: Heavy near trailhead, light beyond Bell Pass

TRAIL SURFACE: Gravel, packed dirt, crushed rock

HIKING TIME: 4.5 hours

WATER REQUIREMENT: 3–4 quarts

DRIVING DISTANCE: 23 miles from Phoenix Sky Harbor Airport

ELEVATION GAIN: 1,720' at trailhead, 3,204' at Bell Pass, 3,031' at Windgate Pass

ACCESS: Sunrise–sunset; no permits or fees required

MAPS: USGS *McDowell Peak;* free maps available at trailhead

FACILITIES: Restrooms, water, horse trailer parking, shaded ramadas, nature trails

WHEELCHAIR ACCESS: Near the beginning around the nature trail

CONTACT: 480-312-7013, scottsdaleaz.gov /preserve

COMMENTS: Dogs must be leashed at all times

tower above the desert foothills. This portion of the hike, an easy warm-up for the hills to come, is also wheelchair accessible. Browse the interpretive signs detailing the Sonoran Desert flora as you pass the amphitheater. A quarter mile from the trailhead, zigzag through a rocky dry wash lined with palo verde and mesquite trees. Soon you'll reach a well-signed trail junction with the Gateway Loop and Saguaro Loop Trails at 0.4 mile from the trailhead.

Turn south (right) to hike the loop counterclockwise. A wide and gently ascending trail, Gateway Loop is a pleasant hike in its own right. One advantage of hiking the McDowells is the seemingly limitless possibilities of forming loops from a vast network of trails and customizing your hike to suit your tastes. If you're worried about getting lost, take a park map with you and navigate using the many signs, which clearly give directions and distance to the next junction. Hike south-southeast, staying left at the next few trail junctions. Pass a fence post 0.8 mile from the Gateway Trailhead, where Crossover Trail branches off to the right. Stay on Gateway Loop Trail and turn east, heading straight toward Thompson Peak (page 126). The trail smooths out as it contours around a hill studded with teddy bear chollas and saguaros. Barrel cacti and creosote bushes complete the desert landscape as you leave the city behind and hike deeper into the preserve.

After passing Paradise Trail and then crossing a significant drainage, you'll reach the signed Bell Pass Trail junction 1.5 miles from the Gateway Trailhead. Bell Pass Trail has one of the steeper sections within the preserve. Here, if desired, you can shorten the hike by following Gateway Loop Trail. To complete our target loop, however, veer right onto Bell Pass Trail and commit to a longer but more picturesque hike.

Soon after turning onto Bell Pass Trail, you'll cross another significant dry wash. Your hike so far has gradually gained 300 feet in elevation since the trailhead, but the slope is noticeably increasing as you hike deeper into the heart of McDowell

Bell Pass and Windgate Pass Loop

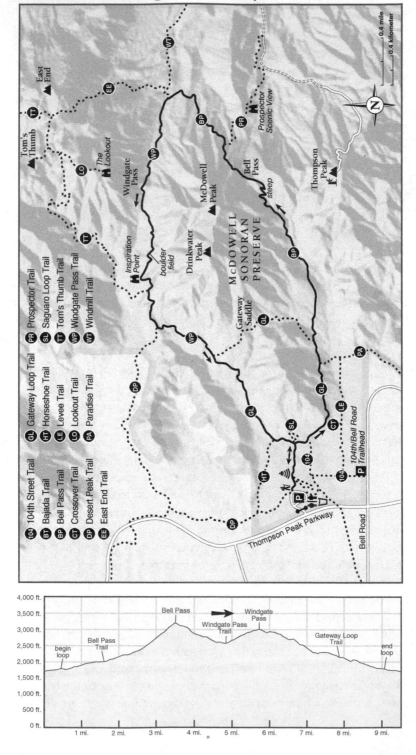

PR Prospector Trail
SL Saguaro Loop Trail
TT Tom's Thumb Trail
WP Windgate Pass Trail
WT Windmill Trail

GL Gateway Loop Trail
HT Horseshoe Trail
LE Levee Trail
LO Lookout Trail
PA Paradise Trail

104 104th Street Trail
BT Bajada Trail
BP Bell Pass Trail
CT Crossover Trail
DP Desert Peak Trail
EE East End Trail

Sonoran Preserve. Signs of housing developments are now gone, and crowds have thinned. The radio towers atop Thompson Peak may be the only remaining sign of civilization. Marvel at the fields of teddy bear chollas and stands of saguaros as you hike toward Bell Pass, the obvious saddle ahead, which is guarded by a rock outcrop.

At 2.4 miles from the trailhead, the trail begins a steep switchbacking ascent. Many hikers use Bell Pass Trail as a training hike: the next mile is a section that can quickly raise your heart rate. The trail runs along a natural shelf to the right of a ravine but eventually crosses to the opposite side. If you need a quick breather, turn around to admire the distant city views and Piestewa Peak (see Hikes 10 and 11, pages 64 and 68) through the gap between hills. Bell Pass Trail continues to climb steeply through a majestic stand of saguaros and up rocky switchbacks. McDowell Peak looms over your left shoulder. Above a series of switchbacks, an unmarked fork in the trail may cause temporary confusion. Taking either branch works, but turn right to stay on the trail proper. The two forks eventually merge as the steep incline gives way to a milder slope, with Bell Pass directly ahead.

Bell Pass sits at 3,204 feet—the highest point of this loop—and 3.5 miles from the Gateway Trailhead. Take a well-deserved break here to savor the views from this vantage point. For the first time on this hike, you can gaze into the eastern half of McDowell Sonoran Preserve, with Mount Ord (see Hike 48, page 246) and Four Peaks (see Hike 46, page 237) on the horizon and the town of Fountain Hills below. Continue on Bell Pass Trail as it gently descends into the tranquil interior basin where the only noise is an occasional airplane overhead. Around a bend, the rugged ridges of the Superstition and Goldfield Mountains come into view, with Weaver's Needle as a prominent landmark.

Contouring around another hill, you'll see the paved road winding its way up toward Thompson Peak. At 3.8 miles from the trailhead, descend a steeper hill amid jojoba, prickly pear cacti, and catclaw acacia. Watch your footing on loose rocky terrain as you pass the junction with the Prospector Trail, staying left at the fork. Notice some desert mistletoe clinging to branches of mesquite and palo verde trees. These parasitic plants feed on their hosts, eventually killing them. The steep downhill section is a mere 0.5 mile; its slope then eases into a smoother trail again.

Bell Pass Trail winds around small hills, turns north, and dives deeper into the eastern basin. East End Peak, a towering pile of boulders and the highest peak within McDowell Sonoran Preserve, comes into view. Even though you're surrounded by cities, hiking this part of the preserve gives you that desert-wilderness experience.

At 4.7 miles from the Gateway Trailhead, you'll cross a sizable drainage, with Windgate Pass now to the left and the greener eastern foothills below. Bell Pass Trail ends here at a three-way trail junction with Windgate Pass Trail and Windmill Trail. This is the halfway point of the loop.

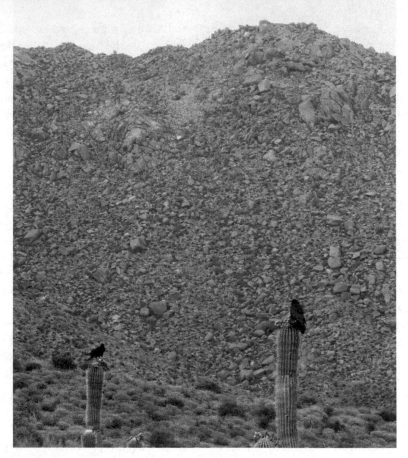

Ravens perch atop budding saguaros along Bell Pass Trail.

Turn left at the signed junction to take Windgate Pass Trail west. Begin an easy and manageable ascent on dark river rock, regaining some of the 620 feet you lost descending from Bell Pass. The trail continues to climb, crosses a dry wash at 5.5 miles from the trailhead, and then straightens out. A quarter mile farther, you'll reach the top of Windgate Pass (3,031'). Aptly named, this pass often sees a stiff but welcoming breeze blowing in from between McDowell Peak and East End Peak. Turn around to enjoy a parting view of the eastern horizon before crossing over Windgate Pass.

Continue hiking west on a gentle downhill, with city views of Scottsdale and Phoenix and rolling hills in the distance. The trail soon hugs a shelf on the hillside, just left of the main basin below. At 6.3 miles from the trailhead, you'll cross a giant talus of rock and then a boulder-ridden gulley. Next, you'll arrive at Inspiration Point, a prominent rest area on Windgate Pass Trail. Take a break on the shady bench to enjoy the mountain scenery. During early-morning hours or at dusk, you may spot some mule deer or families of javelina in these hills.

The Tom's Thumb Trail junction comes next, after you zigzag down a hill. Tom's Thumb Trail offers another enjoyable loop toward East End Peak. For this hike, continue straight, heading west on Windgate Pass Trail. Familiar views from this trail section include the semicylindrical building at West World, the classic profile view of Camelback Mountain (see Hikes 2 and 3, pages 29 and 34), Mummy Mountain, Piestewa Peak, and north Scottsdale. Pass the Desert Park Trail junction, and continue hiking between two hills. Drier west-facing foothills foster a variety of cacti, such as the giant saguaro, barrel cactus, teddy bear cholla, and buckhorn cholla.

At 7.9 miles from the trailhead, Windgate Pass Trail ends at the Gateway Loop Trail junction. Consider this the home stretch of our loop; you can now see the Gateway Trailhead in the distance. Follow Gateway Loop Trail west, resuming a mile-long descent on rocky terrain. Behind you is an excellent view of Tom's Thumb, perched atop the ridge.

You'll reach level ground at 8.8 miles from the original trailhead, leaving all the rocky hills behind. Since this is a lengthy loop, your aching feet will appreciate the gravelly surface here. Pass through one more junction, for Horseshoe Trail, to finally return to Saguaro Trail, where our counterclockwise loop hike began. Turn right to follow Saguaro Trail the final 0.4 mile back to the Gateway Trailhead.

NEARBY ACTIVITIES

McDowell Sonoran Preserve boasts many hiking opportunities, including **Brown's Mountain Loop** (see Hike 17, page 100), **Tom's Thumb** (see Hike 25, page 134), **Thompson Peak** (see Hike 23, page 126), and **Sunrise Peak** (see Hike 21, page 116). **McDowell Mountain Regional Park,** on the eastern flanks of the preserve, offers excellent mountain-biking trails. **Pinnacle Peak** (see Hike 20, page 112) and **Black Mountain** (see next hike) are farther north. **Cave Creek** and **Bartlett Reservoir** are located nearby.

• •

GPS TRAILHEAD COORDINATES N33° 38.968' W111° 51.502'

DIRECTIONS From Loop 101 and Bell Road, travel east 1.7 miles to Thompson Peak Parkway. Turn north (left) onto Thompson Peak Parkway; then continue 0.4 mile to the Gateway Trailhead's entrance gate.

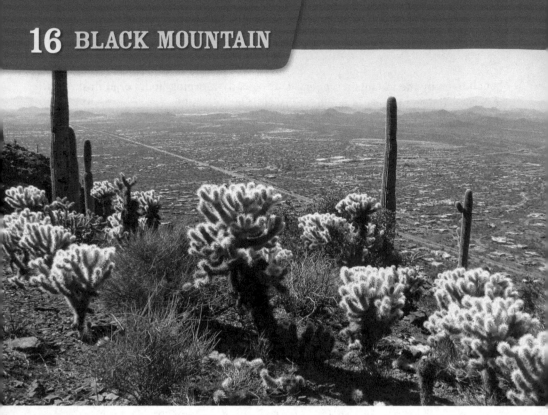

Teddy bear chollas and saguaros accentuate an open view of Cave Creek from Black Mountain.

HIKERS IN NORTH PHOENIX have a number of nearby options for regular exercise. Black Mountain ranks first on that list for the quick workout and the splendid view from its summit.

DESCRIPTION

Looming over the northern outposts of Cave Creek and Carefree like a dark fortress, Black Mountain is as forbidding as it is inviting. To unfamiliar hikers, Black Mountain presents some challenges in terms of finding a suitable trailhead, adequate parking, and acceptable access to the summit. However, once you overcome those challenges, the short but challenging hike up Black Mountain rivals the best short hikes in Phoenix.

Named for the black slate and phyllite that form much of the mountain, Black Mountain has long been the pride of the twin communities. Cave Creek and Carefree were once separated from urban sprawl and held a distinct mystique for city dwellers. As new development blurred the lines between Western outposts and suburbia, these communities have grown to embrace change. Black Mountain has often been caught in the middle of that change—a struggle between the old and the new, seclusion and development, preservation and growth.

DISTANCE & CONFIGURATION: 2.4-mile out-and-back

DIFFICULTY: Strenuous

SCENERY: Black Mountain, city panorama, desert, unique geology

EXPOSURE: Completely exposed

TRAIL TRAFFIC: Light–moderate

TRAIL SURFACE: Gravel, packed dirt, crushed rock

HIKING TIME: 1.5 hours

WATER REQUIREMENT: 1.5 quarts

DRIVING DISTANCE: 33 miles from Phoenix Sky Harbor Airport

ELEVATION GAIN: 2,180' at trailhead, 3,398' on Black Mountain summit

ACCESS: Sunrise–sunset; no permits or fees required

MAPS: USGS *Cave Creek*

FACILITIES: Restrooms, water, horse-trailer parking, shaded ramadas, nature trails

WHEELCHAIR ACCESS: None

CONTACT: 480-488-6601

COMMENTS: Summit park is owned by Maricopa County, access is managed through town of Cave Creek; dogs must be leashed at all times

Though the top of Black Mountain is a preserve, there is no officially sanctioned way for hikers to reach the summit at this writing. Land owners, conservationists, and various municipalities continue to struggle over access, while hikers patiently await a resolution so they can enjoy the sweeping views from Black Mountain's ridges and crest. Over the years, however, a de facto trail and easement have emerged on the north side of Black Mountain, along School House Road, so that's where we begin our hike.

Walk south on School House Road with the mountain in sight. Beyond Military Road/Mark Way, begin a gentle ascent past homes in the area. As you approach the foothills, the pavement gives way to a packed-dirt road and eventually a jeep trail up the northern flanks of Black Mountain. Don't be discouraged by this bit of road hiking; there's plenty of pristine desert ahead.

A third of a mile past Military Road, veer right at the entrance to a private driveway; you'll find a small trail to the left of the main dirt road (which is intermittently closed to hikers). Turn away from the road here and hike the narrow trail next to the private driveway. Sonoran Desert flora abounds here, where jojobas, triangle-leaf bursage, mesquite trees, and saguaros line the trail. You'll feel your pulse rise in proportion to the slope.

A half mile past Military Road, the trail becomes rockier and steeper as it steadily climbs. Smooth gravel and packed dirt degrade into broken rock, and a variety of cacti encroach on the narrow trail. At 0.6 mile, a marker carved into rock indicates that you are crossing into a Maricopa County park. Soon after the sign, the narrow trail reaches a wide lookout and meets the extension of the dirt road you left earlier. This is roughly the halfway point of the hike and a good place for a short rest. Turn around to gaze back down the trail to see how far you have already hiked. On the northern horizon, the New River Mountains frame the town of Cave Creek.

Black Mountain

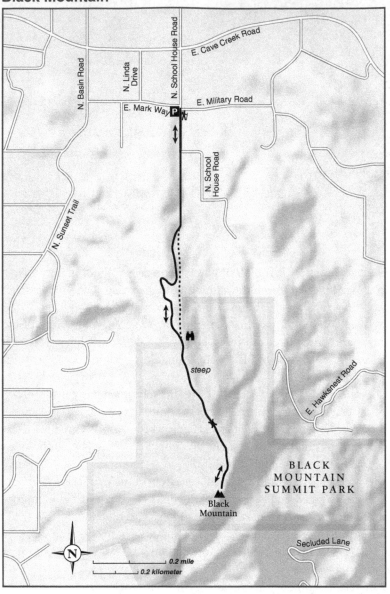

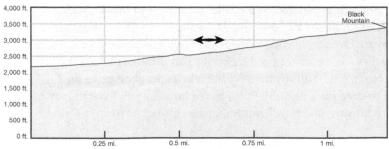

Resume your ascent along a wide ridge toward the summit of Black Mountain. Watch your footing on the sharp rocks along this rugged trail. Jojoba, buckhorn cholla, and flat-top buckwheat thrive here. At 0.75 mile the trail steepens formidably to ascend a rocky staircase made for giants. Take your time laboring up these steep inclines, knowing that a summit panorama awaits.

Nearly 1 mile past the starting point at Military Road, you'll reach the summit ridge as the trail levels slightly. Here, you have the best opportunity for an up-close view of the black metamorphic rock that gave the mountain its name. Actually, these dark ancient stones occur only in the western half of Black Mountain; the eastern half consists of much younger granite. The black slate and phyllite are some of the oldest exposed rocks in the state, rivaling those found at the bottom of the Grand Canyon in age.

Finish the last quarter mile enjoying expansive views of the surrounding cityscape and distant mountain ranges. The summit of Black Mountain (3,398') is considerably higher than those of Camelback Mountain (see Hikes 2 and 3, pages 29 and 34) and Piestewa Peak (see Hikes 10 and 11, pages 64 and 68). Your arduous climb is rewarded with a panoramic view that will take your breath away. To the east the horizon presents familiar silhouettes of Four Peaks, the McDowell Mountains and Tom's Thumb (see Hike 25, page 134), and the Superstition Mountains. To the west lie the Bradshaws and the White Tanks. To the south, metropolitan Phoenix stretches as far as the eye can see.

Take your time enjoying the views before you retrace your steps to descend Black Mountain.

NEARBY ACTIVITIES

North of Cave Creek, **Spur Cross Ranch Conservation Area** offers several hikes through pristine desert in the shadow of **Elephant Mountain** (page 232). **Cave Creek Regional Park** (page 241) is 3 miles due east of Black Mountain. **Bartlett Reservoir** and **Seven Springs Recreation Area** are both accessible via Cave Creek Road.

• •

GPS TRAILHEAD COORDINATES N33° 49.792' W111° 56.598'

DIRECTIONS *From East Valley:* Take Loop 101 to Scottsdale Road. Drive north 12 miles to Cave Creek Road. Turn west (left) on Cave Creek, and follow it 1.25 miles to School House Road. Turn south (left) on School House Road, drive 0.2 mile, and turn right on Mark Way, where you'll find a small parking area immediately on your right.

From Phoenix: Take Loop 101 to Cave Creek Road, and drive 13 miles north to School House Road, crossing AZ 74/Carefree Highway at 10 miles. Turn right (south) on School House Road, drive 0.2 mile, and turn right on Mark Way, where you'll find a small parking area immediately on your right.

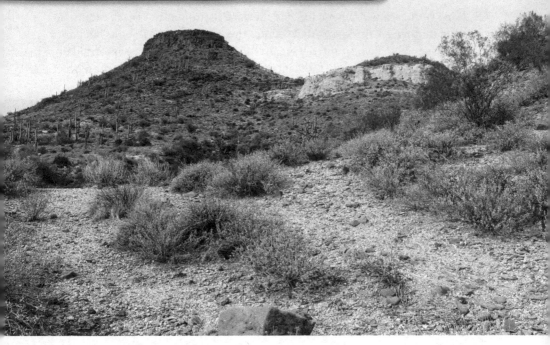

Brown's Mountain looms like a dark fortress over surrounding desert foothills.

BROWN'S MOUNTAIN LIES within the relatively new and relatively flat northern section of McDowell Sonoran Preserve. A mild loop takes hikers around Brown's Mountain, with a spur trail to its summit for a bird's-eye view.

DESCRIPTION

McDowell Sonoran Preserve encompasses a vast area of 35,000 acres of pristine desert, permanently protected from development. The preserve's southern section boasts mountainous terrain studded with high peaks reaching 4,000 feet in elevation, while the northern half covers mostly desert foothills with a few smaller mountains. The northern section also holds the newest of trailheads and trails within the preserve.

Then Brown's Ranch Trailhead opened in 2013, providing access into historic Brown's Ranch, an area that was established by E. O. Brown and partners for cattle grazing more than 100 years ago. The City of Scottsdale purchased and annexed Brown's Ranch to the preserve in 1999. Anchoring Brown's Ranch is Brown's Mountain, his namesake peak and the objective of this hike.

Begin this loop from behind the Brown's Ranch Trailhead's building area. The trail follows Brown's Ranch Road, a wide, packed-dirt thoroughfare, toward the north. Brown's Mountain, a cone-shaped hill with a flat summit, lies ahead in the distance. The northern section of McDowell Sonoran Preserve sits at 2,700 feet elevation, significantly

DISTANCE & CONFIGURATION: 4.1-mile loop

DIFFICULTY: Easy

SCENERY: Brown's Mountain, McDowell Sonoran Preserve, desert, Scottsdale

EXPOSURE: Mostly exposed

TRAIL TRAFFIC: Moderate

TRAIL SURFACE: Gravel, packed dirt, rock

HIKING TIME: 2 hours

WATER REQUIREMENT: 1.5 quarts

DRIVING DISTANCE: 32 miles from Phoenix Sky Harbor Airport

ELEVATION GAIN: 2,710' at trailhead, 3,253' on Brown's Mountain summit

ACCESS: Sunrise–sunset; no permits or fees required

MAPS: USGS *Cave Creek*

FACILITIES: Restrooms, water, horse-trailer parking

WHEELCHAIR ACCESS: Section near trailhead passable by wheelchair

CONTACT: 480-312-7013, scottsdaleaz.gov /preserve

COMMENTS: Dogs must be leashed at all times

higher than the City of Phoenix, which averages 1,200 feet. The desert flora found here is noticeably greener than that of the southern deserts. Soap-tree yuccas, teddy bear chollas, jojoba bushes, and palo verde trees are common along the trail.

At 0.4 mile from the trailhead, pass under some power lines to cross Power-line Road. Continue hiking the wide dirt road until 0.6 mile, where there's a marked intersection with Brown's Mountain Trail. At this junction, leave the dirt road to turn left onto a narrower but still smooth trail, with Brown's Mountain to your left. Though gravel, this trail is still navigable by two people hiking abreast. A short distance on, you'll arrive at the Wrangler Trail junction. Go straight through this junction to begin a gradual climb. To your right is Granite Mountain, another prominent feature of the northern McDowells (there is, however, no official trail to its summit). On the horizon, you can see Four Peaks (see Hike 46, page 237) above the power lines. If you look toward the McDowell range, you can see Tom's Thumb (see Hike 20, page 134), Pinnacle Peak (see Hike 25, page 112), and Troon Mountain.

Brown's Mountain Trail begins a series of switchbacks at 0.9 mile from the trailhead. As you turn, the Superstition Mountains appear on the horizon. The trail becomes rocky after the second switchback, and the hill steepens. Take your time on this section; it's the only significant uphill of the loop. You will pass some cliff bands of yellow sandstone and a field of teddy bear cholla. You'll then arrive at a prominent saddle surrounded by jojoba bushes and more teddy bear cholla, 1.2 miles from the trailhead. Give teddy bear cholla a wide berth—the slightest breeze can send a cluster of painful needles in your direction, hence the cactus's nickname, "jumping cholla."

Reach the summit spur trail and overlook junction at 1.4 miles from the trailhead. After a quick visit to the overlook, take the summit spur trail to the top of Brown's Mountain. The spur, steep with poor footing, comprises loose dirt and volcanic rock—take care not to slip here. Tall grasses line the trail, while Brown's Mountain looms like a hilltop fortress. Continue hiking the narrow trail to the top of Brown's Mountain (3,253'), which offers panoramic views of the entire preserve. From this vantage point,

Brown's Mountain Loop

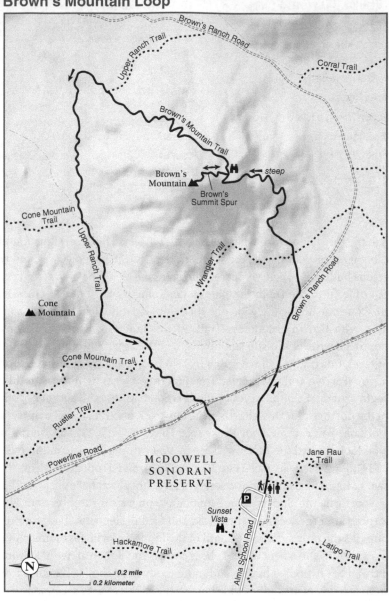

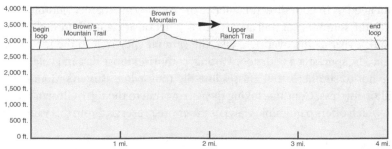

you can clearly see the trailhead buildings, Pinnacle Peak, the McDowell Mountains, and Tom's Thumb. To the northeast you can see most of the Mazatzal Range, and to the east Weaver's Needle and the Superstition Mountains. Imagine what it might have looked like to E. O. Brown as he surveyed his ranch and grazing cattle 100 years ago.

Visiting the summit adds 0.3 mile round-trip to the hike. After resting atop Brown's Mountain, retrace your steps down to the overlook, turn left, and resume hiking along Brown's Mountain Trail. The backside of the loop sees fewer visitors, thus offering greater solitude. Begin a gentle descent on the north side of the mountain. Cooler than the southern exposure, this hillside fosters tall grasses, Mormon tea (also known as ephedra), and buckhorn cholla. As the trail rounds the northwest side of Brown's Mountain, the town of Cave Creek comes into view, with Black Mountain (see previous hike) in the distance. Continue to descend Brown's Mountain Trail until it ends at a T-intersection with Upper Ranch Trail at 2.3 miles from the trailhead.

Keep left and turn onto Upper Ranch Trail. Brown's Ranch is also known as the Upper Ranch; DC Ranch, another historic property in the area, is referred to as the Lower Ranch. This section of Upper Ranch Trail heads northwest, then south toward the Brown's Ranch Trailhead. At 2.4 miles, cross a dry wash as the trail transitions back to gravel and rock. Follow this trail as it undulates gently up and down, passing between Cone Mountain and Brown's Mountain. Pass another dry wash at 2.8 miles from the trailhead to arrive at the first junction with Cone Mountain Trail, which encircles its namesake peak, but for this hike, continue straight on Upper Ranch Trail.

The trail, lined by soap-tree yucca, creosote bushes, and brittlebush, becomes mostly flat and wide again. During spring, the plants' brilliant yellow blossoms add a dash of color to the scenery. Continue hiking Upper Ranch Trail as it passes the second junction with Cone Mountain Trail and Wrangler Trail. Next, cross the trail junction with Rustler Trail; then continue through the intersection with Powerline Road. Finally, return to Brown's Ranch Road and make a right to return to the trailhead.

NEARBY ACTIVITIES

The new **Fraesfield** and **Granite Mountain Trailheads** in the northern half of McDowell Sonoran Preserve, along with the **Tom's Thumb Trailhead** (see Hike 25, page 134) to the south, serve many excellent trails in the area. **Black Mountain** (see previous hike), in the town of Cave Creek, to the north, is another popular hike.

• •

GPS TRAILHEAD COORDINATES N33° 45.692' W111° 50.542'

DIRECTIONS From Loop 101, take Exit 36 for Pima Road and drive north 6.5 miles. Turn right (east) onto Dynamite Road, and drive 2.8 miles. Turn north (left) onto Alma School Road, and follow it 1 mile to the Brown's Ranch Trailhead.

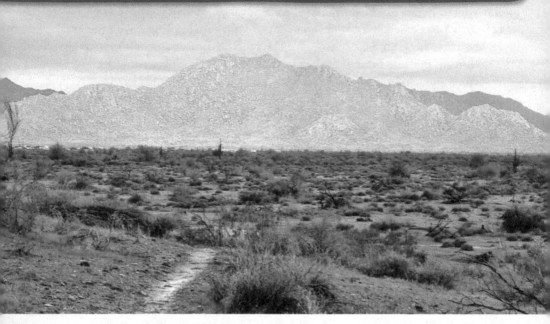

A view toward the rugged McDowell Mountains from Scenic Trail

MCDOWELL MOUNTAIN REGIONAL PARK covers more than 21,000 acres of desert wilderness at the base of the McDowell Mountains. Take the easy Scenic Trail to enjoy expansive views of the surrounding mountains and plains.

DESCRIPTION

Though named for the McDowell Mountains, this large regional park doesn't actually encompass much of its namesake mountain range. Instead, the park spans 21,099 acres of mostly low-lying desert plains encircled by Tonto National Forest, Fort McDowell Indian Reservation, Fountain Hills, and the McDowell Mountains. What the park lacks in altitude it makes up for in variety: more than 50 miles of multiuse trails offer hikers, equestrians, and bikers plenty of recreational opportunities. A competitive track and youth camps round out the park's diverse offerings.

Scenic Trail is the perfect introductory hike to McDowell Mountain Regional Park. Winding around Lousley Hills at the park's eastern edge, this pleasant loop trail takes visitors through a sandy wash and then atop a ridge with grand views of the surrounding mountains and plains. Beginner hikers and families especially appreciate this trail for its gentle slopes and varied scenery.

From the large trailhead staging area, begin by hiking north on Pemberton Trail, the park's longest. At the Scenic Trail junction, turn right and leave Pemberton Trail.

DISTANCE & CONFIGURATION: 4.5-mile loop

DIFFICULTY: Easy

SCENERY: McDowell Mountains, Four Peaks, desert

EXPOSURE: Completely exposed

TRAIL TRAFFIC: Light

TRAIL SURFACE: Gravel, packed dirt, sand

HIKING TIME: 2.5 hours

WATER REQUIREMENT: 1.5 quarts

DRIVING DISTANCE: 30 miles from Phoenix Sky Harbor Airport

ELEVATION GAIN: 1,860' at trailhead, 2,020' at highest point

ACCESS: Park open 6 a.m.–8 p.m. (till 10 p.m. Friday–Saturday); trail closes at sunset; $6/vehicle entry fee

MAPS: USGS *Fort McDowell;* park map available at entrance and maricopacountyparks.net/maps

FACILITIES: Restrooms, drinking water, picnic areas, visitor center, horse corral, competitive track, youth camp

WHEELCHAIR ACCESS: Section near trailhead passable by wheelchair

CONTACT: 480-471-0173, maricopacountyparks .net/mcdowell-mountain-regional-park

COMMENTS: Excellent mountain bike trails within park; dogs must be leashed at all times

The smooth and level Scenic Trail meanders across sparsely vegetated plains toward Lousley Hills, a series of rambling slopes to the east. Stroll past jojoba bushes, triangle-leaf bursage, and mesquite trees; then cross a dry wash at 0.3 mile from the trailhead. Behind you, the McDowell Mountains span the southwestern skyline. The rocky East End Peak and the antenna-studded Thompson Peak (see Hike 23, page 126) stand out against the horizon. You can even see the steep service road to the saddle, left of Thompson Peak. McDowell Sonoran Preserve offers many miles of superb trails within its boundaries. See other hikes in this book for details.

Continue past the remnants of an old fence, and hike toward Lousley Hills, which are covered in brittlebush, and accented by occasional saguaros. At 0.5 mile turn left to enter a wide, sandy wash; the soft sand cushions your every step but can also take the spring out of your stride. Follow the wash 0.2 mile southeast through some old driftwood. There, a trail marker directs you to leave the wash and head right. Continue hiking into the gap between the hills, toward the distant Superstition Mountains. Triangle-leaf bursage and canyon ragweed shrubs line the trail, and many drooping cadaverous trees and limbs litter the landscape. It's hard to imagine how these plants can perish along the wash while their brethren on the drier slopes seem to thrive.

At a fork in the trail near 0.9 mile, bear left and follow the triangular trail markers mounted on stubby rebar posts. The trail returns to the dry wash shortly thereafter. Watch for strategically placed tree limbs blocking off errant paths. Continue along the streambed until a sign directs you away from it at 1.2 miles. In one-tenth of a mile, the trail crosses another dry wash near some metal posts at the Cinch Trail junction before climbing the left bank of the basin.

At 1.5 miles, you'll round the tip of the hill and continue your gradual ascent north among fields of brittlebush, with Four Peaks to the east. Taking this loop counterclockwise saves the best scenery for last. As you gain elevation, views widen

McDowell Mountain Regional Park: Scenic Trail

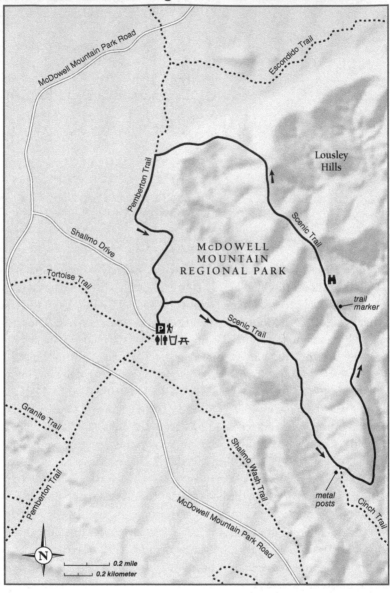

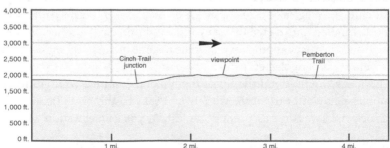

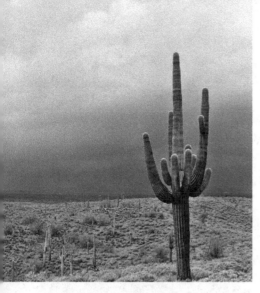

A lone saguaro in McDowell Mountain Regional Park braves the approaching storm.

until you reach a ridgetop at 1,975 feet. The basin and wash you came from lie below. Here you enjoy open views of the McDowell Mountains.

The next 1.5-mile section of Scenic Trail is my favorite. As you walk along the ridgeline of Lousley Hills, it seems the views get better around every corner and over every little bump. It's amazing how much perspective you gain in just 300 feet of elevation. The McDowell Mountains, especially the jagged East End Peak, stand in sharp contrast to the desert plains at their feet. Observe Black Mountain and New River Mesa to the northwest, and the massive Mazatzal Mountains to the northeast. Picturesque basins flank the trail as you hike along the ridgeline.

Near 3.3 miles, the trail begins to descend a winding path with wide-open plains ahead. Cacti are conspicuously absent here. Scenic Trail terminates at a second junction with Pemberton Trail. Turn left here to return to the trailhead along Pemberton Trail for a total hiking distance of 4.5 miles.

NEARBY ACTIVITIES

McDowell Mountain Regional Park offers superb trails for mountain biking. **Pemberton, Stoneman Wash, Tonto Tank,** and **Bluff Trails** form large loops that cover the plains and hills inside the park. Another idyllic setting for a casual hike is nearby **Fountain Hills,** whose main attraction is a 600-foot man-made fountain.

· ·

GPS TRAILHEAD COORDINATES N33° 41.448' W111° 43.105'

DIRECTIONS From Loop 101, exit onto Shea Boulevard. Drive east on Shea Boulevard for 9 miles; then turn north (left) onto Fountain Hills Boulevard. Follow Fountain Hills Boulevard, which eventually becomes McDowell Mountain Park Drive, 7.5 miles to McDowell Mountain Regional Park. Turn west (left) into the park, and pay the entrance fee at the gate. Continue on the park's main road for 3 miles; then turn east (right), onto Shallmo Drive, which terminates at the large trailhead staging area.

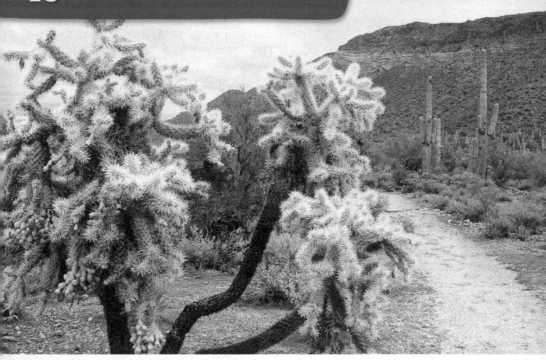

A trailside chain fruit cholla (also known as jumping cholla) frames a view of Pass Mountain.

PASS MOUNTAIN TRAIL forms a large loop around its namesake landmark in the East Valley. This pleasant and easy trail offers grand views of the Goldfield Mountains, Four Peaks, and Superstition Mountains.

DESCRIPTION

Usery Mountain Regional Park borders Tonto National Forest and encompasses 3,648 acres of mountain preserves at the western end of the Goldfield Mountains. Wind Cave Trail (see Hike 26, page 139) is the main attraction in the park, but those who take the time to explore Pass Mountain Trail—one of the best loop hikes in the area— will enjoy expansive views to the east that easily outshine Wind Cave's panoramas.

Pass Mountain Trail begins in Usery Park but runs mostly through Tonto National Forest. Encircling the mountain of the same name, it takes visitors from the desert floor through dry washes, across mountainsides, and up to a saddle with outstanding views. The trail is gentle on the lungs and legs, making it ideal for a family day hike.

I prefer to start from the Wind Cave Trailhead for this loop, though the official trailhead is at the horse staging area. Those in the know may also use the alternate trailhead off Meridian Road to avoid paying the park's entrance fee (there are no restrooms or other services here, however). Hiking the loop clockwise allows you to avoid a steep climb and renders the 730 feet of elevation gain nearly insignificant.

DISTANCE & CONFIGURATION: 7.5-mile loop

DIFFICULTY: Easy but long—good family hike, but older children would likely have more stamina than younger ones on this trail.

SCENERY: Desert, mountain views, city views

EXPOSURE: Mostly exposed

TRAIL TRAFFIC: Light

TRAIL SURFACE: Gravel, packed dirt, rock

HIKING TIME: 3.5 hours

WATER REQUIREMENT: 2.5 quarts

DRIVING DISTANCE: 26 miles from Phoenix Sky Harbor Airport

ELEVATION GAIN: 2,000' at trailhead, 2,620' at highest point

ACCESS: Park open 6 a.m.–8 p.m. (till 10 p.m. Friday–Saturday); trail closes at sunset; $6/vehicle entrance fee

MAPS: USGS *Apache Junction;* park map available at entrance and maricopacountyparks.net/maps

FACILITIES: Restrooms, drinking water, picnic areas, visitor center, camping, archery range; no services at alternate trailhead

WHEELCHAIR ACCESS: Section near trailhead passable by wheelchair

CONTACT: 480-984-0032, maricopacountyparks .net/park-locator/usery-mountain-regional-park

COMMENTS: A portion of Pass Mountain Trail is part of the Maricopa Trail, a county-based trail system that spans 315 miles. Dogs must be leashed at all times.

Find Pass Mountain Trail at the signed junction just north of the Wind Cave Trailhead restrooms. Turn left here to begin a clockwise loop. The first stretch runs north along the park boundary in the shadows of Pass Mountain. As you hike across dry washes and through typical Sonoran Desert scenery, note the huge west-facing P H O E-N I X sign on Usery Mountain, which the Air Explorers Boy Scout Post built in the 1950s to guide lost pilots. We can only hope that no pilot ever needed the sign to navigate.

The trail climbs almost imperceptibly as it traverses the valley floor and goes in and out of dry washes. Look for typical desert plants such as the giant saguaro, teddy bear cholla, brittlebush, and jojoba. Red chuparosa flowers display their tubular shapes along sandy wash bottoms and often attract hummingbirds. Literally translated as "rose sucker," the word *chuparosa* also means "hummingbird" in Spanish.

At 0.9 mile, the trail nears the park's boundary fence. Soon after reaching the fence, you'll descend into a deep drainage and climb the other side to the top of a mound. If you happen to be here on the hour, look northwest into the gap between Usery and One Mountains to see Fountain Hills' famous geyser sending a jet high into the air. The trail bends east and crosses the fence into Tonto National Forest at 1.5 miles from the trailhead. Continue hiking east along the desert floor and cross a wide wash bed into a stand of chain fruit cholla. Along with teddy bear cholla, chain fruit cholla is also known as "jumping cholla," indicating that the slightest wind can blow their sharp needles onto you. Don't worry; the path leaves plenty of buffer space.

The trail ascends gently from the valley floor to a mound about 2 miles from the trailhead; here, a stunning vista of Goldfield Mountains springs into view. A wide, lush valley opens in front of you; to the northeast, you can see the greater Salt River basin; and after winter storms, you can see snow atop Four Peaks. Head east along the trail with the yellowish volcanic Goldfield Mountains directly in front of you, and then descend slowly into a large basin at 2.4 miles.

Pass Mountain Trail

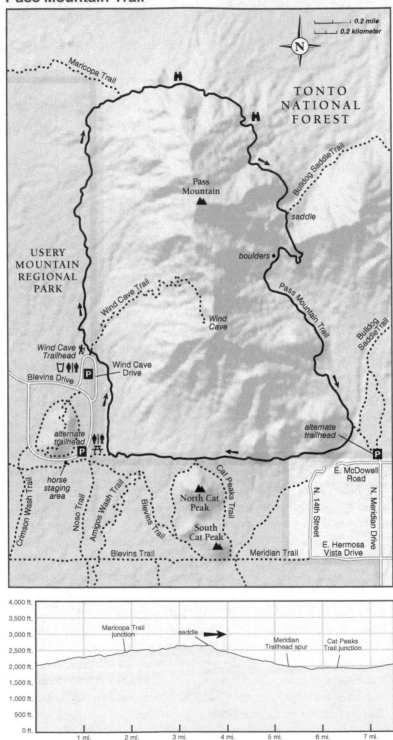

The next mile or so along Pass Mountain Trail is the most spectacular stretch on the entire circuit, offering ever-expanding views at every turn as it hugs the steep northeastern slopes of Pass Mountain. Look for plant life such as palo verde, brittlebush, and jojoba, whose flowers paint the slopes a brilliant gold after a wet winter.

The trail eventually bends south and comes to a wide, flat saddle at 3.6 miles and 2,600 feet elevation. A spur trail takes off east along the northern side of the next hill, but stay on the main trail, heading south. A wide view of east Mesa and Apache Junction opens straight ahead. Just over the saddle, the trail dives steeply into the next basin near some large rock outcroppings. Notice the brilliant contrast of colors here: green plants, chartreuse lichen, yellowish volcanic tuff, and rust-colored rocks.

At 4 miles, you'll pass between two large boulders where the western Superstition Mountains come into view. The trail slowly curves around the basin and heads southeast toward the sprawling city, exposing more and more of the view toward the Superstitions. At 5.3 miles, a cairned spur trail branches east, crosses a deep wash, and leads to the alternate trailhead at the end of Meridian Road. If you parked at that trailhead, note that you'll pass several small side trails, so take care not to get lost.

Otherwise, remain on the main trail at the spur junction; then bend west on noticeably rockier terrain to skirt the southern end of Pass Mountain. Cross a dry wash at 5.8 miles; then continue along a fence marking the Usery Park boundary. Pass the Cat Peaks Trail junction 0.5 mile later. After more wash crossings, you'll come to a sign pointing to the Pass Mountain Trailhead at 6.8 miles. Going left here leads to the horse staging area and the official trailhead—follow Pass Mountain Trail north (right) another 0.6 mile to where it reenters the park to complete the loop near the Wind Cave Trailhead.

NEARBY ACTIVITIES

The popular **Wind Cave Trail** (see Hike 26, page 139) begins at the same trailhead in Usery Park. The **Superstition Mountains,** to the east, present many excellent hiking opportunities, a number of which are outlined in this book.

* *

GPS TRAILHEAD COORDINATES N33° 28.444' W111° 36.441' (Wind Cave Trailhead), N33° 27.977' W111 34.853' (Meridian Trailhead)

DIRECTIONS *Wind Cave Trailhead:* Exit US 60 onto Ellsworth Road and drive north 6.5 miles; then turn east (right) into Usery Mountain Regional Park. Pay at the entrance station; then proceed 1 mile and turn north (left) onto Wind Cave Drive. Park at the Wind Cave Trailhead to access Pass Mountain Trail.

Meridian Trailhead: Exit US 60 onto Signal Butte Road and drive north 0.5 mile; then turn east (right) on Southern Avenue, travel 1 mile, and turn north (left) on Meridian Road. The trailhead is 5 miles ahead, at the end of Meridian Road.

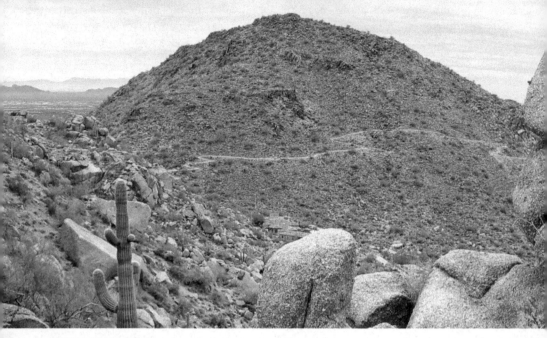

Pinnacle Peak Trail winds along the hillside in Pinnacle Peak Park.

PINNACLE PEAK TRAIL offers residents of north Scottsdale a wonderful place to exercise after work or to spend a weekend afternoon with family. The trail is beautiful and well maintained, and it has just enough elevation gain to be considered moderately difficult.

DESCRIPTION

The 3,170-foot Pinnacle Peak rises from the desert floor like a needle. It is a distinctive landmark in the Phoenix area, and many resorts have situated themselves in its shadows. Once the rustic fringe of civilization, this area is now a thriving suburbia replete with affluent new homes and golf courses. This interesting contrast between the Old West and new development, raw desert and urban sprawl, gives the Pinnacle Peak foothills an alluring charm.

For those living in the northeastern part of the valley, Pinnacle Peak is the analogue of Camelback Mountain or Piestewa Peak. Pinnacle Peak Park and its main trail belong to the City of Scottsdale, which has done a superb job of packaging the desert experience into a 3.5-mile out-and-back hike. When you arrive at the park, stop by the visitor center to pick up a trail map and a copy of the native-plant guide, which identifies the desert flora along the way.

DISTANCE & CONFIGURATION: 3.5-mile out-and-back

DIFFICULTY: Moderate

SCENERY: Pinnacle Peak, desert, golf courses, city views, desert plants

EXPOSURE: Mostly exposed

TRAIL TRAFFIC: Heavy

TRAIL SURFACE: Packed dirt

HIKING TIME: 1.5 hours

WATER REQUIREMENT: 1.5 quarts

DRIVING DISTANCE: 29 miles from Phoenix Sky Harbor Airport

ELEVATION GAIN: 2,570' at trailhead, 2,889' at highest point

ACCESS: 5 a.m.–7 p.m. summer, 7 a.m.–5:30 p.m. winter (click "Hours" at the website below for additional seasonal hours); no permits or fees required

MAPS: USGS *McDowell Peak;* trail map available from visitor center

FACILITIES: Restrooms, drinking water, ramada, picnic area, visitor center

WHEELCHAIR ACCESS: yes

CONTACT: 480-312-0990, scottsdaleaz.gov /parks/pinnacle-peak-park

COMMENTS: Nature trail near entrance with native plants display; rock-climbing access; no dogs allowed

This interpretive trail tries to be all things to all people and for the most part succeeds. Hikers share the trail with joggers, rock climbers, tourists, families, and, on rare occasions, even equestrians.

Begin the hike near the visitor center at a well-marked trailhead in the shadows of Pinnacle Peak. The wide, manicured trail circles the base of the mountain, showcasing a rich assortment of desert flora that any arboretum would be proud to own. Numbered signs identify various plants, such as Christmas cholla and desert mistletoe, two of the most interesting species. The Christmas cholla is a cactus but looks like a shrub, and desert mistletoe is a parasitic plant that lives in leguminous host trees—such as mesquite, acacia, and palo verde—plants that, along with the giant saguaro cactus, define the Sonoran Desert. Refer to your plant guide for more-detailed explanations.

After a quarter mile, the trail, which begins to ascend via switchbacks, overlooks the visitor center, parking lot, and northern Scottsdale. The silhouette of Four Peaks graces the eastern horizon. At 0.4 mile the trail levels and then heads northwest. A small side trail on the left allows rock climbers with ropes and harnesses to access the craggy summit of Pinnacle Peak. If you're not feeling like Spider-Man, remain on the main trail and head toward the smaller hills in front of you. Another rock-climbing access trail splits off to the right, near the northernmost part of the trail.

Pinnacle Peak Trail makes a 180-degree turn to climb south to the Grandview lookout at 0.65 mile. Rest here while you survey the landscape below. Lush green golf courses and blue lakes contrast sharply with the brown desert and sand-colored houses. Embedded in the circular brickwork like tick marks on a clock face, etched wooden logs point to numerous landmarks, such as Four Peaks and Granite Mountain. Shortly after Grandview, the trail climbs to its highest point at 2,889 feet.

Pinnacle Peak Trail

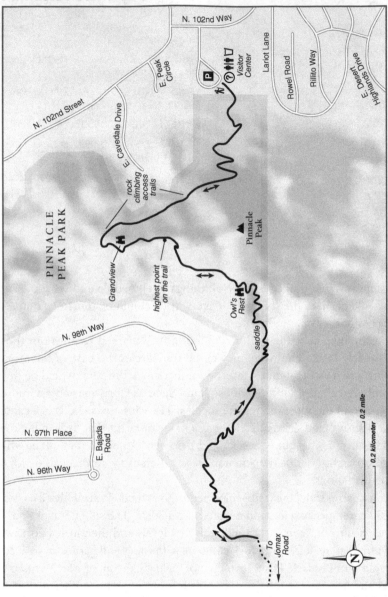

N. 102nd Way

Lariot Lane

Rowel Road

Rillito Way

E. Desert Highlands Drive

E. Peak Circle

Visitor Center

N. 102nd Street

E. Cavedale Drive

rock climbing access trails

PINNACLE PEAK PARK

Pinnacle Peak

Grandview

highest point on the trail

Owl's Rest

saddle

N. 98th Way

0.2 mile

0.2 kilometer

N. 97th Place

E. Bajada Road

N. 96th Way

To Jomax Road

N

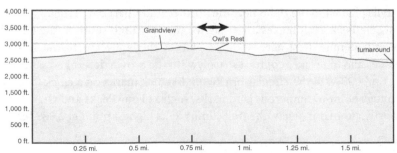

Grandview

Owl's Rest

turnaround

4,000 ft.
3,500 ft.
3,000 ft.
2,500 ft.
2,000 ft.
1,500 ft.
1,000 ft.
500 ft.
0 ft.

0.25 mi.   0.5 mi.   0.75 mi.   1 mi.   1.25 mi.   1.5 mi.

At 0.9 mile, you'll pass Owl's Rest lookout, with its nautilus-shaped brickwork. Perched above a steep hill, it provides a convenient rest stop on the return hike. West of Owl's Rest, you'll descend view-studded switchbacks and duck around large boulders to reach a saddle point at 2,625 feet elevation. The trail climbs once again, up the flank of an unnamed 3,000-foot hill west of Pinnacle Peak. Gauge your progress by the conspicuous distance markers every 0.25 mile. Near the 1.25-mile marker, the trail reaches its second crest, at 2,725 feet, and then flattens.

The final 0.5 mile of Pinnacle Peak Trail is the steepest part of your hike. It drops 400 feet via switchbacks to a shady rest spot at the western boundary of Pinnacle Peak Park. Should you choose to continue hiking in that direction beyond the park boundary another 0.3 mile, you would end up on Jomax Trail, which is behind a housing development on Jomax Road. After a good rest, most people turn around at the park boundary because the first 0.5-mile climb on the return trip will test your endurance. Return to the visitor center along the same trail.

NEARBY ACTIVITIES

Rock climbers with proper equipment can scale Pinnacle Peak by taking a special climber's access trail at the 0.4-mile mark on Pinnacle Peak Trail. **Tom's Thumb** (see Hike 25, page 134) in the McDowell Mountains presents a challenging hike to another popular rock-climbing destination. To the north, **Brown's Ranch Trailhead** (see Hike 17, page 100) leads to still more hiking trails.

• •

GPS TRAILHEAD COORDINATES N33° 43.670' W111° 51.620'

DIRECTIONS From Loop 101, exit at Princess Drive. Drive east, then north, on Pima Road 4.5 miles; then turn east (right) onto Happy Valley Road. Continue 2 miles, and then turn north (left) on Alma School Road. Drive 1 mile, and then turn west (left) on Pinnacle Peak Parkway. Drive 0.5 mile farther to Pinnacle Peak Park.

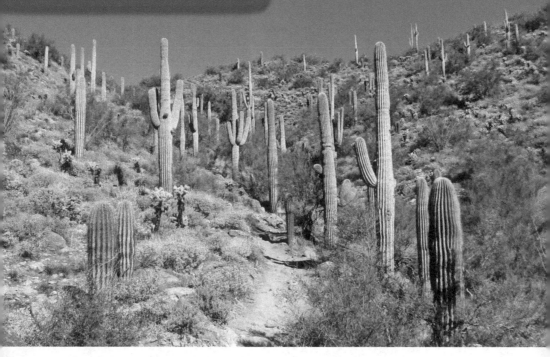

Saguaros flourish on south-facing slopes of Sunrise Peak.

ONE OF THE Phoenix area's most popular in-town hikes, Sunrise Trail is a treat. Enjoy unspoiled desert in the beautiful McDowell Sonoran Preserve, take in fantastic views of Scottsdale and Fountain Hills, and challenge yourself on the superbly maintained trail to the 3,069-foot Sunrise Peak.

DESCRIPTION

Constructed in 2004, Sunrise Trail was one of the first trails in McDowell Sonoran Preserve. Since its creation, Sunrise has been steadily gaining popularity, first with nearby residents in Scottsdale and Fountain Hills and then, as word spread, with Phoenicians in general. The trail's success comes as no surprise. Its ease of access, proximity to town, multiple trailheads, stunning scenery and views, and perfect balance between challenge and enjoyment appeal to a wide range of hikers. If you can't find something to love about this trail, you might be having a really bad day.

Located on the southeastern tip of McDowell Sonoran Preserve, Sunrise Peak straddles the mountainous divide between Scottsdale and Fountain Hills. The trail skirts this summit to span a significant portion of the southern McDowells, overlooking heavily populated suburbs. Four trailheads service this trail, offering numerous options for a customized hike.

DISTANCE & CONFIGURATION: 5-mile point-to-point, 6-mile out-and-back to/from summit from Lost Dog Wash Traihead, 4-mile out-and-back to/from summit from Sunrise Trailhead

DIFFICULTY: Moderate

SCENERY: Sunrise Peak, city panorama, desert

EXPOSURE: Completely exposed

TRAIL TRAFFIC: Moderate–heavy

TRAIL SURFACE: Packed dirt, gravel, rock

HIKING TIME: 3 hours

WATER REQUIREMENT: 2 quarts

DRIVING DISTANCE: 22 miles from Phoenix Sky Harbor Airport

ELEVATION GAIN: 1,755' at Lost Dog Wash Trailhead, 3,069' at Sunrise Peak

ACCESS: Sunrise–sunset; no permits or fees required

MAPS: USGS *Sawik Mountain;* map available at trailhead

FACILITIES: *Lost Dog Wash Trailhead:* restrooms, water, ramada, trail volunteers on weekends; *Sunrise Trailhead:* water, ramada

WHEELCHAIR ACCESS: Nature trail at Lost Dog Wash Trailhead

CONTACT: 480-312-7013, scottsdaleaz.gov/preserve

COMMENTS: Dogs must be leashed at all times

This hike covers a complete west-to-east traversal of Sunrise Trail, including a detour to Sunrise Peak. Of course, one drawback to hiking one-way is that it requires a car shuttle. Park one car at the Sunrise Trailhead; then drive the other to the well-appointed Lost Dog Wash Trailhead, located at the end of 124th Street north of Shea Boulevard.

Lost Dog Wash, the first major trailhead built for the preserve, provides access to the southern McDowells. On weekends, volunteers from McDowell Sonoran Conservancy greet visitors there and offer general information, trail maps, helpful advice, safety tips, and even organized hikes. The conservancy is a nonprofit organization that drove the creation of McDowell Sonoran Preserve and partnered closely with Scottsdale's government to fund, acquire, build, and manage the preserve, which has designated 36,000 acres of desert wilderness for conservation. McDowell Sonoran Preserve is now the largest municipal park or nature preserve in the United States.

Begin your hike from behind the building area, striking out on Lost Dog Wash Trail amid Sonoran Desert flora. Brittlebush and palo verde line the wide dirt path. The trail turns north next to a small hill to head toward the distant antenna-studded Thompson Peak. At 0.2 mile you'll cross a dry creekbed; then turn right to reach the official start of Sunrise Trail. Trail signs in the preserve are easy to find, easy to read, and very informative.

The west half of Sunrise Trail takes a gentle approach to Sunrise Peak, meandering through open desert before climbing toward the summit. You'll hike along the dry wash for a short distance before the trail gently inclines. At the next trail junction, with Anasazi Spur, keep left to remain on Sunrise Trail, and then head northeast toward a saddle between rugged peaks. All signs of city life disappear ahead, as you are engulfed in the desert hiking experience. Hardy creosote bushes, barrel cacti, and thorny ocotillos dominate the landscape.

Sunrise Trail

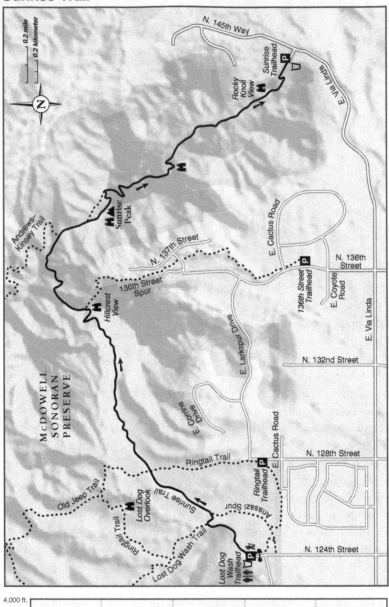

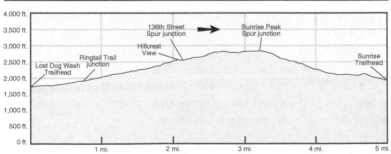

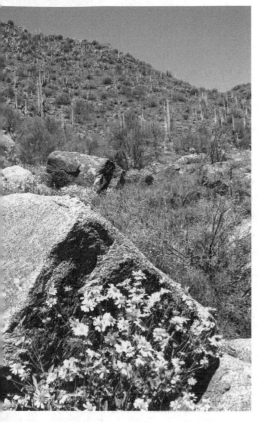

Brittlebush flowers add a splash of gold to desert hills.

Reach Ringtail Trail at 0.7 mile from the trailhead. The second trailhead with access to Sunrise Trail can be found 0.5 mile south of this junction, on 128th Street. Continue straight through the trail junction to hike deeper into the preserve, leaving behind fine views of Scottsdale and distant Camelback Mountain (see Hikes 2 and 3, pages 29 and 34). The slope remains gentle as you gain an elevated ridge at 1.3 miles. After good spring rains, brittlebush blossoms paint these hills a golden yellow, followed by brightly colored cactus and ocotillo flowers a month later. A springtime hike on Sunrise Trail can be an exquisite experience.

At 1.8 miles, you follow sharp switchbacks to climb out of the drainage and then reach a wide overlook at 2,550 feet elevation. Sunrise Peak comes into view in the distance, and you can trace the trail's profile as it cuts across the hill to the north. A narrower trail, called the 136th Street Spur, can take you down to the housing subdivision where you'll find the third trailhead for this hike. But for now, remain on Sunrise Trail as it crosses the hillside, affording an open view toward Camelback, Piestewa Peak (see Hikes 10 and 11, pages 64 and 68), and the downtown Phoenix skyline. After steadily climbing 1,000 vertical feet, the trail finally levels off as it approaches the base of Sunrise Peak.

Find a signed junction with Sunrise Peak Spur at 2.8 miles from the trailhead. This spur trail forms a 0.25-mile detour to the summit of Sunrise Peak and then rejoins Sunrise Trail at another junction. Take the spur trail here and head south toward the summit. The spur trail is narrow, rough, and steep, but mercifully short. Once you gain the summit, you'll revel in a magnificent panoramic view. To the east, Four Peaks (see Hike 46, page 237) towers over Fountain Hills. If you arrive just past the hour, you'll be treated to a fountain show. Weaver's Needle (see Hike 34, page 179), the Superstition Mountains, and Red Mountain are all visible. To the south and west, metropolitan Phoenix stretches for many miles. Other rugged McDowell peaks complete the panorama.

The eastern half of Sunrise Trail differs greatly from the western half. It's considerably steeper and more mountainous, and it runs through a narrow canyon instead of open desert, yielding a more intimate setting for your descent. For those looking for a more challenging climb, consider starting from the eastern end instead; be careful, though, as gravel and steep slopes require you to step judiciously. Follow the spur trail east until it intersects Sunrise Trail once more; then turn right and head down a cactus-studded hill. Tall stands of saguaro and clusters of fuzzy teddy bear cholla line the trail here.

Pass an overlook at 3.8 miles from the trailhead. (This would be a great place for a rest if you hiked up the eastern side.) Teddy bear chollas frame a distant view of the city. Below the overlook, Sunrise Trail forks for a short distance, but soon the forks rejoin. The steep descent soon gives way to rolling hills; lift your gaze to admire the scenery again. You'll reach the smaller Sunrise Trailhead at the end of Via Linda Street, a distance of 5 miles from the Lost Dog Wash Trailhead. If you planned well, your shuttle vehicle is waiting for your arrival.

NEARBY ACTIVITIES

Lost Dog Wash and **Ringtail Trails** in the southern McDowells are also accessible from the Lost Dog Wash Trailhead. Frank Lloyd Wright's **Taliesin West** studio (12621 N. Frank Lloyd Wright Blvd.; 888-516-0811, franklloydwright.org/taliesin -west) is just a short distance from these trails. Other trails in McDowell Sonoran Preserve offer longer excursions into the preserve's interior. **Tom's Thumb** (see Hike 25, page 134), in the northern part of the preserve, is a popular rock-climbing destination. Nearby **McDowell Mountain Regional Park** (see Hike 18, page 104) contributes even more options for hiking and biking.

• •

GPS TRAILHEAD COORDINATES
N33°35.762' W111°46.065' (Sunrise Trailhead)
N33° 36.028' W111° 48.704' (Lost Dog Wash Trailhead)

DIRECTIONS *Sunrise Trailhead:* Exit Loop 101 at Shea Boulevard, and drive east on Shea for 6 miles to 136th Street. Turn north (left) onto 136th Street, drive 0.5 mile, and then turn east (right) onto Via Linda. Follow Via Linda east 1.5 miles to the access area.

Lost Dog Wash Trailhead: From the Sunrise Trailhead, drive west 3.5 miles on Via Linda Road; then turn north (right) onto 124th Street and follow it 1 mile to the Lost Dog Wash Trailhead.

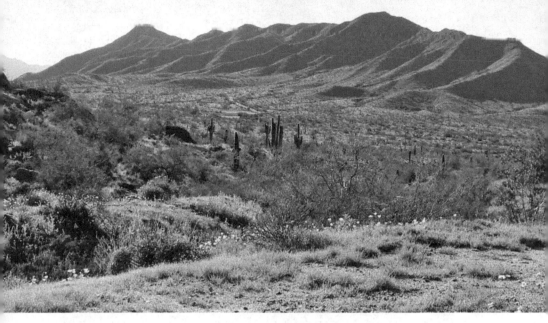

Lush vegetation covers the interior of South Mountain Park/Preserve after strong winter rains.

SERVED BY ONE of two trailheads on the south side of South Mountain, Telegraph Pass is popular among Ahwatukee residents. It begins as a gentle stroll along the foothills and climbs to the top of Telegraph Pass, with Hohokam petroglyphs along the way.

DESCRIPTION

To reach Phoenix from the suburb of Ahwatukee requires a lengthy and traffic-congested drive on I-10 around South Mountain. Sometimes, in fact, it seems quicker to hike into downtown rather than drive to it. Silly as that option may be, I'm sure that many frustrated Ahwatukee commuters must have contemplated it while sitting in traffic.

The hypothetical hiking shortcut they would take through South Mountain Park/ Preserve is via Telegraph Pass, which bisects the 11-mile mountainous barrier at a point in line with Phoenix's Central Avenue. In fact, during the 1800s, the Army Signal Corps chose this very pass as the optimal route for a telegraph line from Maricopa Wells to Phoenix and then on to the territorial capital, Prescott. Today, Telegraph Pass is still a prominent and popular saddle in the park.

DISTANCE & CONFIGURATION: 2.4-mile out-and-back (add 2.4 miles for Kiwanis Trail)

DIFFICULTY: Easy–moderate

SCENERY: South Mountain, city panorama, desert, petroglyphs

EXPOSURE: Early-morning and late-afternoon shade, otherwise exposed

TRAIL TRAFFIC: Heavy on Telegraph Pass Trail, light on Kiwanis Trail

TRAIL SURFACE: Pavement, gravel, crushed rock

HIKING TIME: 1.5 hours (add 1 hour for Kiwanis Trail)

WATER REQUIREMENT: 1.5 quarts

DRIVING DISTANCE: 20 miles from Phoenix Sky Harbor Airport

ELEVATION GAIN: 1,490' at Telegraph Pass Trailhead, 2,010' at Telegraph Pass, 1,570' at Kiwanis Trailhead

ACCESS: Gates open 5 a.m.–7 p.m.; trails open until 11 p.m.; no permits or fees required

MAPS: USGS *Lone Butte;* trailhead plaque

FACILITIES: Water but no restrooms

WHEELCHAIR ACCESS: First paved section only

CONTACT: 602-262-7393, phoenix.gov/parks /trails/locations/south-mountain

COMMENTS: Dogs permitted on leash except when temperatures exceed 100°F

Telegraph Pass Trailhead is one of two entrances on South Mountain Park/Preserve's southern side, making this hike extremely popular among Ahwatukee residents. On weekends, expect to see a steady stream of people, bikes, pets, and strollers on the trail. Don't let the crowds put you off, though—Telegraph Pass Trail is an excellent short hike. The trail leaves the edge of suburbia, runs through desert foothills and up a canyon, and eventually ends at its namesake saddle. Views from Telegraph Pass make the 1.2-mile climb worth it; as a bonus, you also get a history lesson, thanks to the Hohokam petroglyphs along the way. If you have extra time, consider hiking over the saddle and down Kiwanis Trail to visit the interior basin of South Mountain Park/Preserve. From Telegraph Pass, you can also choose to hike National Trail in either direction for a higher vantage point.

Trailhead parking can be scarce during peak hours, but the trail's short length ensures high turnover so you never have to wait too long for a parking spot. From the parking area, start out north on wide, level pavement that meanders along the fringes of neighborhoods. Mount Suppoa and its forest of antennas loom directly ahead. There is a low hill, or, more accurately, a berm, on the west side of the sidewalk-like trail. In season, Coulter's lupine and phacelia blanket this hill, adding a dash of blue. Near 0.2 mile, you'll pass a fence that marks the park boundary and then cross a dry wash a bit farther on. The pavement ends where Desert Classic Trail begins, at a wide spot 0.4 mile from the trailhead. A popular mountain-biking trail, Desert Classic runs east 9 miles through the foothills and terminates in Pima Canyon at the east end of South Mountain.

Turn left at the trail junction to continue hiking Telegraph Pass Trail, which heads northwest into the hills. Now gently climbing on a dirt and gravel trail, aim for a gap left of the mountaintop. At 0.75 mile, stop to visit petroglyphs left by the Hohokam people more than 600 years ago. South Mountain Park/Preserve contains

Telegraph Pass Trail and Kiwanis Trail

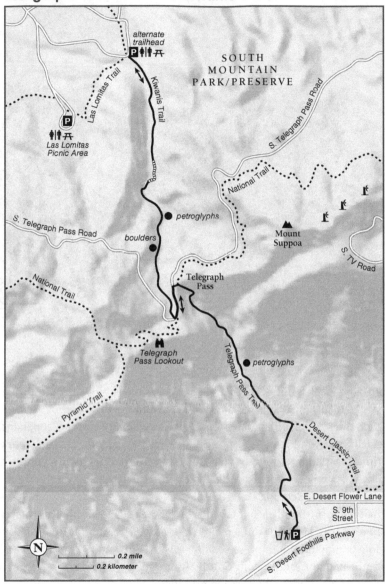

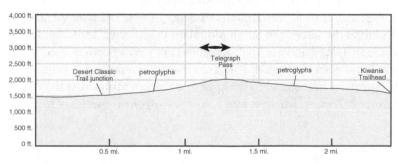

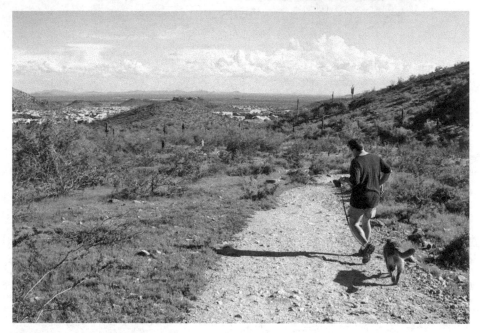

A trail-runner jogs Telegraph Pass Trail with his best friend.

many petroglyph sites, but perhaps none as accessible as this one; a trailside interpretive sign explains the history of the Hohokam and their culture.

Beyond the petroglyph pullout, Telegraph Pass Trail becomes steeper and rockier, especially after trail marker 4. As you hike up the canyon, crossing a dry wash
several times, watch for ambitious trail runners who dart up and down this narrow
path daily. At 1.1 miles, begin ascending a few final switchbacks on the right side of
the canyon to reach Telegraph Pass (2,010').

A major hub in South Mountain Park/Preserve, Telegraph Pass bisects two
mountain ranges and touches three major trails as well as Summit Road. This prominent saddle commands an impressive view toward Ahwatukee. National Trail runs
east–west through the saddle along South Mountain's spine, whereas Telegraph Pass
and Kiwanis Trails straddle the pass longitudinally.

Though many people turn around at Telegraph Pass, consider spending an extra
hour exploring the interior of South Mountain via Kiwanis Trail. Similar in length
and profile to Telegraph Pass Trail, Kiwanis Trail heads north toward the heart of
the park. From where Telegraph Pass Trail meets Summit Road at the saddle, turn
left and walk next to the road to the apex of a hairpin turn. Cross the road here to
access Kiwanis Trail, which dives into a narrow canyon on a series of stony steps.

Kiwanis Trail descends steeply at first but soon levels considerably. At 0.2 mile beyond Telegraph Pass, buildings in downtown Phoenix come into view in a V-shaped gap between the hills. Directly behind you on the hill is a stone lookout tower built by the Civilian Conservation Corps. The trail follows the canyon north past large rock outcroppings that offer some afternoon shade. Though not as prominent as those found on Telegraph Pass Trail, some petroglyphs are visible under a palo verde tree near trail marker 5.

A half mile from the saddle, descend into and cross a dry wash. Next, negotiate some stairs at a steep section a bit farther on the trail, which soon flattens as it follows the dry wash north. Look for a rusted wreck in the wash just before the trail enters a small meadow—how the vehicle landed amid these rugged hills is a mystery. About 1 mile from Telegraph Pass, you'll reach the Kiwanis Trailhead in the interior basin of South Mountain, where you face the Ma Ha Tauk Range and the massive Sierra Estrella Mountains to the west. Though you could shuttle a vehicle to this trailhead through South Mountain Park/Preserve's Central Avenue entrance for a one-way hike, the relatively short trail hardly justifies such a long drive. Return to Ahwatukee the way you came.

NEARBY ACTIVITIES

South Mountain hosts many hiking and biking trails, including **Alta, Desert Classic, Holbert** (see Hike 6, page 47), **Mormon** (see Hike 5, page 43), **Ranger,** and **National** (see Hike 14, page 82). Picnicking here is popular, and there's even a go-kart-racing track. The **Environmental Education Center,** near the Central Avenue entrance, has a superb visitor center, complete with a three-dimensional model of the entire park.

• •

GPS TRAILHEAD COORDINATES N33° 19.065' W112° 03.998'

DIRECTIONS Exit I-10 onto either Chandler Boulevard or Ray Road. Drive west 3.3 miles until these roads intersect; then continue west on Chandler Boulevard 1.75 miles to Desert Foothills Parkway. Turn north (right) onto Desert Foothills Parkway, and follow it 1.2 miles to the trailhead parking lot.

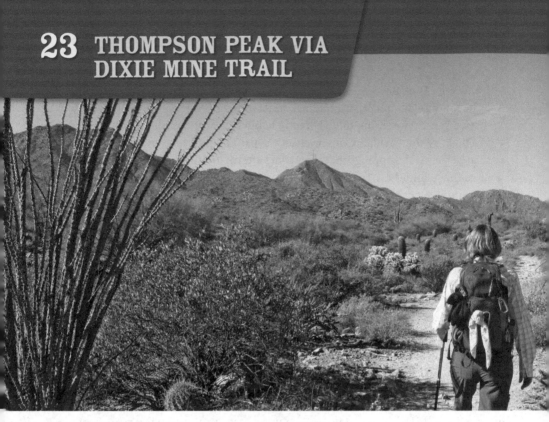

Kelly Liu of Mesa hikes toward Thompson Peak along Dixie Mine Trail.

ONE OF THREE prominent peaks in McDowell Sonoran Preserve, Thompson Peak rises to nearly 4,000 feet. Enjoy a leisurely hike from the town of Fountain Hills through Sonoran Desert foothills; then make the invigorating climb up a steep service road to Thompson Peak's summit.

DESCRIPTION

One can see Thompson Peak and its radio towers from nearly anywhere in Phoenix. It's the only major peak in the McDowell Mountains with the summit access that hikers live for. The view from Thompson Peak, which overlooks the McDowell Mountains and north Scottsdale, rivals that from any vantage point near Phoenix.

The most direct route to Thompson Peak begins from the Golden Eagle Trailhead, which serves McDowell Mountain Regional Park. Begin by walking around the housing development's entrance gate, making sure to stay on the sidewalk and follow the designated signs for the trailhead. Turn right at Desert Tortoise Trail to reach the trailhead proper, on the boundary of McDowell Mountain Regional Park, 0.5 mile from the parking area.

Notice a sign-in kiosk at the park gate, where you'll find self-pay envelopes. Be sure to deposit the requisite $2-per-person entrance fee. (If you have an annual pass to Maricopa County Parks, you may enter without additional payment.) Strike

DISTANCE & CONFIGURATION: 9.4-mile out-and-back

DIFFICULTY: Strenuous

SCENERY: McDowell Sonoran Preserve, Thompson Peak, Dixie Mine, city views

EXPOSURE: Mostly exposed

TRAIL TRAFFIC: Light

TRAIL SURFACE: Gravel, packed dirt, pavement

HIKING TIME: 4 hours

WATER REQUIREMENT: 3 quarts

DRIVING DISTANCE: 29 miles from Phoenix Sky Harbor Airport

ELEVATION GAIN: 2,135' at trailhead, 3,969' on Thompson Peak summit

ACCESS: Sunrise–sunset; free parking; $2/person entry fee

MAPS: USGS *McDowell Peak;* maricopacounty parks.net/maps or at entrance booth

FACILITIES: Water, restrooms

WHEELCHAIR ACCESS: None

CONTACT: 480-471-0173, maricopacountyparks .net/mcdowell-mountain-regional-park

COMMENTS: Dogs must be leashed at all times

out on Dixie Mine Trail, heading north on the wide, packed-dirt path. The surface quickly becomes rocky and uneven as the trail turns west.

Signs of housing developments quickly fade as you hike deeper into the park, immersed in the Sonoran Desert landscape. Thompson Peak and its radio towers lie directly ahead. This arid environment hosts many hardy plants, such as buckhorn cholla, jojoba, and creosote. In the morning and at dusk, you can see cottontail rabbits hopping from one bush to another.

About 0.9 mile from the parking area, you'll crest a little hill and then descend the other side. Dixie Mine Trail undulates up and down over minor drainages but does not gain significant elevation. Enjoy the relatively easy stroll amid the desert foothills. If you look behind you, you can see Four Peaks (see Hike 46, page 237) and Weaver's Needle (see Hike 34, page 179) on the eastern horizon. Cross a dry creekbed and make the steep climb up the opposite side; then hike along a little ridge next to the creek.

You'll reach a trail junction with Sonoran Trail at 1.2 miles from the parking area. Sonoran Trail branches left and leads into Fountain Hills McDowell Mountain Preserve—stay on Dixie Mine Trail and continue straight; then cross another dry wash. Continue hiking northwest as the trail levels briefly amid a field of triangle-leaf bursage and brittlebush. Next, you'll pass a rock outcrop on the left, and then climb another hillock, marked by white quartz rocks. At 2.1 miles from the parking area, you'll cross a wide, dry wash and climb a short but steep hill, a prelude to the ascent of Thompson Peak.

Dixie Mine Trail meets the wide service road for Thompson Peak at 2.5 miles. To your right, on the opposite hill, lies Dixie Mine, with a pile of spent ore called tailings clearly visible from this junction. The mine is worth a detour, but be sure to return to the trail after your exploration. Established in the late 1800s, Dixie Mine held the promise of gold and silver for dozens of miners. Ownership changed hands numerous times over the years; unfortunately, the mine produced very little tangible

Thompson Peak via Dixie Mine Trail

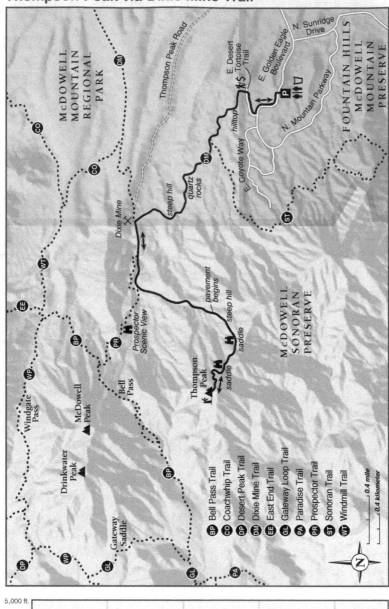

McDOWELL MOUNTAIN REGIONAL PARK

Thompson Peak Road

N. Sunridge Drive

E. Desert Tortoise Trail

E. Golden Eagle Boulevard

N. Mountain Parkway

E. Coyote Way

hilltop

FOUNTAIN HILLS

McDOWELL MOUNTAIN PRESERVE

Dixie Mine

steep hill

quartz rocks

pavement begins

steep hill

saddle

Prospector Scenic View

McDOWELL SONORAN PRESERVE

Bell Pass

Thompson Peak

saddle

saddle

McDowell Peak

Windgate Pass

Drinkwater Peak

Gateway Saddle

BP Bell Pass Trail
CO Coachwhip Trail
DP Desert Peak Trail
DM Dixie Mine Trail
EE East End Trail
GL Gateway Loop Trail
PA Paradise Trail
PR Prospector Trail
ST Sonoran Trail
WT Windmill Trail

0.4 mile
0.4 kilometer

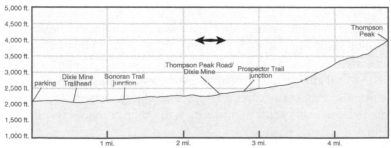

5,000 ft.
4,500 ft.
4,000 ft.
3,500 ft.
3,000 ft.
2,500 ft.
2,000 ft.
1,500 ft.
1,000 ft.

Thompson Peak

parking

Dixie Mine Trailhead

Sonoran Trail junction

Thompson Peak Road/ Dixie Mine

Prospector Trail junction

1 mi.   2 mi.   3 mi.   4 mi.

minerals. However, the main mineshaft remains, visible from behind a locked gate. Nearby, look for some Hohokam petroglyphs carved into the surrounding rocks by ancient desert dwellers.

Dixie Mine Trail continues northeast into McDowell Mountain Regional Park. For this hike, return to the Thompson Peak service road and follow it toward the prominent peak. The graded dirt road climbs to meet a marked junction with Prospector Trail, which leads toward Bell Pass Trail (see Hike 15, page 90). Stay on the service road and continue hiking west.

Three miles from the parking area, the road turns south. Now you can see the final stretch of the hike: it climbs steeply to a ridge and then sweeps right, toward the summit. The road remains fairly level for another 0.5 mile before crossing a dry wash and beginning its uphill climb in earnest. Soon the dirt road transitions into paved concrete as you climb the relentlessly steep hill. This section of the hike is as steep as any major trail in town.

You'll reach the summit ridge at 4.1 miles from the parking area. Here, views to the south open up at a wide overlook. Take a break to enjoy the scenery. Can you identify Camelback Mountain, Mummy Mountain, South Mountain, the Sierra Estrellas, and Table Top Mountain (see Hike 59, page 298)? The road levels and contours around the ridge for 0.25 mile; then the steep climb resumes for the final pitch toward the summit.

You'll summit Thompson Peak at 4.7 miles from the parking area—this is the highest vantage point from any major peak within the Phoenix area. Your toils up the steep incline are rewarded with spectacular panoramic views of the city below and all the mountain ranges around Phoenix. Take your time to enjoy the scenery, and then return via the same route.

NEARBY ACTIVITIES

McDowell Sonoran Preserve hosts many miles of hiking trails. **Bell Pass Trail** (see Hike 15, page 90), **Tom's Thumb Trail** (see Hike 25, page 134), and **Sunrise Trail** (see Hike 21, page 116) are local favorites. McDowell Mountain Regional Park offers excellent mountain-biking opportunities.

• •

GPS TRAILHEAD COORDINATES N33° 38.146' W111° 46.113'

DIRECTIONS From Loop 101, take Exit 41 for Shea Boulevard. Drive east on Shea for 8 miles to Palisades Boulevard. Turn north (left) onto Palisades and continue 3 miles to Golden Eagle Boulevard. Turn northwest (left) at Golden Eagle; then drive 2.8 miles to a small parking lot next to a gated entrance.

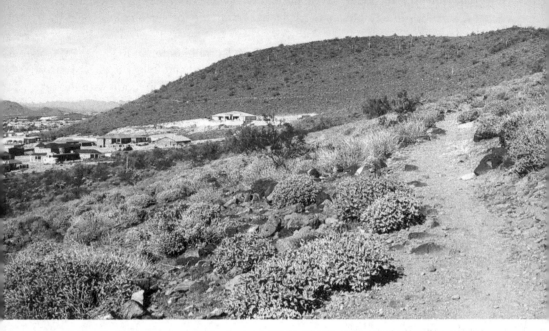

Cholla Loop Trail winds around brittlebush-covered Hedgpeth Hills and overlooks Glendale.

CHOLLA LOOP TRAIL in Thunderbird Park offers a great beginner's hike, taking visitors up the northernmost Hedgpeth Hill and providing ample open views of the city and surrounding mountains. Sometimes in spring, golden brittlebush blossoms completely cover the Hedgpeth Hills.

DESCRIPTION

The City of Glendale acquired land around Hedgpeth Hills in the 1950s and then created Thunderbird Conservation Park (known informally as Thunderbird Park), which was named after a nearby WWII fighter-training facility. Maricopa County improved the park and managed it until 1984, when the City of Glendale took over its operation. Today the park is a hotbed of activity for northwest-Valley residents.

Thunderbird Park offers 1,185 acres of mountain preserves and approximately 20 miles of hiking trails. These hills are named after Robert Hedgpeth, an early settler of the area. Cholla Loop Trail and a section of Coach Whip Trail form a convenient loop that is particularly popular among Thunderbird Park patrons. The loop traces a heart-shaped path over and around the northernmost Hedgpeth Hill and presents picturesque panoramic views of the park and surrounding housing developments.

Located east of the amphitheater and just south of the first parking area inside the park, the information plaque near the main entrance to Thunderbird Park on

DISTANCE & CONFIGURATION: 3.6-mile loop

DIFFICULTY: Easy–moderate

SCENERY: City panoramas, Thunderbird Park, Hedgpeth Hills, desert

EXPOSURE: Completely exposed

TRAIL TRAFFIC: Moderate

TRAIL SURFACE: Gravel, packed dirt, rock

HIKING TIME: 1.5 hours

WATER REQUIREMENT: 1 quart

DRIVING DISTANCE: 27 miles from Phoenix Sky Harbor Airport

ELEVATION GAIN: 1,340' at trailhead, 1,833' at highest point

ACCESS: Sunrise–sunset; no permits or fees required

MAPS: USGS *Hedgpeth Hills;* trailhead plaque

FACILITIES: Water, restrooms, picnic areas, wildlife-viewing areas

WHEELCHAIR ACCESS: Available elsewhere in the park but not on this trail

CONTACT: 623-930-2820, glendaleaz.com/parks andrecreation/thunderbirdpark.cfm

COMMENTS: Dogs must be leashed at all times

59th Avenue is the ideal place to begin the loop. Strike out northeast from the plaque with 59th Avenue on your right; then cross the paved access road inside the park. About 100 yards from the starting point, you'll find a marked trail junction. Turn left to begin hiking Cholla Loop Trail.

Hike northwest on a wide and gentle packed-dirt trail overlooking housing developments in the Arrowhead area. Typical Sonoran Desert vegetation, including palo verde trees, creosote bushes, barrel cacti, and saguaros, surrounds the trail. At 0.3 mile, the trail becomes much rockier. Notice the patina, or desert varnish, giving trail-side rocks a volcanic look. This thin layer of manganese, iron, and clay is only a surface phenomenon; preferring hot and dry desert climates, colonies of microscopic bacteria have built the dark coating over thousands of years. The Hohokam, who inhabited central Arizona hundreds of years ago, created petroglyphs on large boulders by etching designs in the desert varnish, exposing the lighter-colored core of the rock.

Generally heading north, Cholla Loop Trail makes a short uphill zigzag at 0.5 mile. Numerous brittlebush plants cover the hillside, and new suburbs encroach on the base. Follow the trail as it bends west and then rounds the western end of Hedgpeth Hills, overlooking several horse stables and equestrian training facilities. You can see Pilcher Hill and Ludden Mountain directly to the north as the trail begins to ascend some switchbacks at 1 mile.

Climb mildly sloping switchbacks for 0.2 mile to gain the top of a ridge, where you'll have an impressive view of neighboring housing developments and distant mountains. Continue climbing a moderate hill to the top of a small mound and a cluster of boulders at 1.5 miles from the start. Vegetation atop the ridge is somewhat different than on the hillsides, with noticeably more cacti nestled among lush grasses and not as many brittlebushes.

The gentle ascent resumes after you pass the small mound. Hike up the spine of the hill to a false summit with an old fire ring. Finish the climb along a view-studded ridge to the 1,833-foot summit, 1.9 miles from the start. You'll want to take a breather

Thunderbird Park: Cholla Loop

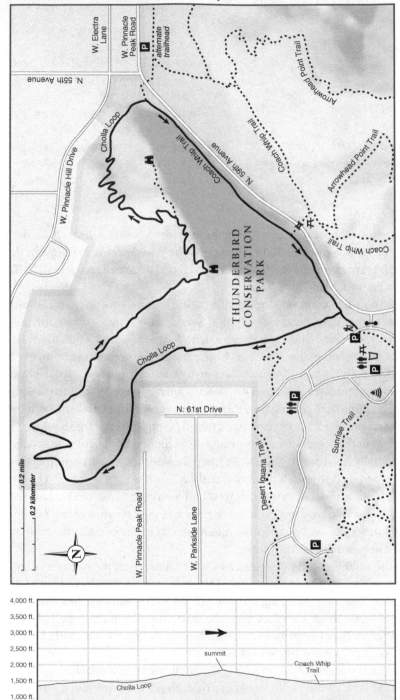

here to admire the scenery, including the tallest Hedgpeth Hill, which lies across 59th Avenue to the southeast. Thousands of brittlebush blossoms cover these hills like a golden fleece in spring, while a blanket of tiled roofs covers the valley. View the White Tank Mountains on the southwestern horizon. The Bradshaw Mountains and New River Mesa span the northern skyline, and you can see the McDowell Mountains, Four Peaks, and even Weaver's Needle in the Superstitions to the east.

From the summit, Cholla Loop Trail switchbacks down to the northeast. At 2.1 miles, you'll pass a trail junction with a spur trail heading due east to a vista point. Check out the view if you wish; then return to this junction. Veer left and continue hiking down switchbacks toward a large housing development at the base of the hill. The trail comes so close to houses at one point that you can see right into their living rooms. Once on the valley floor, the trail circles around the eastern edge of the hill and terminates where it joins Coach Whip Trail at 2.8 miles from the start of the loop.

Turn southwest (right) onto Coach Whip and hike along 59th Avenue between the two Hedgpeth Hills. Traffic whizzes alongside the level trail. Pass, but do not cross, a pedestrian bridge at 3.3 miles; then pass the initial trail junction with Cholla Loop 0.2 mile farther on. Finish this pleasant loop just inside the main entrance of Thunderbird Park for a grand total of 3.6 miles.

NEARBY ACTIVITIES

Thunderbird Park offers a bird-watching area and an amphitheater; its trails also cater to equestrians and mountain bikers. **Adobe Dam Recreation Area,** on the eastern side of the Hedgpeth Hills, presents additional opportunities for outdoor activities: a water park, a sports complex, and a golf course, along with go-kart racing and even model-airplane flying. **White Tank Mountain Regional Park** (see Hikes 54 and 55, pages 276 and 280), west of Phoenix, also offers excellent hiking trails.

• •

GPS TRAILHEAD COORDINATES N33° 41.426' W112° 11.326'

DIRECTIONS Exit Loop 101 onto 59th Avenue. Drive north on 59th Avenue 1.5 miles to the main entrance of Thunderbird Park, just past a hillside amphitheater. Turn west (left) into the park, and leave your car in any of the lots near the amphitheater.

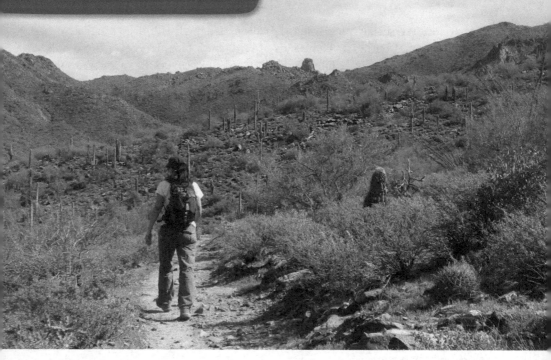

Paila Cherkofsky of Phoenix hikes toward Tom's Thumb in McDowell Sonoran Preserve.

VISIT A POPULAR landmark in the McDowell Mountains, enjoy commanding views of Fountain Hills and north Scottsdale, and hike through rugged and rocky desert. If you enjoy rock climbing, the Tom's Thumb area also offers challenging climbs.

DESCRIPTION

Look up from most places in Scottsdale and the East Valley, and you'll see the McDowell Mountains and their undulating peaks against the horizon. Look closely and you might find a thimblelike protrusion known as Tom's Thumb perched high on the ridgeline. That tiny thimble—named not after the fairy-tale character but after local climber Tom Kreuser's thumb—is actually a 150-foot granite spire that's popular with local rock climbers. The Tom's Thumb area boasts many technical routes to challenge a climber's skills.

You need not be a climber to seek out this famous McDowell landmark, however. Hikers find plenty of reasons to make a short trek to visit this rock. The Tom's Thumb Trailhead provides easy access and ample parking, and a short but challenging trail takes visitors right to the base of Tom's Thumb.

McDowell Sonoran Preserve comprises more than 30,000 acres of mountain wilderness, making it the largest city preserve in the United States. Funded by

DISTANCE & CONFIGURATION: 4.4-mile out-and-back

DIFFICULTY: Strenuous

SCENERY: City panorama, Tom's Thumb, desert, McDowell Sonoran Preserve

EXPOSURE: Completely exposed

TRAIL TRAFFIC: Heavy

TRAIL SURFACE: Loose gravel, packed dirt

HIKING TIME: 2.5 hours

WATER REQUIREMENT: 2 quarts, more if you plan to rock-climb

DRIVING DISTANCE: 33 miles from Phoenix Sky Harbor Airport

ELEVATION GAIN: 2,813' at trailhead, 3,925' at Tom's Thumb

ACCESS: Sunrise–sunset; no permits or fees required

MAPS: USGS *McDowell Peak;* maps available at trailhead and on trailhead plaque

FACILITIES: Restrooms, horse-trailer parking, shaded ramada, but no water

WHEELCHAIR ACCESS: Near trailhead area

CONTACT: 480-312-7013, scottsdaleaz.gov/preserve

COMMENTS: Dogs must be leashed at all times

taxpayers, this ambitious project sets aside one-third of Scottsdale's total landmass for conservation. Completion of the Tom's Thumb Trailhead and the Brown's Ranch Trailhead (see Hike 17, page 100) allows hikers to easily explore the newest parts of McDowell Sonoran Preserve.

The 5-mile Tom's Thumb Trail takes hikers through the northern flanks of the McDowell Mountains. This trail runs from the parking area to the base of Tom's Thumb, then descends into the heart of the McDowells and terminates at Windgate Pass Trail (see Hike 15, page 90). We'll explore the northern half of the trail in this trip description, although you can also take a much longer hike to reach Tom's Thumb from the Gateway Trailhead.

From behind the trailhead building area, hike west on a well-groomed path through the foothills. The trail begins on relatively level ground, with the tip of Tom's Thumb visible to the west. It may be hard to believe, but you're already at an elevation higher than Camelback Mountain (see Hikes 2 and 3, pages 29 and 34), the highest point within Phoenix city limits. Jojoba bushes dot the arid landscape, and you may notice the peculiar absence of saguaros and other large cacti. Interpretive signs highlight various types of cholla cacti and other desert plants.

Go straight through the Mesquite Canyon Trail junction, and continue approaching the base of the mountain. After you hike through a couple of sandy dry washes at 0.3 mile, you'll reach a signed junction for Feldspar Trail. Continue past that junction and the Half and Half Wall and Lost Wall climbing access path. This is the first of many rock-climbing areas accessible from Tom's Thumb Trail. Stay left and begin climbing. Large boulders flank the trail as you ascend. The trail steepens, and loose gravel may prove slippery if you're not careful. Trekking poles may help, especially on the descent.

For the next quarter mile, you'll climb steep switchbacks and cross several ridges, from which you begin to see the full height of Tom's Thumb to the west. If you need a break, stop at an overlook 0.6 mile from the trailhead to admire distant

Tom's Thumb

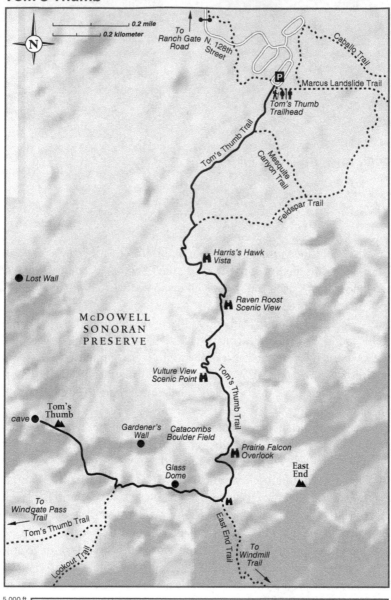

N

0.2 mile
0.2 kilometer

To
Ranch Gate
Road

N. 128th
Street

Caballo Trail

P

Marcus Landslide Trail

Tom's Thumb
Trailhead

Tom's Thumb Trail

Mesquite
Canyon
Trail

Feldspar Trail

Harris's Hawk
Vista

Lost Wall

Raven Roost
Scenic View

McDOWELL
SONORAN
PRESERVE

Vulture View
Scenic Point

Tom's Thumb Trail

cave

Tom's
Thumb

Gardener's
Wall

Catacombs
Boulder Field

Prairie Falcon
Overlook

East
End

Glass
Dome

To
Windgate Pass
Trail

Tom's Thumb Trail

Lookout Trail

East End Trail

To
Windmill
Trail

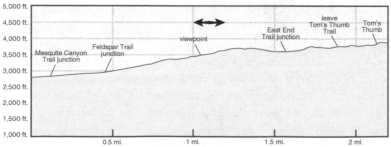

5,000 ft.
4,500 ft.
4,000 ft.
3,500 ft.
3,000 ft.
2,500 ft.
2,000 ft.
1,500 ft.
1,000 ft.

Mesquite Canyon
Trail junction

Feldspar Trail
junction

viewpoint

East End
Trail junction

leave
Tom's Thumb
Trail

Tom's
Thumb

0.5 mi.
1 mi.
1.5 mi.
2 mi.

views of Four Peaks, Bartlett Reservoir, and the Cave Creek Mountains to the north. The trail then contours around the hillside and crosses a wash, with Pinnacle Peak (see Hike 20, page 112) to the right.

At 0.9 mile, you'll pass the signed junction to Gardener's Wall, one of several ways to reach this popular climbing destination. You can see Gardener's Wall, a massive granite slab on the hilltop, where many rock climbers go to test their mettle, below Tom's Thumb. You might even see some climbers clinging to cracks on that rock face.

The steep ascent resumes, not relenting until you reach a 3,680-foot hillcrest about 1.2 miles from the trailhead. Take a well-deserved rest here as the trail levels off. As you've now passed the colder northern face of the mountain and reached a warmer hilltop, you'll notice teddy bear cholla growing here. At 1.4 miles, you'll descend 100 feet into a wide, grassy basin, with the Catacombs boulder field off to your right. Before this new trail was constructed, the only way to access Tom's Thumb was through that treacherous gulley. You'll find a variety of wildflowers in this basin in spring and early summer. Some species, such as the Arizona caltrop and black-foot daisy, bloom well into September. Reach the signed junction with East End Trail atop a prominent view-studded saddle at 1.6 miles. East End Peak towers above your left shoulder and Fountain Hills lies below. If you happen to arrive at this point on the hour, you'll see the fountain's signature plume in the distance. Red Mountain, Pass Mountain (see Hike 19, page 108), and Superstition Mountain (see Hike 39, page 201) stand along the southeastern horizon. East End Trail dives steeply to the south and eventually meets Windmill Trail, but stay on Tom's Thumb Trail and head west.

From the saddle, pass some banana yuccas and jojoba bushes; then climb a moderately steep, gravelly hill. Pass the Glass Dome climbing access path, and then go through a gap between two large boulders on top of the hill. Odd rock formations abound atop the McDowells; if you use your imagination, you might see the rocky profile of an old man facing left, with droopy eyes and nose. Pass to the left of this rock to reach another saddle, this one overlooking north Scottsdale, at 1.9 miles from the trailhead.

From this saddle, leave Tom's Thumb Trail and turn right, following the climbing access path toward Tom's Thumb and Gardener's Wall. You can see Tom's Thumb from here, but the trail first skirts the left side of a large rock outcropping in front of you. You will pass one more junction to access a climbing area called Slip and Slide—and you might wonder why anyone would climb that!

Snaking around huge boulders atop the McDowell ridgeline, you finally come to a stunning view of Tom's Thumb 2.2 miles from the trailhead. It's hard to imagine that this 150-foot monolith is actually the little thimble visible from town. Approach the base of this spire to get an appreciation for its true height. From this 3,830-foot vantage point, you can also view Camelback Mountain and Piestewa Peak (see Hikes 10 and 11, pages 64 and 68) to the southwest, and the town of Carefree and Bartlett Dam to the northeast.

For an even more spectacular view, you might try climbing to the top of Tom's Thumb. Doing so, however, requires proper climbing equipment and an expert lead climber. Routes range in difficulty from 5.7 to 5.12a on the Yosemite Decimal System, a rating system developed for technical climbing (see Glossary, page 311). Consult a rock-climbing guidebook for further details. Needless to say, you shouldn't attempt to climb Tom's Thumb without safety gear and rock-climbing experience.

Nonclimbers will find another point of interest worth visiting near Tom's Thumb. Work your way around the massive rock tower by ducking through a crevice at the left side of Tom's Thumb. Bushwhack down past some dense shrubs; then turn right and climb back up to the ridge behind Tom's Thumb. You've now reached the other side of Tom's Thumb. Find and follow a faint trail approximately 200 feet northwest, and then veer left off the trail to find a cave. Past visitors have left some trinkets, a makeshift memorial, a notebook, and even some artwork on the walls. Once satisfied with the cave and Tom's Thumb, return to the trailhead by retracing your steps.

For a slightly longer hike, consider turning right when you return to Tom's Thumb Trail at the second saddle. You'll soon come to a junction with Lookout Trail. Hiking that trail adds about 1 mile to the trip but takes you to another view-studded vantage point called the Lookout. If you set up a car shuttle in advance, you can descend Tom's Thumb Trail to its terminus, then follow Windgate Pass Trail west toward the Gateway Trailhead—an 8.5-mile hike one-way.

NEARBY ACTIVITIES

The nearby **Pinnacle Peak Trail** (see Hike 20, page 112) offers a hike similar in distance to Tom's Thumb. Many popular McDowell trails are accessible from the south side of the mountain range; see **Sunrise Trail** (Hike 21, page 116) and **Bell Pass Trail** (Hike 15, page 90) for details. **Brown's Mountain Loop** (see Hike 17, page 100) lies within the newest part of the preserve, north of Tom's Thumb.

• •

GPS TRAILHEAD COORDINATES N33° 41.638' W111° 48.129'

DIRECTIONS Exit Loop 101 at Pima/Princess Drive, and turn northeast onto Pima Road. Follow Pima 4.5 miles to Happy Valley Road. Turn east (right), and drive 4.3 miles on Happy Valley Road, following its bend to the north. Turn east (right) onto Ranch Gate Road; then continue 1.3 miles to 128th Street. Turn south (right) and drive another 1.3 miles to the Tom's Thumb Trailhead.

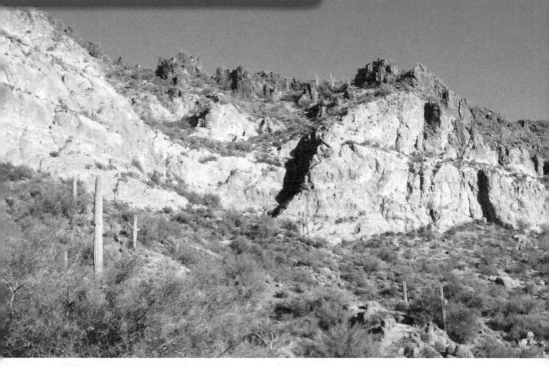

Lichen-covered cliffs of Pass Mountain dominate the view from Wind Cave Trail.

WIND CAVE TRAIL is the most popular attraction in Usery Mountain Regional Park. This moderate hike takes visitors across the desert valley floor, through a dry wash, up the slopes of Pass Mountain, and across a strip of volcanic tuff, and ends at a wind-eroded overhang called Wind Cave.

DESCRIPTION

Two obvious features stand out in the Usery Mountain range east of Mesa: a huge PHOENIX sign on the side of Usery Mountain pointing toward town, and a distinctive yellow stripe of volcanic tuff across Pass Mountain. The latter can be seen from most places in Phoenix. Though Pass Mountain isn't as tall as the Superstition Mountains behind it, the yellowish horizontal stripe snaking halfway up its western slope makes the otherwise ordinary mountain one of the most recognizable landmarks in the East Valley. Wind Cave—really only an eroded overhang—sits at the southern tip of the volcanic tuff and draws many visitors to Usery Mountain Regional Park. In addition to the cave and superb views from its lofty setting, Wind Cave Trail offers a desert experience the entire family can enjoy. My 5-year-old nephew relished the opportunity to learn about various kinds of cacti and to climb over the rocks. He even spotted a tarantula next to the trail!

DISTANCE & CONFIGURATION: 3.2-mile out-and-back

DIFFICULTY: Moderate

SCENERY: Wind Cave, Usery Mountains, desert, city panorama

EXPOSURE: Some early-morning shade, otherwise exposed

TRAIL TRAFFIC: Heavy

TRAIL SURFACE: Gravel, packed dirt, boulders

HIKING TIME: 1.5 hours

WATER REQUIREMENT: 1 quart

DRIVING DISTANCE: 26 miles from Phoenix Sky Harbor Airport

ELEVATION GAIN: 2,015' at trailhead, 2,840' at Wind Cave

ACCESS: Park open 6 a.m.–8 p.m. (till 10 p.m. Friday–Saturday); trail closes at sunset; $6/vehicle entry fee

MAPS: USGS *Apache Junction;* maps available at park entrance and maricopacountyparks.net /maps

FACILITIES: Restrooms, drinking water, picnic areas, camping, archery range

WHEELCHAIR ACCESS: Near trailhead area

CONTACT: 480-984-0032, maricopacountyparks .net/park-locator/usery-mountain-regional-park

COMMENTS: Dogs must be leashed at all times

Wind Cave Trail begins at a picnic area on Wind Cave Drive, a paved loop 1 mile inside Usery Mountain Regional Park. The guard at the park entrance provides everyone with a detailed map of the park, but this trail is easy to follow, and conspicuous signs make navigation a cinch. Almost immediately, Wind Cave Trail crosses Pass Mountain Trail (see Hike 19, page 108) and shoots northeast into the desert. About 450 feet into the hike, you'll cross an equestrian barrier and enter Tonto National Forest. The trail continues to meander along the desert floor. The first half of the trail is a gentle path along the base of the mountain, where you can take time to study the flora. Typical Sonoran Desert plant life, such as saguaros, chollas, palo verdes, and creosotes, dominate the region, but the variety of cacti is especially rich here. See if you can identify all of the following: giant saguaro, buckhorn cholla, teddy bear cholla, chain fruit cholla, strawberry hedgehog, prickly pear, beaver tail, and fishhook barrel.

At 0.2 mile, the trail crosses a dry creek and continues gently uphill along a wide and nicely graded gravel path. As you approach the base of Pass Mountain, the going gets steeper and slightly rougher. Look toward the mountain to find Wind Cave at the right edge of a band of volcanic tuff. On weekends many hikers dot the distant trail like ants on a tree trunk. Stands of saguaros cover the hillside, and palo verde trees add a splash of color to the scene. (Many of these palo verde trees contain dark clumps of desert mistletoe, a parasitic plant that saps nutrients from its gracious host, eventually killing it.) While enjoying the serene scenery, you might be surprised to hear barrages of gunfire breaking the silence. Don't be alarmed: the gunshots originate at the Usery Mountain Shooting Range across the main road and pose no threat, although they may annoy.

Near 0.8 mile, the trail begins to ascend a series of switchbacks. Neatly graded gravel degenerates into crushed rock; you'll occasionally encounter steps so tall that a small child would have to scale them on all fours. Still, the trail is by no means difficult or unmanageable. If you require a break during the steep ascent to catch your

Wind Cave Trail

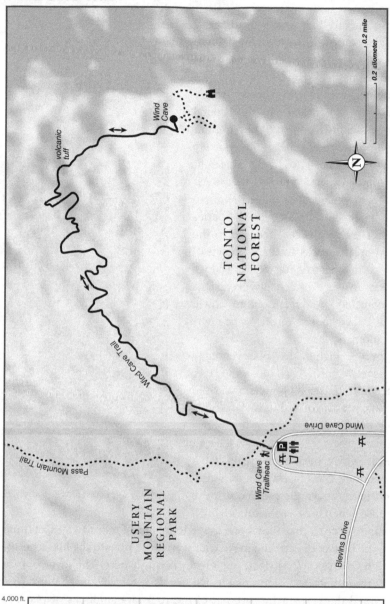

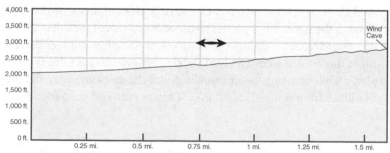

breath, turn and look west toward Usery Mountain. Notice the huge arrow painted on its side where the tail of the arrow spells out and points to Phoenix.

You might wonder why this seemingly needless sign exists, and why the Federal Aviation Administration would even grant a pilot's license to anyone so directionally challenged as to need it. The sign was built as a community-service project by the Air Explorers Boy Scout Post under the direction of an eccentric pilot named Charles Merritt. They constructed the sign in the 1950s from large rocks and several coats of whitewash in order to guide wayward pilots. Whether anyone ever actually needed its help—or cared to admit it—is unknown. The PHOENIX sign is nevertheless an interesting landmark.

Climbing higher, the trail eventually draws level with the base of a wide layer of volcanic tuff. This 25-million-year-old formation consists of compacted volcanic ash and debris, quite different in composition from the rocky granite and basalt found elsewhere on the mountain. High quartz content gives this layer a shimmering glow in the afternoon sun. A coating of chartreuse lichen finishes the tuff, giving it

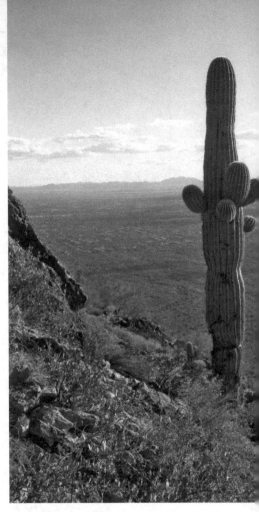

A hardy saguaro stands on the hillside near Wind Cave.

the distinctive color that allows one to see it dozens of miles away. Continue by traversing the base of the tuff and make your way south toward the hike's destination.

Wind Cave sits at 2,840 feet, and it really is windy here. The shape of Pass Mountain forces air masses to slide along its western face toward the south; this phenomenon carved the C-shaped alcove out of the rock over millions of years. Moisture seeping through the smooth but porous walls feeds clusters of rock daisy, which seem to grow downward from the ceiling like chandeliers. On a hot summer day, the shade and breeze in this eroded alcove feel absolutely heavenly. Wind Cave is a wonderful place to picnic while enjoying the surroundings and the awesome view, but prepare to defend your lunch from resident chipmunks. They're cute and quite friendly.

Though the official trail ends at Wind Cave, adventure seekers can hike to the top of Pass Mountain via an unmaintained path at the south end of the cave. The ridge is only 200 feet higher than Wind Cave but offers superb views toward the east, where you'll see the Superstition Mountains in all their glory. Consider taking an extra half hour to hike up to the ridgetop and back, but be careful with your footing on the rougher access trail. The tallest point on Pass Mountain is 0.6 mile to the north along the ridge, but reaching it requires significant bushwhacking and is not recommended; it's only another 100 feet higher anyway. Once satisfied with the expansive views from atop Pass Mountain, return to the trailhead the same way you came. Be careful descending on the trail's slippery, loose gravel.

NEARBY ACTIVITIES

Usery Mountain Regional Park offers many other popular trails, such as **Blevins Trail** and **Pass Mountain Trail** (see Hike 19, page 108). Other recreational activities available at the park include archery, camping, and picnicking. Fans of firearms can discharge their weapons at **Usery Mountain Shooting Range** (3960 N. Usery Pass Road; 480-984-9610, rsscaz.com), at the base of Usery Mountain. The **Superstition Wilderness** to the east is a hiker's dream; many hikes in this book explore the Superstition Mountains. River rats can visit the **Salt River** north of the Usery Mountains to swim or to float downstream in an inner tube, a favorite pastime among Phoenix residents; a good outfitter to try is **Salt River Tubing** (9200 N. Bush Highway, Mesa; 480-984-3305; saltrivertubing.com).

• •

GPS TRAILHEAD COORDINATES N33° 28.444' W111° 36.441'

DIRECTIONS From US 60, exit onto Ellsworth Road. Drive north 6.5 miles, and turn east (right) into Usery Mountain Regional Park. Pay at the entrance station. Once inside the park, proceed 1 mile, and then turn north (left) onto Wind Cave Drive. Parking and restrooms are located at the picnic area.

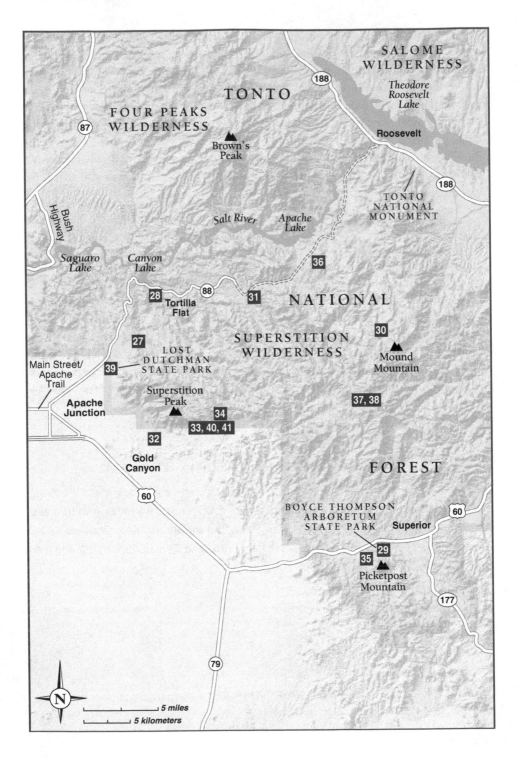

EAST
(Including Superstition Wilderness)

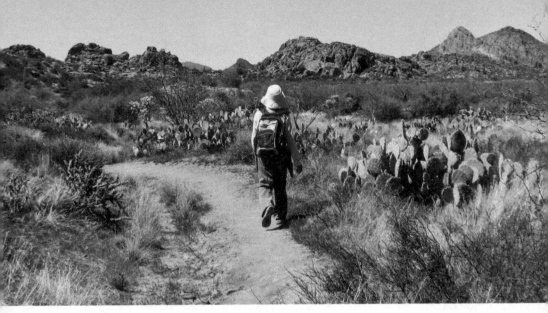

Patricia Ewanski of Phoenix hikes along Black Mesa Trail in Superstition Wilderness.

A MODERATE BUT lengthy loop, this combination of three popular trails takes visitors through the stunning foothills of the Superstition Wilderness. Notable sights include Weaver's Needle, Black Mesa, the Goldfield Mountains, and a variety of desert flora and unique rock formations.

DESCRIPTION

The Superstition Wilderness, anchored by the massive Superstition Mountains (locally nicknamed "The Supes"), encompasses the southwestern corner of Tonto National Forest. Dozens of trails totaling hundreds of miles within the Superstitions delight Phoenicians with a plethora of hiking and backpacking opportunities. The fabled Lost Dutchman's gold is rumored to lie hidden in these hills. Many prospectors have come to seek the elusive treasure over the years, and some have even perished in their quest.

This loop hike takes visitors through these beautiful yet mysterious foothills, offering glimpses of the major landmarks associated with the Lost Dutchman's legend and mentioned on supposed treasure maps. Stumbling upon lost treasure is unlikely, but this hike will certainly delight your senses.

Begin your hike from the popular First Water Trailhead, at the northern terminus of Dutchman's Trail. Hike 0.3 mile on a wide and level trail to a prominent

DISTANCE & CONFIGURATION: 9.1-mile loop

DIFFICULTY: Moderate

SCENERY: Superstition Mountains, Weaver's Needle, Four Peaks, seasonal creeks

EXPOSURE: Mostly exposed

TRAIL TRAFFIC: Moderate

TRAIL SURFACE: Rock, gravel, packed dirt, seasonal shallow creek crossings

HIKING TIME: 4.5 hours

WATER REQUIREMENT: 3 quarts

DRIVING DISTANCE: 36 miles from Phoenix Sky Harbor Airport

ELEVATION GAIN: 2,290' at trailhead, 2,760' at the highest point on Black Mesa

ACCESS: Park open 6 a.m.–8 p.m. (till 10 p.m. Friday–Saturday); trail closes at sunset; $6/vehicle entry fee

MAPS: USGS *Goldfield*; USFS *Superstition Wilderness* (see nationalforestmapstore.com/product-p/az-18.htm)

FACILITIES: Restrooms and horse-trailer parking, but no water

WHEELCHAIR ACCESS: None

CONTACT: 480-610-3300, www.fs.usda.gov/activity/tonto/recreation/hiking

COMMENTS: Dogs must be leashed at all times. Scenic loop hike in the Superstition Wilderness, highlighted by stunning views of Weaver's Needle, Superstition Mountains, and seasonal pools and running water after rains.

fork, the signed junction of Dutchman's Trail 104 and Second Water Trail 236. Veer right to hike this loop counterclockwise. Shortly after the junction, you'll reach First Water Creek, a dry creek of river rock and occasional pools that you'll cross numerous times. During the rainy season and after seasonal monsoons, First Water Creek is especially pleasant as it turns into a babbling brook.

Desert flora around First Water Creek tends to be greener than the usual desert plants, with species such as hopbush and Fremont barberry mixed with the typical prickly pear and jojoba. As in much of the Goldfield and Superstition Mountains, yellowish volcanic tuff peppered with bright lichen dots the landscape. A thin coat of desert varnish paints large boulders and cliffs dark brown.

Follow Dutchman's Trail along the creekbed as it winds around a rocky hill. About a mile into the hike, you'll arrive at some interesting rock outcrops on the hillside. The trail crosses First Water Creek several more times in the next half mile. Seasonal pools and occasional puddles, an unexpected sight in our desert environment, reflect the sun. The Flatiron (see Hike 39, page 201) and Superstition Ridgeline (see Hike 40, page 206) lie to the right, and the tip of Weaver's Needle comes into view just as you leave First Water Creek.

At 1.7 miles, you'll climb to a chalky hilltop saddle and viewpoint. Here you can turn to see the Goldfield Mountains behind you and the profile of Weaver's Needle ahead. Gentle slopes and chalky terrain define this next section of the hike, while palo verde trees, prickly pear cacti, and chain fruit chollas line the trail. Volcanic tuff bluffs and distant ridgelines fill out the scene. The trail extends southeast, winding along the hillside, and arrives at Parker Pass about 2.5 miles from the trailhead. At 2,660 feet in elevation, this saddle offers another stunning view of Weaver's Needle and the wide meadow before you.

Black Mesa Loop

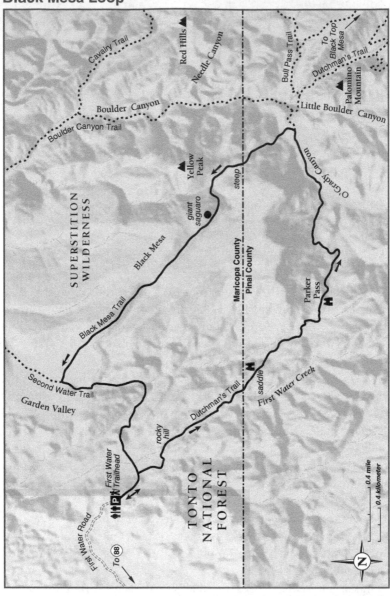

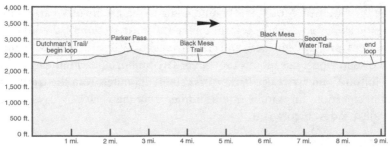

Descending from Parker Pass, the trail drops 150 feet over the next 0.5 mile. You're now walking on the right side of a hill with limestone rock formations to the left. At 3 miles from the trailhead, make a sharp hairpin turn; then continue wending your way downhill through a canyon framed by multicolored cliff bands, hopbush trees, and plenty of saguaros. Tight turns and rocky terrain force you to watch your step to avoid a fall.

The canyon soon yields to an open area, where the trail crosses two dry creekbeds with seasonal pools and maybe even trickling water. Look for cairns while crossing these creeks as the trail may be difficult to follow. Continue hiking down toward a wide flat basin covered in palo verdes, jojobas, and creosote bushes. Weaver's Needle has disappeared from view; a ring of hills and small peaks surround the tranquil basin. At a wide spot in the trail, find the signed junction for Black Mesa Trail 241. Dutchman's Trail meanders through the Superstition Wilderness another 15 miles, but you'll turn left at this junction to hike northwest.

Black Mesa Trail is less rocky but narrower, and it may seem confusing at first as it snakes around a dry creekbed. The trail turns sharply left, then bends back to the right. Incorrect paths are often blocked by stacked river rocks, so be sure not to step over them. Look for cairns to guide you across a wide creekbed while staying on the trail. Hike through the basin and approach a steep, rocky hill on the way up to Black Mesa. This next section is the steepest part of our loop, gaining roughly 400 feet in less than 0.5 mile. If you need a break as you ascend, turn to catch Weaver's Needle darting in and out of view, playing hide-and-seek behind the hills around this valley.

Reach the top of Black Mesa at 4.9 miles from the trailhead. The dark volcanic rocks to your left give this plateau its name. Notice a definite change in the plants here, compared to those in the basin below. Agaves grow in abundance, flaunting their showy stalks. Small Christmas chollas with bright-red fruit thrive in the shade of palo verde and ironwood trees. The trail flattens as it follows a valley between two hills, with Yellow Peak to the right.

At 5.1 miles from the trailhead, there's an unmarked fork in the trail—veer left and climb onto a small ridge before descending again into a side canyon. The trail turns left into this canyon and ascends the left side of the drainage. About halfway up the hill, cross over to the right side and into dense brush. The trail levels off at 2,700 feet elevation, at the base of a giant saguaro. Notice a forest of saguaros to your right, on the sunny south-facing slopes, while there are very few to your left. At mile 6, the trail passes through a grassy, wide-open area covered with teddy bear chollas. This is the highest point of the entire loop, and some hikers have apparently chosen to camp here.

Begin descending from Black Mesa at 6.2 miles from the trailhead, crossing a drainage and following the trail on the right side of the ravine. Through the gap between two hills, you can see colorful mountains on the horizon. Follow the downhill slope 0.5 mile; views open again as you hike through a pass between the hills.

Garden Valley stretches out below your vantage point. Finish your descent into Garden Valley, a wide, flat, grassy plain, with the Superstition Mountains to the left and Four Peaks to the right between the hills. Black Mesa Trail ends at a signed junction with Second Water Trail 236, 7.3 miles from the trailhead.

Turn left here onto Second Water Trail to finish the loop. Chain fruit chollas dot the landscape, while the level packed-dirt trail is a welcome respite from rocky terrain. A short distance on, you'll begin another descent on a rocky trail section, the last significant downhill of the loop. At an open area where a use trail splits off to the right, stay left to remain on Second Water Trail and continue heading downhill. The trail reaches the bottom of this hill, crosses a drainage, and immediately climbs the opposite side. There are a couple more ups and downs as the trail bisects two hills and contours to the right of another.

At 8 miles from the trailhead, you'll hike up a short but moderately steep hill among beautiful sandstone rocks tilted by shifting tectonic plates. Pass through the sandstone landscape for another 0.5 mile; the view opens again and the trail reaches level ground one final time. Cross First Water Creek, the same creek that crisscrossed Dutchman's Trail earlier on the hike; then return to the initial trail junction between Second Water Trail and Dutchman's Trail. From here, it's a short jaunt back to the First Water Trailhead to complete this tour of the Superstition Wilderness, at 9.1 total miles.

NEARBY ACTIVITIES

Many attractions can be reached via AZ 88/Apache Trail: **Lost Dutchman State Park** (6109 N. Apache Trail; 480-982-4485, azstateparks.com/lost-dutchman); **Goldfield Ghost Town** (4650 N. Mammoth Mine Road; 480-983-0333, goldfieldghosttown .com); **Superstition Mountain Museum** (4087 N. Apache Trail; 480-983-4888, super stitionmountainmuseum.org); and **Canyon, Apache,** and **Roosevelt Lakes.** Hiking opportunities abound as well along this famous road, including **Siphon Draw Trail** (see Hike 39, page 201), **Boulder Canyon Trail** (see next hike), **Fish Creek** (see Hike 31, page 165), and **Reavis Falls** (see Hike 36, page 18).

• •

GPS TRAILHEAD COORDINATES N33° 28.799' W111° 26.581'

DIRECTIONS From central Phoenix, drive east on US 60 and take Exit 196 north onto Idaho Road. After 2.25 miles, turn northeast (right) onto AZ 88, and continue 5.25 miles (0.25 mile past Lost Dutchman State Park). Turn right, onto First Water Road. Follow the dirt road 2.5 miles to the First Water Trailhead.

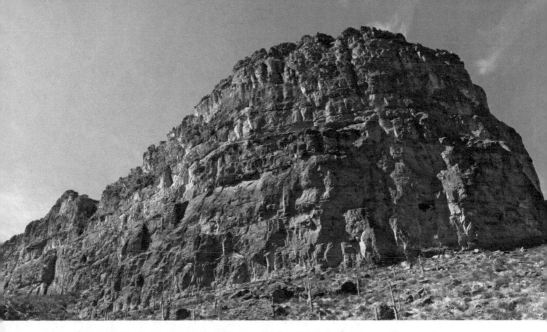

The sheer cliffs of Battleship Mountain tower above Boulder Canyon Trail.

THIS SUPERB ROUTE through the Superstition Wilderness packs plenty of scenery into a 10-mile hike. If close-up views of Canyon Lake, Battleship Mountain, Weaver's Needle, and the Superstition Ridgeline aren't enough to motivate you, then tranquil pools and an enticing swimming hole in LaBarge Canyon ought to do the trick. An optional thrilling scramble up Battleship Mountain can also delight hardy adventurers.

DESCRIPTION

In addition to legendary lost gold, the Superstition Wilderness harbors treasures of a different kind. Rugged and surreal mountains, tranquil valleys, and trickling springs entertain outdoor enthusiasts seemingly to no end. Dozens of trails and even more unnamed routes cover the 160,200-acre wilderness area. The striking juxtaposition of a harsh desert environment with hidden streams and emerald pools intrigues all who venture into the depths of the wilderness.

Boulder Canyon Trail 103 exemplifies the exceptional beauty of this unique landscape. Offering stunning hills, rocky streams, panoramic views, and even an abandoned mine, this trail has something for everyone. Easy access from Canyon Lake Marina also makes this trail one of the most popular hikes around. However,

DISTANCE & CONFIGURATION: 10.5-mile balloon (plus an optional 1.5 tough miles to climb Battleship Mountain)

DIFFICULTY: Strenuous

SCENERY: Canyon Lake, Battleship Mountain, Weaver's Needle, LaBarge Canyon, pools, swimming holes, cliffs

EXPOSURE: Mostly exposed; some shade inside LaBarge Canyon's mouth

TRAIL TRAFFIC: Light

TRAIL SURFACE: Rock, gravel, sand, boulder-hopping and scrambling

HIKING TIME: 6 hours, 8–10 if climbing Battleship Mountain

WATER REQUIREMENT: 4 quarts, 5–6 quarts if climbing Battleship Mountain

DRIVING DISTANCE: 43 miles from Phoenix Sky Harbor Airport

ELEVATION GAIN: 1,670' at trailhead, 2,360' at highest point, 2,700' on Battleship Mountain

ACCESS: Sunrise–sunset; no permits or fees required

MAPS: USGS *Mormon Flat Dam;* USFS *Superstition Wilderness* (see nationalforestmapstore.com /product-p/az-18.htm)

FACILITIES: Restrooms, water, restaurant, and campground at Canyon Lake Marina

WHEELCHAIR ACCESS: None

CONTACT: 480-610-3300, www.fs.usda.gov /activity/tonto/recreation/hiking

COMMENTS: Dogs must be leashed at all times; route-finding skills required; optional climb up Battleship Mountain requires scrambling skills on exposed ledges.

only a very small percentage of people venture off trail to visit the LaBarge Box, truly a hidden treasure in the Superstitions, or dare to climb Battleship Mountain, a hair-raising wild scramble.

This hike describes an adventurous route to visit these landmarks. Minutes off the main trail, LaBarge Canyon features a narrow rocky gorge framed by sheer cliffs and a large pool suitable for swimming. The route described here begins on Boulder Canyon Trail, takes a detour along LaBarge Creek to LaBarge Canyon, and then crosses over a saddle to loop back on Boulder Canyon Trail. From this saddle, those who are unafraid of heights can also reach the summit of Battleship Mountain via a thrilling exposed scramble.

Upon arrival at Canyon Lake Marina, be sure to park in the designated trailhead parking area against the fence. Cross AZ 88 and begin the hike from a signed trailhead east of the one-lane bridge. The rocky trail hugs the roadside fence and heads east. Keep right at an unsigned fork in the trail, and then turn south heading up a moderately steep hill. Desert plants dominate the hillside, but in spring, you can find colorful wildflowers, such as desert mariposa lilies, bluedicks, and Mexican gold poppies, here. As you climb, turn often to survey Canyon Lake behind you and expect to enjoy this view again upon your return.

A series of vista points line this part of the trail. At 0.4 mile, you'll arrive at a mound with a bird's-eye view of Boulder Recreation Site to the right. A bit farther, a wooden sign marks the wilderness boundary at a point overlooking Boulder Canyon. The trail turns left uphill, where it reaches yet another vista point, this time affording views of the Salt River basin and of Apache Trail to the east. At 1.2 miles,

Boulder Canyon Trail to LaBarge Box and Battleship Mountain

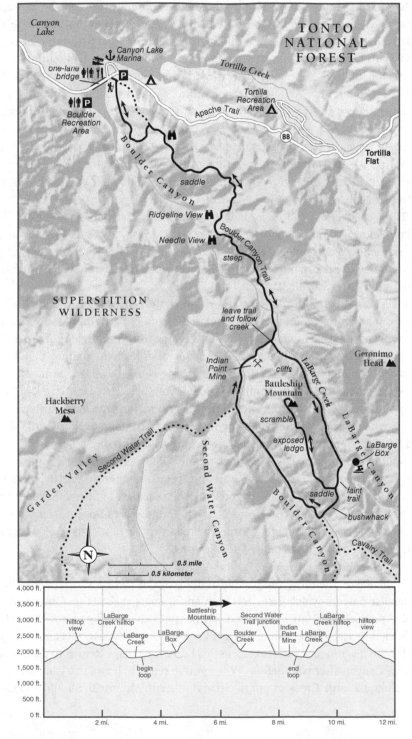

Canyon Lake

Canyon Lake Marina

one-lane bridge

Boulder Recreation Area

Tortilla Creek

TONTO NATIONAL FOREST

Apache Trail

Tortilla Recreation Area

88

Tortilla Flat

Boulder Canyon

saddle

Ridgeline View

Needle View

Boulder Canyon Trail

steep

leave trail and follow creek

SUPERSTITION WILDERNESS

Indian Paint Mine

cliffs

Battleship Mountain

scramble

exposed ledge

LaBarge Creek

Geronimo Head

LaBarge Box

Hackberry Mesa

Garden Valley

Second Water Trail

Second Water Canyon

Boulder Canyon

saddle

faint trail

bushwhack

LaBarge Canyon

Cavalry Trail

N

0.5 mile
0.5 kilometer

Elevation profile:

4,000 ft. / 3,500 ft. / 3,000 ft. / 2,500 ft. / 2,000 ft. / 1,500 ft. / 1,000 ft. / 500 ft. / 0 ft.

hilltop view — LaBarge Creek hilltop — LaBarge Creek — LaBarge Box — begin loop — Battleship Mountain — Boulder Creek — Second Water Trail junction — Indian Paint Mine — end loop — LaBarge Creek — LaBarge Creek hilltop — hilltop view

2 mi.   4 mi.   6 mi.   8 mi.   10 mi.   12 mi.

you'll reach the summit of a 2,360-foot hill with panoramic views of the entire area. Weaver's Needle lies straight ahead, with the entire Superstition Ridgeline to its right. To its left, a boxy formation called Battleship Mountain flaunts its sheer cliffs. Believe it or not, there's a way to reach its seemingly insurmountable summit.

Past the hilltop, the trail descends slightly and follows a ridge to the east. Cross a flat saddle point at 1.7 miles and then contour around the hills. The trail bobs up and down, never finding a comfortable path across the slopes. Jagged rocks loom above you on the left, and a deep valley stretches out to the right. At 1.9 miles, you'll cross a drainage carved by seasonal rains. Another 0.25 mile farther, the trail rounds a bend to reveal a stunning view of the Superstition Ridgeline. From here, you'll ascend switchbacks to reach another high point at 2,300 feet, with closer views of Weaver's Needle and Battleship Mountain.

Turn left over a small rocky saddle to see the entire LaBarge Creek drainage directly below. Dropping 500 feet, the next trail section descends a steep and slippery slope down to the creek and then crosses it at 3.25 miles from the trailhead. *Note:* LaBarge Creek can flow dangerously strong after major storms. Do not attempt to ford it if it's overflowing.

Once on the western side of the creek, follow the trail over a small hill, but break away from it before it climbs toward a saddle in front of Battleship Mountain. If you pass remnants of a makeshift campsite, you've gone too far. Turn left off the trail and into wide, boulder-strewn LaBarge Creek at 3.5 miles from the trailhead. Make your way south along LaBarge Creek, sandwiched between massive Battleship Mountain on your right and towering Geronimo Head on your left. There is no trail, but negotiating the rocky creek bottom should present no major problems. A quarter mile after leaving the trail, you should begin to see a sharp mountain ahead and a flat hill to its left. LaBarge Box lies between these landmarks.

Boulder-hopping up LaBarge Creek requires light scrambling and some trial and error. If you encounter a troublesome area, you can often find an easy bypass nearby. About 4.5 miles from the trailhead, you'll arrive at the base of the arête. You'll hardly believe your eyes: LaBarge Box features an emerald-colored pool at its mouth and a narrow stone passage farther in, guarded by towering vertical cliffs. Welcome to one of the most beautiful places in the Superstitions!

A slickrock area next to the pool is the ideal setting for a picnic. Spend some time lounging on the rocks and playing in the water. It's worth further exploring the spectacular canyon, which first curves left and then right. LaBarge Canyon features massive boulders and large pools and can be quite challenging to negotiate. If you aren't used to scrambling, you won't get very far. Nevertheless, this area is worth a visit for the magnificent cliffs that form this narrow passage. Return to the mouth of LaBarge Canyon after your detour. When you're ready to leave, you can either backtrack along LaBarge Creek or opt to circle Battleship Mountain. Should you choose the latter option, you'll need some route-finding tips. First, find a faint trail beginning at the western end of the pool. Marked by occasional cairns, this narrow use trail zigzags up a steep hill to the saddle at Battleship Mountain's southern tip, where you'll have an unobstructed view of Weaver's Needle.

With its sheer cliffs, Battleship Mountain presents an irresistible temptation for daring adventure-seekers. Be aware, however, that climbing it requires nerves of steel, a healthy respect for airy exposure, and solid scrambling skills. The optional scramble up Battleship Mountain adds 1.5 miles round-trip and 2 hours to your trek. Should you choose to tackle this challenge, make sure that you have sufficient daylight and are prepared with extra water.

Climbing Battleship Mountain isn't for everyone. The recommended route begins at its southern tip, on the left side as you face the summit. You'll need to clamber up several rocky obstacles to reach and stay on its ridgeline. In general, stay on the ridge and occasionally descend on the left when needed. Cairns are sparse, and route-finding can be a challenge. A narrow, exposed ledge in the middle of the ridge will test your tolerance for heights; nevertheless, reaching the summit of Battleship Mountain can be a thrilling experience. Consider also bushwhacking to its northern tip for a dizzying view down its vertical cliffs. Carefully work your way back to the saddle when finished. Once again, you can backtrack down to LaBarge Creek, or choose to go over the saddle and link up with Boulder Canyon Trail.

As you traverse the saddle at Battleship Mountain's tail, the trail is sometimes difficult to find. Follow the faint foot trail down a steep slope, and then veer right, toward Boulder Creek. Once at the bottom, look for cairns in the creekbed marking Boulder Canyon Trail; then turn right to hike north on a much more navigable trail.

Boulder Canyon Trail crisscrosses its namesake creek many times and runs along the basin lined by tall chain fruit cholla. Pass a large pool at 1.4 miles from LaBarge Box; then find the signed junction with Second Water Trail 236 a half mile ahead, on the left side of Boulder Creek. Continue north on Boulder Canyon Trail, and cross Boulder Creek a final time at 2.2 miles from LaBarge Box. Next, climb a hill to the abandoned Indian Paint Mine, nestled among reddish rocks at a saddle just north of Battleship Mountain. Cross this saddle to find the point where you earlier left the trail to enter LaBarge Creek. From there, retrace your steps 3.5 miles to complete the loop. Save some gusto for the 500-foot climb up out of the creekbed.

NEARBY ACTIVITIES

Canyon Lake, the third in a chain of reservoirs in the Salt River Valley, provides many opportunities for water sports. You can even take a steamboat cruise from the marina. On AZ 88/Apache Trail, **Lost Dutchman State Park** (6109 N. Apache Trail; 480-982-4485, azstateparks.com/lost-dutchman) offers many excellent hikes, including **Siphon Draw Trail** to The Flatiron (see Hike 39, page 201). Also on AZ 88,

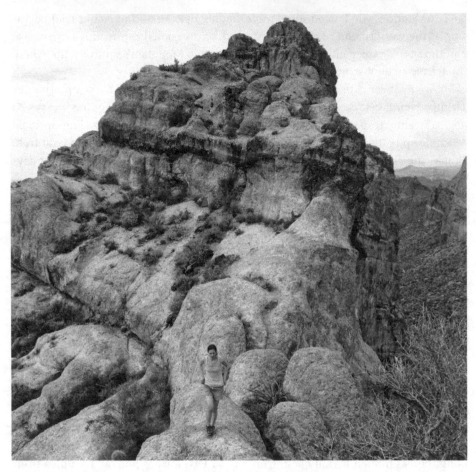

Sara Robinson of Phoenix crosses an exposed, narrow ledge on Battleship Mountain.

Tortilla Flat (480-984-1776, tortillaflataz.com) is a small but charming tourist trap 2 miles east of Canyon Lake Marina.

• •

GPS TRAILHEAD COORDINATES N33° 32.038' W111° 25.373'

DIRECTIONS From central Phoenix, drive east on US 60 and take Exit 196 north onto Idaho Road. After 2.25 miles, turn northeast (right) onto AZ 88/Apache Trail. Drive 14 miles on AZ 88 to Canyon Lake Marina, just past the second one-lane bridge. Turn left into the marina, and park in specially marked trailhead parking spots along the fence closest to AZ 88.

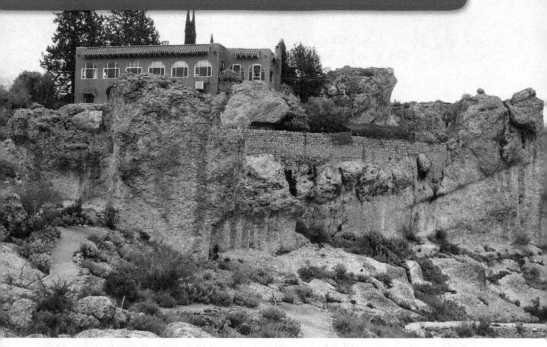

The Picket Post House overlooks Boyce Thompson Arboretum State Park.

IN THE SHADOW of Picketpost Mountain, Boyce Thompson Arboretum State Park showcases a unique collection of native desert flora as well as arid landscape plants from around the world. The park's trail system routes visitors through impressive botanical displays in a scenic natural setting.

DESCRIPTION

Nestled at the base of Picketpost Mountain (see Hike 35, page 183), Boyce Thompson Arboretum State Park houses a wide assortment of plants, specializing in those typically found in deserts and other arid regions of the world. The arboretum was named for Colonel William Boyce Thompson, a wealthy businessman who lived at the turn of the 20th century.

Blandly named and 1.5 miles in length, the Main Trail connects Boyce Thompson Arboretum's major features while many side paths and loops compete for your attention. A typical traversal of the Main Trail ends up being somewhere between 2 and 3 miles in length with all the inviting detours. As you stroll through the plant displays, look for green numbered signs that identify correspondingly numbered plants on the park map. It's a fascinating way to learn about the rich biodiversity of the desert around us.

DISTANCE & CONFIGURATION: 1.5- to 3-mile balloon with many side trails

DIFFICULTY: Easy

SCENERY: Wide variety of desert plants, wild-flowers, Queen Creek, Picketpost Mountain

EXPOSURE: Partly shaded

TRAIL TRAFFIC: Moderate

TRAIL SURFACE: Packed dirt, gravel, pavement

HIKING TIME: 2.5 hours

WATER REQUIREMENT: 1 quart

DRIVING DISTANCE: 56 miles from Phoenix Sky Harbor Airport

ELEVATION GAIN: 2,430' at trailhead, with no significant rise

ACCESS: 8 a.m.–5 p.m. winter, 6 a.m.–3 p.m. summer; last entry 1 hour before closing; admission $12.50 adults, $5 children

MAPS: USGS *Picketpost Mountain;* park map at entrance

FACILITIES: Visitor center, restrooms, water

WHEELCHAIR ACCESS: About 70% of the trail is ADA-accessible.

CONTACT: 520-689-2723, azstateparks.com /boyce-thompson

COMMENTS: Enjoy an educational and scenic family outing. Dogs must be leashed at all times.

Inside the main entrance, pass the gift shop and restrooms to begin your self-guided tour. Notice the view of towering Picketpost Mountain to the south. Be sure to visit the 0.25-mile Sonoran Desert Trail to your left—this loop showcases plants typically encountered on hikes near Phoenix. The Curandero Trail, also on this loop, provides interpretive signs that explain medicinal uses for plants native to the Sonoran Desert (*curandero* is Spanish for "medicine man").

Return to the Main Trail and walk down next to the aloes. You'll soon cross a service road and enter a shaded garden with displays designed to attract humming-birds. Beyond the Hummingbird Garden, follow the signs for the Main Trail toward the Rose Garden and the Smith Interpretive Center. This historic building contains two greenhouses dedicated to cacti and succulents from around the world. The next building on your left is the Gloria Wing Ong Children's Learning Center, where you'll likely find interactive displays and educational programs.

The Main Trail forks beyond the Children's Learning Center—continue east, saving the river walk for last. Near the Cactus Garden, you'll find a boojum tree—it looks like someone uprooted a giant carrot and then planted it upside-down. After the Cactus Garden, walk east toward Ayers Lake, a reservoir that holds water for all the gardens in the park and provides a sanctuary for migrating waterfowl.

East of Ayers Lake, Main Trail becomes rougher as it winds through rocky hills known as the Magma Ridge, the only segment not recommended for wheelchairs. No gardens grace these rocks, but they're naturally beautiful. Several interpretive stations afford superb views of the rocky terrain and the surrounding area. Near Boyce Thompson Arboretum's eastern edge, Main Trail passes below the hilltop perch of the historic Picket Post House, where Colonel Thompson lived in the early 1900s.

After a few more steep turns, Main Trail enters a densely wooded riparian zone on the banks of Queen Creek. This is my favorite part of the entire park. Sandwiched between sheer cliffs on the right and tall trees on the left, the trail heads back west

Boyce Thompson Arboretum: Main Trail

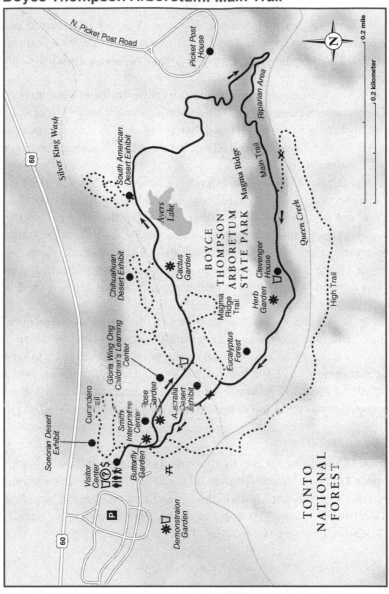

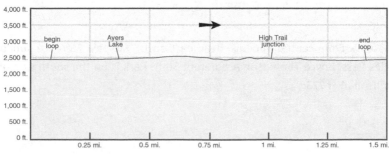

under a canopy of shady branches and leaves. A newly constructed suspension bridge provides access to High Trail, an unimpressive name for an otherwise fine natural trail. There are no plant displays on this trail, and it eventually connects to the picnic area downstream.

Unless you have extra time, I would skip High Trail and head straight for the Herb Garden, where an assortment of fragrant plants delights your senses. Rub some leaves gently between your fingers, and then try to identify their scent without reading the labels. Also inside the Herb Garden, notice the charming Clevenger House, built right into the rocky cliff.

Beyond the Herb Garden, pass through a forest of palms and giant eucalyptus trees. If any section of Main Trail looks unnatural in Arizona, this would be it. The arboretum did an excellent job, however, of putting the tall trees next to Queen Creek, where they would be less conspicuous. Finally, finish your exploration of the park by crossing the whitewashed Outback Bridge and returning via the Australian Walkabout. Along the way, browse the old-fashioned wool-shearing shed, which looks like it might belong to an unkempt groundskeeper whose rusted heap of a pickup truck lies nearby.

Boyce Thompson Arboretum State Park is dedicated to "educational, recreational, research, and preservation opportunities associated with arid land plants." It offers enough diversity of flora, seasonal variations, and special events to keep visitors coming back. Before you leave, browse the Demonstration Garden near the entrance for landscaping ideas and perhaps even buy some desert plants or wildflower seeds for your next home-improvement project.

NEARBY ACTIVITIES

Picketpost Mountain looms directly above Boyce Thompson Arboretum State Park. **Picketpost Trail** (see Hike 35, page 183) is a challenging route to its summit. US 60 also provides access to many hikes in the Superstition Wilderness, including **Peralta Trail** (see Hike 34, page 179), **Rogers Canyon Trail** (see Hike 38, page 196), and **Lost Goldmine Trail** (see Hike 33, page 174).

• •

GPS TRAILHEAD COORDINATES N33° 16.801' W111° 9.543'

DIRECTIONS From central Phoenix, head east on US 60, past Florence Junction and Gonzales Pass. Boyce Thompson Arboretum State Park is on the south side of US 60, near mile marker 223.

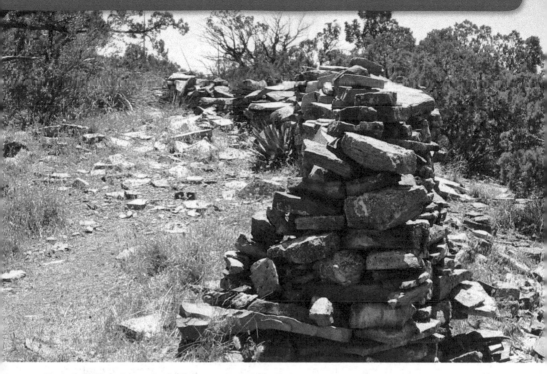

Mysterious Circlestone ruins left by an ancient civilization

WITHIN THE DEPTHS of the Superstition Wilderness, an ancient people built a large ring of stone atop a hill. Circlestone is as remote as it is mysterious. Visitors can ponder its origins in complete solitude while enjoying panoramic views of the surrounding mountains and forests.

DESCRIPTION

Legends of lost gold aside, the Superstition Wilderness contains real treasures of an entirely different kind. Cultural gems like Rogers Canyon's cliff dwellings and Hieroglyphic Canyon's petroglyphs lie hidden throughout the wilderness area. These remnants of ancient cultures add to the amazing natural landscape and make the Superstitions one of the best places in Arizona to explore.

Of all archaeological sites in the Superstition Wilderness, perhaps none is as grand or as mysterious as Circlestone. Its easiest access route requires an hour's drive on primitive roads from the nearest highway, plus a 10-mile one-way hike through mountainous terrain. Likely receiving only a few dozen groups annually, Circlestone's remoteness serves as its own preservation mechanism.

As its name suggests, Circlestone is a nearly circular ring of primitive walls made of stone. It lay undisturbed in the middle of nowhere for centuries, and its origin and

DISTANCE & CONFIGURATION: 6.7-mile out-and-back from Reavis Ranch, 18.7-mile out-and-back from Rogers Trough Trailhead)

DIFFICULTY: Moderate for shorter option, strenuous for longer option

SCENERY: Pine forest, high desert, Superstition Wilderness, Circlestone ruins, Mound Mountain

EXPOSURE: Mostly exposed, some shade available near Reavis Creek

TRAIL TRAFFIC: Very light

TRAIL SURFACE: Packed dirt, gravel, rock

HIKING TIME: 3.5 hours (10 hours from Rogers Trough Trailhead)

WATER REQUIREMENT: 3 quarts (5 quarts from Rogers Trough Trailhead)

DRIVING DISTANCE: 65 miles from Phoenix Sky Harbor Airport

ELEVATION GAIN: 4,880' at Reavis Ranch, 6,010' at Circlestone

ACCESS: Year-round, 24 hours a day; no permits or fees required

MAPS: USGS *Iron Mountain;* USFS *Superstition Wilderness* (see nationalforestmapstore.com /product-p/az-18.htm)

FACILITIES: None; perennial Reavis Creek provides a water source (filter required)

WHEELCHAIR ACCESS: None

CONTACT: 480-610-3300, www.fs.usda.gov /activity/tonto/recreation/hiking

COMMENTS: Best done as a detour from a Reavis Ranch backpacking base camp; dogs welcome

purpose remain a mystery; for these reasons, some have drawn obvious parallels between Circlestone and Stonehenge. Circlestone's walls consist of large rocks of varying sizes, carefully stacked to 5 feet high in places. No mortar was used in the walls' construction—instead, ancient architects relied on the natural fit of the rock surface. The stone circle measures 133 feet in diameter in most places. Within the confines of the outer wall are some smaller structures that resemble rooms and radial spokes.

Scholars have speculated for years about Circlestone's purpose. Some say it was a stock corral, a trading center, or a defensive stronghold, but the fact that the nearest water source is miles away makes all these hypotheses unlikely. The prevailing theory is that it was a place for religious gatherings. No one knows for sure who built Circlestone. Its construction techniques seem to predate the Hohokam and Salado people. The Anasazi or Hopi may have built the structure well over 1,000 years ago.

Situated atop a 6,010-foot hill, Circlestone overlooks nearly everything in sight. Only the adjacent 6,266-foot Mound Mountain offers a better view, but there are no trails to its summit. When you arrive at Circlestone, which is nearly 1,000 feet higher than Superstition Peak, you're practically standing on the roof of the Superstitions.

To reach this archaeological marvel, it's best to start from a backpacking base camp at Reavis Ranch. While you could certainly hike to Circlestone in a day, you'd likely regret it the next morning: it's a nearly 20-mile death march.

From Reavis Ranch (see Hike 37, page 192), head south on Reavis Valley Trail for about half a mile until you reach the signed Fire Line Trail junction. Turn uphill onto Fire Line Trail 118, which begins a moderate climb out of the shady pine forest and onto exposed slopes. Sharp rocks cover this rugged trail, an indication that very few people have ventured this way. Scrub live oaks and manzanita bushes are the dominant plant species along the trail.

Circlestone from Reavis Ranch

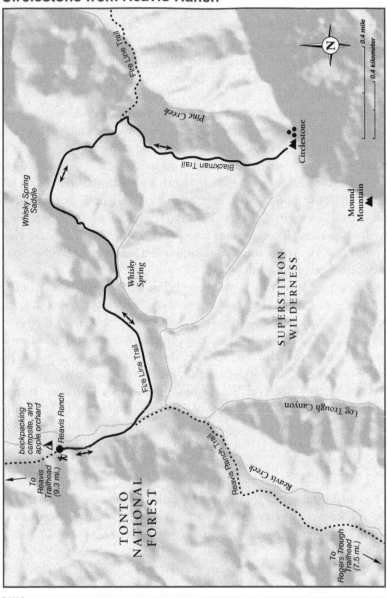

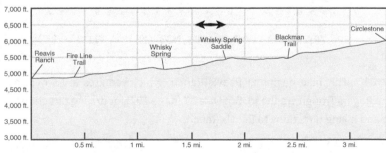

The slope eases near 0.4 mile into Fire Line Trail, where you reach an open plain. Look to your left for the distant outline of Four Peaks. Continue traversing open terrain until you cross the usually dry Whisky Spring at 0.75 mile and reenter a patch of shade. A short distance farther, cross Whisky Spring again and pass a large talus on the side of a hill.

The trail then follows a creekbed up a steep slope near dark-colored volcanic rock. Reach Whisky Spring Saddle at 1.3 miles from the beginning of Fire Line Trail. Pine trees surround this wide, flat saddle, and if you turn back, you can see a wall of large boulders above the trees. The trail swings southeast and descends slightly.

At 1.7 miles and 5,460 feet elevation, the trail runs along the side of a hill with a deep ravine to its left. Look for two large cairns on the right side of the trail before it heads downhill. Leave Fire Line Trail here and turn right, onto the unmarked Blackman Trail, which immediately climbs a steep, rocky slope. Thankfully, the slope levels off after only 0.2 mile. Veer left at a saddle point and keep aiming for the top of a large nondescript mound to the south.

Blackman Trail is actually in great condition for the small amount of foot traffic it receives. As it climbs higher along a gentle ridge, your view steadily improves. Circlestone sits atop the 6,010-foot mound, which is 0.9 mile from the beginning of Blackman Trail. From this high perch, you can clearly see Four Peaks (see Hike 46, page 237), Mound Mountain, and most of the Superstition Wilderness. From the east side of Circlestone, the copper mines in Miami are also visible.

Leave plenty of time to explore the ruins and to soak up the panoramic views. Please take extra care not to topple any of the stones, and leave the site undisturbed.

Consider reading *Circlestone: A Superstition Mountain Mystery* by James A. Swanson before your visit. Better yet, take it along as a reference.

NEARBY ACTIVITIES

Reavis Ranch, the home base for this hike, is itself a popular destination for hikers and backpackers. **Rogers Canyon Trail** (see Hike 38, page 196), which shares a trailhead with Reavis Valley Trail, leads to a Salado cliff dwelling near Angel Basin. North of Reavis Ranch, a spur trail leads to **Reavis Falls** (see Hike 36, page 188), a waterfall nestled in the wilderness. Many other nearby trails crisscross the Superstition Wilderness.

• •

GPS TRAILHEAD COORDINATES N33° 29.481' W111° 9.359'

DIRECTIONS This hike begins at Reavis Ranch, which requires a 7.5-mile hike north from the Rogers Trough Trailhead. See Hike 37 (page 192) for driving directions to Rogers Trough and hiking directions to Reavis Ranch.

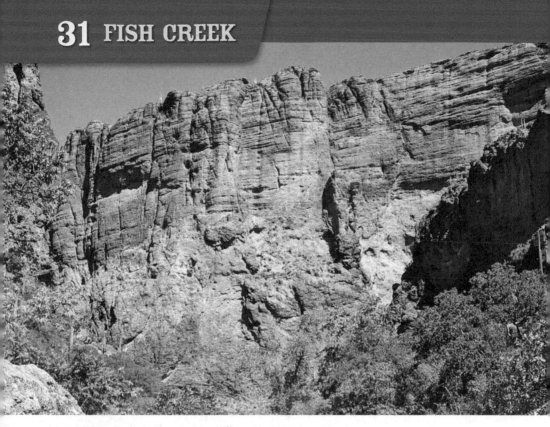

Fish Creek Canyon showcases towering cliffs and lush riparian vegetation.

WITH SPECTACULAR CLIFFS framing a narrow slot canyon, Fish Creek is home to some of the most eye-popping scenery in the Superstitions. The catch: tough scrambling along a tricky creekbed with no trails or route markers.

DESCRIPTION

Fish Creek, or, more appropriately, upper Fish Creek, isn't really a hike. There are no established trails or even route markers such as cairns, flags, or signs. However, Fish Creek does have plenty to offer hikers in terms of beautiful slot canyons bounded by sheer cliffs, intriguing rock formations, and a lush riparian habitat reminiscent of a rainforest. You would never expect to find scenery like this in the middle of a desert wilderness, but that's precisely what makes the Superstitions unique.

Note: Fish Creek flows through a narrow slot canyon, which means there's no place to escape to should you get caught in a flash flood—*do not attempt this hike during or after heavy storms.* Hiking during monsoon season is also risky because of the likelihood of sudden downpours that can trigger flash floods.

The first obstacle you'll face is entering the creek. The Fish Creek Bridge on AZ 88 hangs high above the creekbed, with precipitous drop-offs on all sides. Standing on the bridge, you can see the narrow slot canyon and tall cliffs that rise on either

DISTANCE & CONFIGURATION: 3-mile out-and-back

DIFFICULTY: Moderate in effort but requires advanced route-finding and scrambling skills

SCENERY: Fish Creek Canyon, rainforest-like vegetation, cliffs, pools, wildlife

EXPOSURE: Considerable shade with some clearings

TRAIL TRAFFIC: Very light

TRAIL SURFACE: Heavy scrambling over boulders and along creekbed

HIKING TIME: 4 hours

WATER REQUIREMENT: 2.5 quarts

DRIVING DISTANCE: 54 miles from Phoenix Sky Harbor Airport

ELEVATION GAIN: 2,240' at Fish Creek Bridge, 2,500' at reasonable turnaround point

ACCESS: Sunrise–sunset; no permits or fees required, but parking is very limited

MAPS: USGS *Horse Mesa Dam;* USFS *Superstition Wilderness* (see nationalforestmapstore.com /product-p/az-18.htm)

FACILITIES: None

WHEELCHAIR ACCESS: None

CONTACT: 480-610-3300, www.fs.usda.gov /activity/tonto/recreation/hiking

COMMENTS: Very scenic but can be overgrown; not a good hike for dogs due to scrambling

side. You can also see the pebbly creekbed below, but it's not obvious how to get to it. The trick is to cross back over the bridge from the parking area and find a small trail that leads up to a cave on the western side of the canyon.

It may seem counterintuitive to go up when you're trying to descend, but the safest route into the creek is at the cave. Begin by following a narrow trail up to the large cave, actually an alcove eroded from a massive rock bluff. Incidentally, the cave provides a high vantage point for watching the sometimes-comical shuffling of boat-laden trucks trying to squeeze past each other on the narrow dirt road and bridge below.

Follow an obvious trail from the cave down a steep slope and into the creekbed. Turn right upstream to forge deeper into Fish Creek Canyon. Hop around large boulders to enter a dense forest. Water-loving plants such as cottonwoods and willows thrive here, while desert plants such as giant saguaros sprout from shelves on the cliff walls. Pools of various sizes remaining from the last flood are scattered among large boulders, reflecting the green canopy and an occasional patch of clear sky. Some of these pools stagnate from the lack of fresh water and develop a putrid film of algae and slime, while others remain surprisingly clear. Each pool seems to teem with life—tadpoles, butterflies, spiders, and frogs—until it eventually dries up.

The going gets considerably tougher about 0.2 mile from the cave—here's where your scrambling skills and your imagination come into play. Finding a route through the myriad boulders, pools, and shrubbery isn't easy, but there's usually a way to get through that doesn't require any dangerous moves. Sometimes you have to climb over rocks; at other times you might crawl through an opening under overlapping boulders.

It's difficult to judge distance in Fish Creek, because you will likely make very slow progress upstream, and high-tech gadgets like GPS units don't work here because of the canyon's tall walls. Nevertheless, the canyon opens up near 0.4 mile into the hike, yielding a better view of the imposing cliffs surrounding it. The reddish

Fish Creek

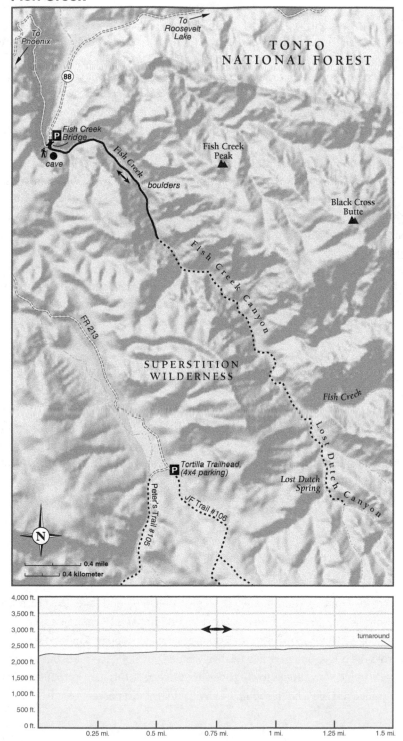

To Phoenix

To Roosevelt Lake

TONTO NATIONAL FOREST

88

Fish Creek Bridge

cave

Fish Creek

boulders

Fish Creek Peak

Black Cross Butte

Fish Creek Canyon

FR 213

SUPERSTITION WILDERNESS

Fish Creek

Lost Dutch Canyon

Tortilla Trailhead, (4x4 parking)

Lost Dutch Spring

Peter's Trail #105

JF Trail #106

N

0.4 mile
0.4 kilometer

turnaround

hue of the rocks contrasts with the abundant green leaves and blue sky. Hoodoos are often found on top of the canyon walls, and if you're lucky, you might see a bighorn sheep or two peeking down from the cliff's edge.

As you venture deeper into Fish Creek Canyon, large boulders give way to more water and dense vegetation. Instead of scrambling over rocks, you are now bush-whacking through thick undergrowth. It helps to stay near canyon walls on the sides, but you'll have to cross the creek often in order to find an optimal route through the brush. The canyon walls exhibit many interesting formations, such as recumbent folds where sedimentary layers of rock have been folded under intense heat and pressure.

You can explore Fish Creek for as long as you'd like. It eventually leads to Lost Dutch Canyon approximately 3.3 miles from the bridge. You could also do a long one-way hike out of Fish Creek by stashing a shuttle vehicle at the Tortilla Trailhead, which requires a four-wheel-drive to reach. Most people, however, simply head upstream from the bridge as far as they'd like and then return the same way. A fairly reason-able turnaround point comes after about 1.5 miles, which takes a first-time visitor roughly 2.5–3 hours to reach. When choosing your turnaround point, remember that the egress takes roughly half the time of the ingress, because you should have solved some of the tricky scrambling problems on your way in.

NEARBY ACTIVITIES

Canyon, Apache, and **Roosevelt Lakes** are a series of reservoirs on the Salt River with marinas that lie on or near AZ 88. The Superstition Wilderness contains hun-dreds of miles of trails, many of which are accessible via this road. The Reavis Trail-head, near Apache Lake, leads to **Reavis Falls** (see Hike 36, page 188) and **Castle Dome. Boulder Canyon Trail** (see Hike 28, page 151) starts from the Canyon Lake Marina and offers choice views toward Weaver's Needle and Superstition Mountain. Other hikes, such as **Siphon Draw** (see Hike 39, page 201) and **Massacre Grounds,** are near **Lost Dutchman State Park.**

• •

GPS TRAILHEAD COORDINATES N33° 31.488' W111° 18.425'

DIRECTIONS From central Phoenix, drive east on US 60 and take Exit 196 north onto Idaho Road. After 2.25 miles, turn northeast (right) onto AZ 88/Apache Trail. Follow scenic and winding AZ 88 for 25 miles to the Fish Creek Bridge, about 0.5 mile past mile marker 223. Cross the bridge and park in a relatively wide spot along the road, but be careful not to impede traffic. Many trucks towing boats routinely take this narrow roadway. Part of AZ 88 is a graded dirt road, but it should be navigable by most passenger cars.

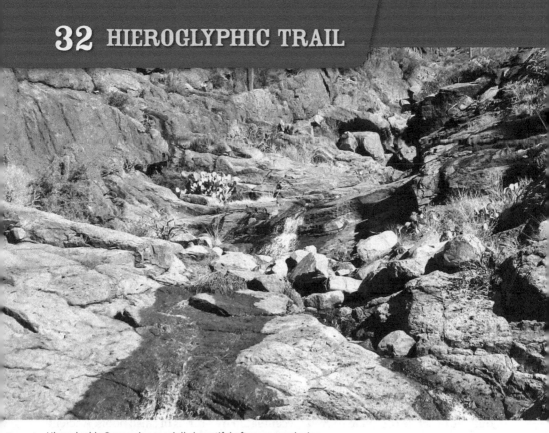

Hieroglyphic Canyon is especially beautiful after seasonal rains.

NESTLED AT THE base of Superstition Mountain, Hieroglyphic Canyon boasts one of the best collections of Hohokam petroglyphs in the state. Venture beyond the petroglyphs and follow Hieroglyphic Canyon up to Superstition Ridgeline for astounding views of Weaver's Needle and the city.

DESCRIPTION

Anchored by a 5,000-foot peak at each end and a long connecting ridge in the middle, Superstition Mountain dominates the East Valley skyline and has some of the best hikes near Phoenix. Hieroglyphic Trail 101 offers an excellent introductory hike for beginners, families, and first-time visitors to the Superstitions. The easily accessible trailhead, relatively short route, and gentle slopes welcome hikers of all levels. Superb views of the majestic Superstitions and a trove of prehistoric Hohokam petroglyphs provide additional incentives for a visit.

Advanced hikers and adventure seekers can continue beyond the petroglyphs and follow Hieroglyphic Canyon up to the Superstition Ridgeline. This optional excursion doubles the hike length and requires scrambling up an additional 1,700 feet. However, the just reward for your toils is an awesome view of the sprawling city below, the interior of the Superstition Wilderness, and Weaver's Needle.

DISTANCE & CONFIGURATION: 3-mile out-and-back; optional hike to Superstition Ridgeline adds 3.3 miles

DIFFICULTY: Easy for main hike, strenuous for optional hike

SCENERY: Superstition Mountains, Hohokam petroglyphs, pools, desert

EXPOSURE: Mostly exposed, limited shade in riparian areas

TRAIL TRAFFIC: Moderate–heavy to petroglyphs, light on optional hike

TRAIL SURFACE: Gravel and rock to petroglyphs, boulders and some scrambling beyond

HIKING TIME: 1.5 hours; optional hike adds 3 hours

WATER REQUIREMENT: 1 quart to petroglyphs; optional hike adds 2 quarts

DRIVING DISTANCE: 39 miles from Phoenix Sky Harbor Airport

ELEVATION GAIN: 2,085' at trailhead, 2,650' at petroglyphs, 4,350' on Superstition Ridgeline

ACCESS: Sunrise–sunset; no permits or fees required

MAPS: USGS *Goldfield*; USFS *Superstition Wilderness* (see nationalforestmapstore.com /product-p/az-18.htm)

FACILITIES: Portable toilets but no water

WHEELCHAIR ACCESS: None

CONTACT: 480-610-3300, www.fs.usda.gov /activity/tonto/recreation/hiking

COMMENTS: Especially scenic after recent rainfall; dogs must be leashed at all times

Hieroglyphic Canyon roughly bisects Superstition Mountain from east to west, culminating in a prominent saddle point high on its ridgeline. Near the canyon's mouth lies a cradle of granite bedrock accentuated by a series of small pools. Ancient Hohokams, who inhabited Central Arizona more than 800 years ago, etched hundreds of petroglyphs here onto a canvas of patina-covered boulders. Modern miners and settlers in the region came upon these primitive drawings and mistook them for Egyptian hieroglyphics. Thus, the canyon's name arose from a simple misunderstanding.

Hieroglyphic Trail and Lost Goldmine Trail (see next hike) share a common trailhead at the northern end of a large parking area at the end of Cloudview Avenue. Begin by climbing a short hill up to a ridge where two wooden signs mark the spot where Lost Goldmine Trail forks to the east. Stay left here, and continue hiking toward the mountain, enjoying clear views of Superstition Peak. To the west, mounds of hoodoos cap sedimentary plateaus like birthday candles atop a layer cake. The Flatiron (see Hike 39, page 201) lies on the higher plateau at the extreme western tip of this mountain range.

Near 0.3 mile, you'll cross the Superstition Wilderness boundary fence, where typical Sonoran Desert vegetation surrounds you. Triangle-leaf bursage, jojobas, and chollas line the trail, while saguaros and palo verde trees blanket the foothills. The trail becomes rocky as it begins a gentle ascent toward the mouth of Hieroglyphic Canyon. When the slope levels out at 0.6 mile, you'll catch an open view of the city. Pass Mountain, Camelback Mountain, and South Mountain all come into view to the west, while Sombrero Butte, a hat-shaped hill, lies to the east.

Hieroglyphic Trail

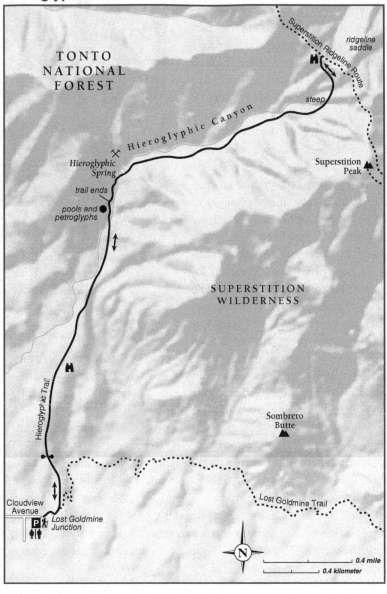

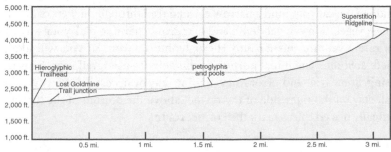

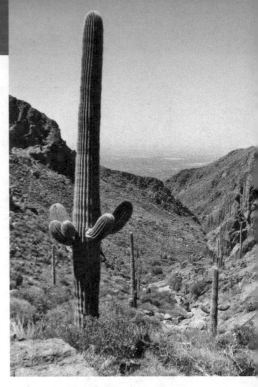

A stunning view of Hieroglyphic Canyon from above

Continue your gentle approach to Hieroglyphic Canyon. Soon, the trail parallels Hieroglyphic Spring and begins a moderate but short climb uphill. Skirt a rocky knoll 1.1 miles from the trailhead to enter the mouth of Hieroglyphic Canyon. Mesquite and ironwood trees provide some shade here on a hot day.

At 1.5 miles from the trailhead, reach a large rocky area where eons of water erosion have polished the granite streambed into natural tubs for several small pools. These aren't quite large enough for taking swim, but there's likely some water here year-round. Large boulders framing the pools provide a natural canvas for hundreds of Hohokam petroglyphs. The ancient Hohokam people etched scenes from their lives into a layer of desert varnish on the rocks, preserving a slice of history for generations to come. The petroglyphs here show a complex range of subjects and are among the finest collections of Hohokam artwork in Arizona; sadly, vandals have also left their marks. Another set of petroglyphs can be found by following the creekbed downstream about 0.1 mile.

After investigating the petroglyphs, turn around and look out toward the city. The slickrock and pools frame a stunning vista to the south. Hieroglyphic Trail ends here; casual hikers should return along the same route. Remember that the return trail is located on the eastern side of the canyon, just above the slickrock and pools.

For adventurous advanced hikers, an optional trek into the upper reaches of Hieroglyphic Canyon leads to some breathtaking views from the Superstition Ridgeline. Note, however, that you'll need some scrambling and route-finding skills to complete the ascent. This optional segment doubles the total distance and more than triples the elevation gain.

Follow Hieroglyphic Spring upstream from the petroglyph site, staying near the right side of the canyon. Find a narrow cairned trail through thickets of desert brush and trees; vegetation can get dense and overgrown here, so pick your way carefully. Hikers rarely venture this far into Hieroglyphic Canyon, so you will likely enjoy complete solitude. The initial portion of this seldom-used trail is perhaps the most confusing. Some trial-and-error route-finding may be necessary to stay on course. In general, stay on the right side of the ravine, above the bottom of the dry creekbed. Strategically placed cairns mark the correct route.

At 2.3 miles from the trailhead, you'll arrive at the apparent confluence of two drainages—take the left fork even though the faint path looks less traveled than the right fork. A few hundred feet farther, you'll reach the top of a wall, where a dark streak of color on the rock indicates there's a waterfall here after significant rainfall. The dense vegetation gives way to open rock faces and porous volcanic tuff as you hover above the right side of the streambed past a few small pools farther up Hieroglyphic Canyon.

At 2.7 miles, you'll arrive at another rocky area and then a fork in the streambed. Route-finding is tricky here, but occasional cairns mark the way. You want to keep right, but there's another short dry waterfall and some thick brush in the way. Work your way upward around these obstacles, and then regain the faint trail. Ascend steeply uphill toward a needlelike rock; then pass along its right side. Above that point, the route climbs a shale-covered slope. A trail on these slopes is marked by sparsely spaced cairns; over the years, this route has seen increasingly more traffic, so it's now easier to find.

The final ascent involves steep but manageable hiking through rocky terrain, still on the right side of the main drainage. A few final switchbacks take you up to a prominent saddle point on the Superstition Ridgeline at 4,340 feet elevation, some 1,700 feet higher than the petroglyph site. The Superstition Ridgeline hike (see Hike 40, page 206) passes through this saddle, and you can see its well-worn use trail. Needless to say, views here are stunning. To the north, a foreshortened Four Peaks (see Hike 46, page 237) tower over the rugged interior of the Superstition Wilderness. Behind you, the city seems very far away. Turn right and walk up the hill for a spectacular profile view of Weaver's Needle, revealing that it actually consists of two rock spires.

The truly masochistic can continue southeast another 0.7 mile to reach Superstition Peak, which is another 700 feet higher. Enjoy the gorgeous views and return via the same route. On the way down, stay left of Hieroglyphic Spring and look for cairns to guide your descent. Remember to veer left around the steep waterfalls.

• •

GPS TRAILHEAD COORDINATES N33° 23.386' W111° 25.477'

DIRECTIONS From central Phoenix, drive east on US 60 about 38 miles to Kings Ranch Road, between mile markers 202 and 203. Turn northeast (left) onto Kings Ranch Road and follow it 2.8 miles. Immediately after crossing a cattle guard, turn east (right), onto Baseline Road, and drive east 0.3 mile. Turn left onto Mohican, and continue north 0.3 mile. Turn left onto Valley View Drive, and follow it as it curves into Whitetail Road. Then turn right, onto Cloudview Avenue, and proceed 0.5 mile to the large trailhead parking lot. This route may sound complicated, but all other turns after Baseline Road are marked with DEAD END signs.

33 LOST GOLDMINE TRAIL

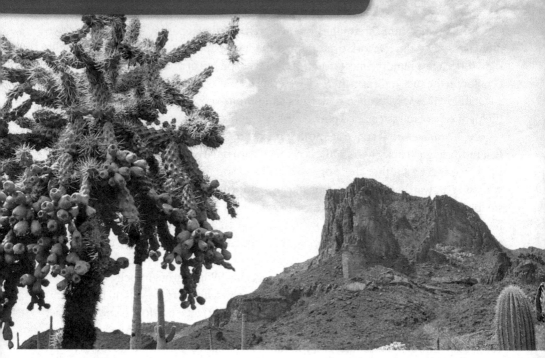

A chain fruit cholla along Lost Goldmine Trail frames a view of the Three Sisters.

TO THOSE WHO wish to enjoy the Superstition Mountains without scaling steep grades, Lost Goldmine Trail offers a nearly level jaunt through scenic foothills. Roughly tracing the Superstition Wilderness boundary, this trail skirts rugged cliffs and tall peaks on the southern flank of the Superstitions.

DESCRIPTION

Constructed by volunteers in 2001, Lost Goldmine Trail is one of the most level trails near the Superstition Mountains. This 6-mile trail runs along an easement just outside the Superstition Wilderness's southern boundary and links Peralta Canyon on the prominent mountain range's eastern end with Hieroglyphic Canyon in the middle. A disjointed section of this trail extends to Jacob's Crosscut Trail near the Broadway Trailhead at the mountain range's western end. Lying in the shadows of massive cliffs and hoodoo-lined ridges, Lost Goldmine Trail showcases the rugged beauty of the venerable Superstitions and its desert foothills. This trail's relatively level elevation profile and proximity to the city also attract a wide range of hikers, bikers, and equestrians.

Lost Goldmine Trail takes its name from the legend of the Lost Dutchman's Mine, an enduring fable that has captured prospectors' imaginations for more than 100 years. Folks with dreams of finding lost treasure have come from all over the

DISTANCE & CONFIGURATION: 6-mile point-to-point

DIFFICULTY: Easy

SCENERY: Superstition Mountains, desert

EXPOSURE: Completely exposed

TRAIL TRAFFIC: Light

TRAIL SURFACE: Gravel, rock

HIKING TIME: 2.5 hours

WATER REQUIREMENT: 2 quarts

DRIVING DISTANCE: 39 miles from Phoenix Sky Harbor Airport

ELEVATION GAIN: 2,280' at trailhead, with no significant rise

ACCESS: Sunrise–sunset; no permits or fees required

MAPS: USGS *Goldfield* and *Weavers Needle*

FACILITIES: None

WHEELCHAIR ACCESS: None

CONTACT: 520-866-6910, pinalcountyaz.gov /openspacetrails/pages/lostgoldminetrail.aspx

COMMENTS: Western trail section to Broadway Trailhead is omitted from description; dogs must be leashed at all times

world to comb this region, but no gold has ever been found. As recently as 2004, the U.S. Forest Service granted a rare Treasure Trove permit to a group of explorers and archaeologists attempting to locate the Lost Dutchman's Mine. They are not the first and certainly won't be the last to try.

With a shuttle vehicle, you can hike Lost Goldmine Trail in either direction. This chapter describes the route from east to west. Begin the one-way trip from the Lost Goldmine Trailhead, at the end of a large parking area just shy of the Peralta Trailhead (see next hike) on Peralta Road. Pinal County manages this trail and has obtained a permanent lease on the trail right-of-way from the Arizona State Land Trust. Therefore, visitors never need a permit to access this trail. Hike west into the dense desert vegetation of triangle-leaf bursage, mesquite, palo verde, and various cacti. Superstition Mountain's eastern end features sheer cliffs and jagged peaks. The vertical face of Dacite Cliffs lies to the north. Turning northwest, you soon reach the wilderness boundary fence at 0.25 mile. A majority of this trail traces the fence, but don't worry, you are still surrounded by wilderness.

Following the fence west, the trail crosses many dry washes and arroyos that drain seasonal rainfall away from the mountain. Near these dry washes, larger bushes thrive in dense clusters. A particularly deep wash lies 0.6 mile from the trailhead. Somewhere north of this spot, at the base of the cliffs, Dacite Cliffs Mine lies hidden from view. Its long, dark mineshaft remains intact and hosts many bats and other nocturnal creatures. Finding the mine and exploring it will be left as an exercise for the adventurous reader. Continuing west along the fence, the trail intersects a dirt road at 0.8 mile, crosses another major wash, and then meets the unmarked Carney Springs Trail at 1.1 miles. For ambitious hikers seeking the ultimate challenge, a torturous traversal of Superstition Ridgeline (see Hike 40, page 206) begins here and ends inside Lost Dutchman State Park on the other side of the mountain range. A shorter side trip to the Wave Cave (see Hike 41, page 211) is also possible from this point.

Lost Goldmine Trail

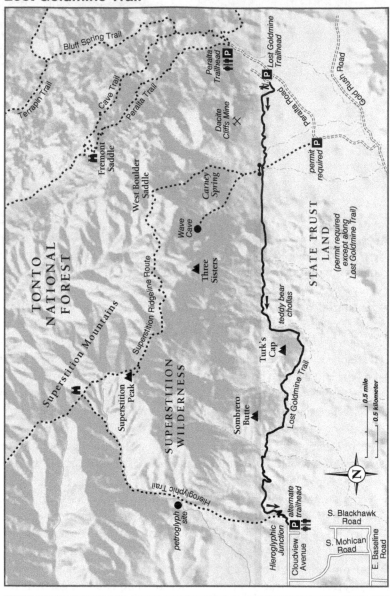

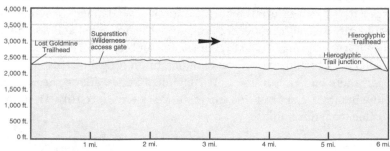

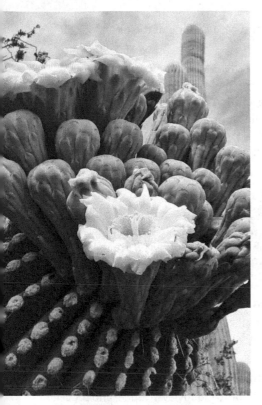
Arizona's state flower is the giant saguaro blossom.

Pass the remains of an old stock tank, and then cross Carney Spring. At 1.5 miles, go through a gated fence to reach a flat mound from which expansive views abound. The jagged rock formations on top of the mountain to your right are the Three Sisters; the hoodoo-covered 5,057-foot Superstition Peak lurks behind them. Directly west lie Turks Cap and Sombrero Butte. Majestic saguaros dot the landscape, while clusters of bristly cholla glow in the sunlight. In spring, a variety of wildflowers add a splash of color to the harsh Sonoran Desert landscape. Not bad for a place only minutes from the city.

Continue hiking west amid forests of saguaros and fields of cholla, through picturesque valleys and across gentle slopes. The trail remains fairly level, but there are enough ups and downs to keep you on your toes. At 3 miles from the trailhead, turn south to circumnavigate a craggy hill called Turks Cap. Vegetation thins out on the south side of Turks Cap, giving a sense of airiness to the hike. Once past Turks Cap, cross a surprisingly wide, smooth dirt road that heads straight into the hills. Superstition Peak is clearly visible now. The trail then rounds Sombrero Butte, a hill in the shape of an inverted hat.

A series of dry washes cuts across the trail, which returns to the wilderness boundary at 4.8 miles from the Lost Goldmine Trailhead. Look for a seasonal waterfall and a cave high up on the mountainside. By now you can see the western end of Superstition Mountain in the distance. Siphon Draw Trail (see Hike 39, page 201), inside Lost Dutchman State Park, takes hikers to a prominent feature called The Flatiron, on the western tip of Superstition Mountain.

Descend into a small valley at 5 miles from the trailhead. Housing developments begin to come into view, a sign that the trail's end is near. The Superstitions' dramatic western end seems to get closer and closer. Cross a few more washes as the trail approaches a tall berm. The trail curves south, paralleling the berm for a short distance before climbing a few switchbacks to the top of the berm. There you'll find the well-marked intersection with Hieroglyphic Trail (see previous hike).

The Hieroglyphic Canyon Trailhead lies on the western side of the berm, a total of 6 miles from the Lost Goldmine Trailhead.

NEARBY ACTIVITIES

Hieroglyphic Trail takes hikers into **Hieroglyphic Canyon,** where they can view some of the finest Hohokam petroglyphs in the state. The popular Peralta Trailhead provides access to **Peralta Trail** (see next hike), **Dutchman's Trail,** and **Bluff Spring Trail.** The grueling **Superstition Ridgeline** hike (see Hike 40, page 206) is also accessible from the Lost Goldmine Trailhead.

• •

GPS TRAILHEAD COORDINATES
N33° 23.386' W111° 25.477' (Hieroglyphic Canyon/Cloudview Trailhead)
N33° 23.589' W111° 21.242' (Lost Goldmine Trailhead)

DIRECTIONS *Hieroglyphic Canyon Trailhead:* From central Phoenix, drive east on US 60 about 38 miles to Kings Ranch Road, between mile markers 202 and 203. Turn northeast (left) onto Kings Ranch Road and follow it 2.8 miles. Immediately after crossing a cattle guard, turn east (right), onto Baseline Road, and drive east 0.3 mile. Turn left onto Mohican and continue north 0.3 mile. Turn left onto Valley View Drive, and follow it as it curves into Whitetail Road. Then turn right onto Cloudview Avenue, and proceed 0.5 mile to the large trailhead parking lot. This route may sound complicated, but after Baseline Road, all other turns are marked with DEAD END signs.

Lost Goldmine Trailhead: Return to US 60 and continue east. Past mile marker 204, turn northeast onto Peralta Road. *Reset your odometer at this turn.* Peralta Road becomes a dirt road after 1 mile, but most cars can safely pass, except after heavy storms. Keep left when the road forks at 5.5 miles from the turnoff. Turn into the signed parking lot for the Lost Goldmine Trailhead when your odometer reads 7.1 miles—if you've reached the Peralta Trailhead, you've gone too far.

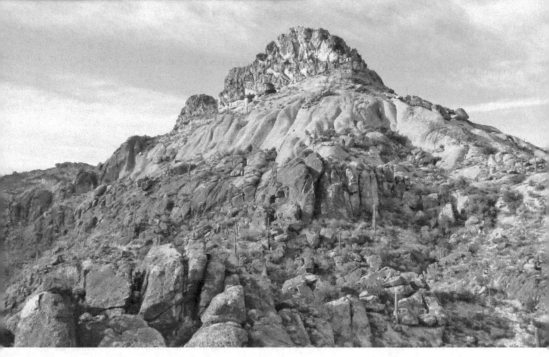

A layer of volcanic tuff and Geronimo's Cave loom above Peralta Trail.

THIS MODERATE HIKE introduces you to the rugged beauty of the Superstition Mountains without taxing your abilities to their limits. Fremont Saddle, your destination, rewards you with a spectacular view of Weaver's Needle, the most famous landmark in the Superstition Wilderness.

DESCRIPTION

The mysterious Superstition Mountains hold the legend of Lost Dutchman's Mine, one of the most enduring tales of lost gold. Legend has it that the Peralta family from Mexico owned mining operations in the Superstition Mountains in the 1850s but fled after Apaches massacred their miners near present-day Lost Dutchman State Park.

The Dutchman—actually a German immigrant named Jacob Waltz—supposedly came upon a map to a Peralta mine and found hidden caches of gold. He died in 1891 and left a legacy of maps and tales, but to this day no gold has been found. Weaver's Needle, a 1,220-foot-tall rock spire in the Superstitions, figures prominently in most stories and various maps related to the Lost Dutchman's Mine.

Peralta Trail takes visitors 2.3 miles up Peralta Canyon to Fremont Saddle, the best overlook from which to view Weaver's Needle. If you haven't yet caught gold fever on the drive to the trailhead, the mysterious hills will capture your imagination

DISTANCE & CONFIGURATION: 4.6-mile out-and-back; optional return on Cave Trail adds 0.6 mile

DIFFICULTY: Moderate for main hike, strenuous if returning via Cave Trail

SCENERY: Desert, riparian plants, unique rock formations, Weaver's Needle

EXPOSURE: Partial shade during early morning and late afternoon; otherwise exposed

TRAIL TRAFFIC: Heavy on Peralta Trail, light on Cave Trail

TRAIL SURFACE: Gravel, rock, boulders

HIKING TIME: 3 hours for main hike, 3.5 hours if returning via Cave Trail

WATER REQUIREMENT: 2.5 quarts

DRIVING DISTANCE: 44 miles from Phoenix Sky Harbor Airport

ELEVATION GAIN: 2,430' at Peralta Trailhead, 3,760' at Fremont Saddle

ACCESS: Sunrise–sunset; no permits or fees required

MAPS: USGS *Weavers Needle;* trailhead plaque; USFS *Superstition Wilderness* (see nationalforest mapstore.com/product-p/az-18.htm)

FACILITIES: Restrooms but no water

WHEELCHAIR ACCESS: None

CONTACT: 480-610-3300, www.fs.usda.gov /activity/tonto/recreation/hiking

COMMENTS: Excellent introduction to Superstition Wilderness; dogs must be leashed

the moment you step out of the car. As you make your way to the trailhead at the end of the parking area, the Dacite Cliffs tower ominously above you on the left.

Begin by taking a left at the trailhead and following the signs for Peralta Trail 102. The trail starts fairly level through a desert riparian landscape full of triangle-leaf bursage, canyon ragweed, jojoba, and cactus. At 0.25 mile, cross the dry Peralta Creek and begin a gradual climb along the eastern bank of the canyon. Sugar sumacs and other brush provide some shade at 0.5 mile from the trailhead. At 0.8 mile, the trail seemingly splits—keep to the right to loop back and rejoin the creekbed. At 0.9 mile, another shady thicket with many smooth boulders beckons you to stop and rest.

The trail ascends cactus-lined switchbacks to the east at 1 mile from the trail-head. Turn around to catch a glimpse of the ridge atop the western side of the canyon. Perhaps the ghost of Lost Dutchman lurks among the hoodoos here? Look for his horse in the form of a rearing-steed-shaped rock.

At 1.3 miles and an elevation of 3,050 feet, the trail crosses the dry creek again and switchbacks up the western side of the canyon. As the trail straightens into a gentle ascent around 1.5 miles, notice nearby jojoba bushes with their teardrop leaves pointing upward. Native Americans used these plants and their almondlike fruits for food and medicine. Peer across the canyon to see a layer of pale green volcanic tuff, and Geronimo's Cave just above it. On the eastern side, look for grotesquely eroded rock formations such as a ghostly face with hollow eye sockets and a gaping mouth. Peralta Trail crosses the creekbed again and switchbacks up to multicolored volcanic bedrock.

At 2 miles, the trail passes the entrance to a deep cave. The ceiling is extremely low, making it difficult to explore, but you can turn around and enjoy a great view of Peralta Canyon below and Picketpost Mountain in the distance. From the cave, continue another 0.3 mile to Fremont Saddle (3,760') for a jaw-dropping view of Weaver's

Peralta Trail

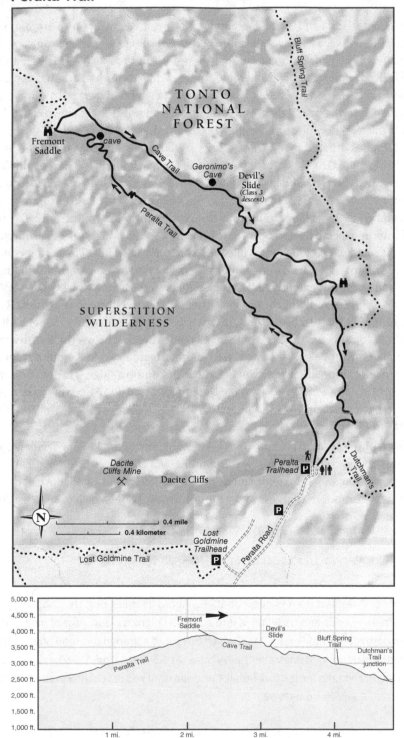

Needle. Peralta Trail continues 4 more miles, but most day hikers turn around here. Rest and ogle Weaver's Needle some more before returning the way you came.

If you're feeling adventurous, consider returning on the much less traveled Cave Trail, which requires scrambling and route-finding skills—bring a map and compass or GPS. Depart Fremont Saddle heading east, following a faint trail marked by cairns. Cave Trail first goes northeast and then loops around to head south along the volcanic ridge you saw earlier. Follow the cairns carefully, and don't descend into Peralta Canyon.

At 1.1 miles from Fremont Saddle, Cave Trail descends steeply at the end of the volcanic ridge. This Class 3 descent (see Glossary, page 311) follows a steep drainage that some call the Devil's Slide, which runs down a slickrock face—*do not attempt this route when it's wet outside*. At the end of the slide is an even scarier drop-off: take care while shimmying down here, using your hands and butt for extra traction. The trail then climbs unexpectedly and bears east in several spots. Watch for cairns marking the trail; if you don't see one for a while, backtrack and try again. The middle mile of this 3-mile return route is the most confusing, so allow extra time for route-finding.

At 2 miles from Fremont Saddle, reach a hillcrest with views of a wide, obvious trail below. While descending the hill, check out Miner's Needle to the northeast. Cave Trail joins Bluff Spring Trail at an unsigned junction 2.1 miles from Fremont Saddle— turn right to continue south. At 2.3 miles, take a quick break at an overlook with a view into Peralta Canyon before the trail makes another bend east. At 2.6 miles from the saddle, make a hairpin turn where you see a huge cairn atop a ridge. The trail descends southwest from here and merges with the Dutchman's Trail just before the parking lot.

NEARBY ACTIVITIES

The **Lost Goldmine Trail** (see previous hike) is just shy of the Peralta Trailhead and also grants access to the **Superstition Ridgeline** and the **Wave Cave** (see Hikes 40 and 41, pages 206 and 211). **Lost Dutchman State Park,** on the northwestern side of the Superstitions, offers access to the **Siphon Draw Trail** (see Hike 39, page 201).

• •

GPS TRAILHEAD COORDINATES N33° 23.858' W111° 20.872'

DIRECTIONS Drive east from Phoenix on US 60. About 23 miles past the Loop 101 junction, the freeway ends and US 60 turns into a divided highway. Just east of mile marker 204, turn north (left) onto Peralta Road, which turns into a graded dirt road after 1 mile— watch out for stream crossings after heavy rains. At 5.5 miles from US 60, follow a conspicuous sign, and take the left fork uphill. Continue until you reach the Peralta Trailhead parking area, 7.5 miles from US 60.

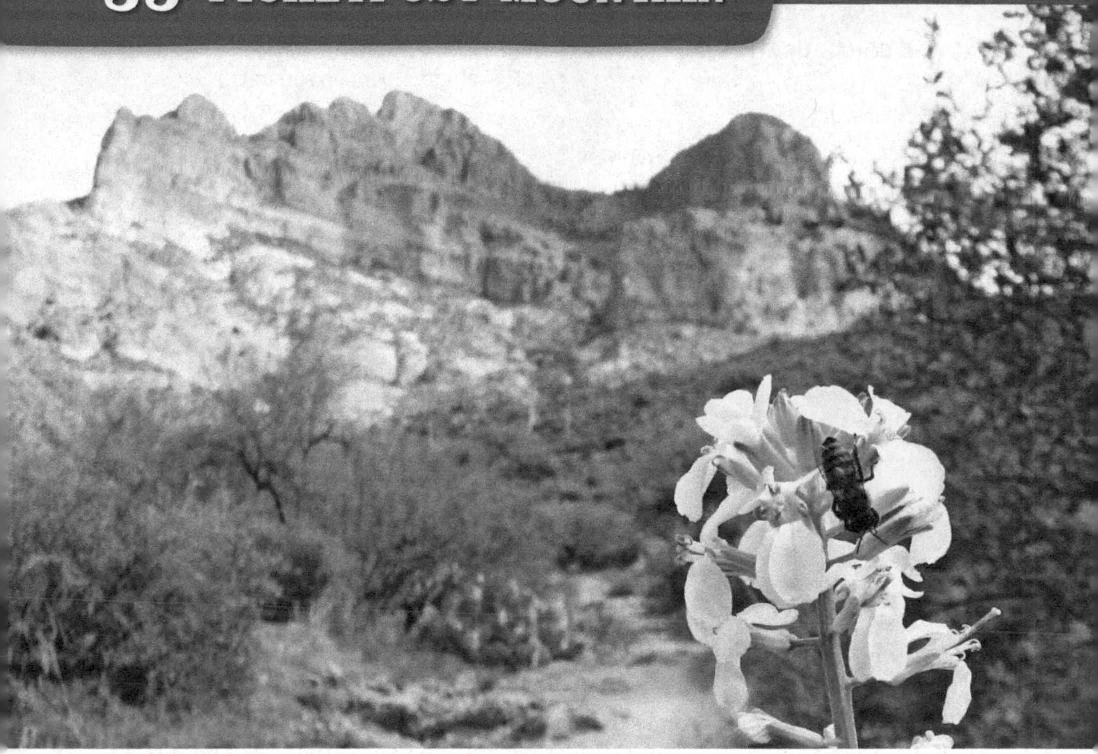

A honeybee browses western wallflowers below picturesque Picketpost Mountain.

THE DAUNTING ANGULAR shape of Picketpost Mountain intrigues all who drive along US 60 between Phoenix and Superior. A short but challenging trail on the northwest side of the mountain takes hikers 2,000 feet above the valley floor to a wide summit where, of all things, a mailbox and steel bench await occasional visitors.

DESCRIPTION

Drivers heading east on US 60 toward Superior must cross the 2,651-foot-high Gonzales Pass. From its apex, an amazing view of Picketpost Mountain almost assaults the spectator. Rugged, daunting, and fortresslike, Picketpost Mountain rises sharply from the desert floor. Its chiseled features and steep cliffs pique the imaginations of passersby. Many wonder if it is possible to hike to its summit, and the answer, of course, is a resounding yes.

Despite its imposing appearance, Picketpost Mountain has a well-established and fairly popular trail to its summit. Picketpost Trail approaches from the northwest and runs up a steep chute cut from sheer cliffs by millennia of erosion. Sweeping panoramic views abound on the summit. The top of Picketpost Mountain is actually quite wide and flat, but getting there is tough. Despite being relatively short,

DISTANCE & CONFIGURATION: 4.3-mile out-and-back

DIFFICULTY: Strenuous

SCENERY: Picketpost Mountain, panoramic views, desert

EXPOSURE: Mostly exposed; limited shade in chute

TRAIL TRAFFIC: Light

TRAIL SURFACE: Gravel, rock, loose dirt, some scrambling

HIKING TIME: 3.5 hours

WATER REQUIREMENT: 2.5 quarts

DRIVING DISTANCE: 55 miles from Phoenix Sky Harbor Airport

ELEVATION GAIN: 2,400' at trailhead, 4,375' on Picketpost Mountain summit

ACCESS: Sunrise–sunset; no permits or fees required

MAPS: USGS *Picketpost Mountain;* USFS *Superstition Wilderness* (see nationalforestmap-store.com/product-p/az-18.htm)

FACILITIES: Toilet but no water

WHEELCHAIR ACCESS: None

CONTACT: 928-402-6200, www.fs.usda.gov/activity/tonto/recreation/hiking

COMMENTS: Hike shares a segment with the Arizona National Scenic Trail; dogs must be leashed at all times

this trail packs in plenty of elevation gain. Some route-finding and scrambling skills are also necessary in order to navigate a steep section in the chute. Hardy hikers who conquer this mountain love the challenging ascent and usually return to Picketpost Mountain regularly.

The name "Picketpost" comes from a military camp that General George Stoneman built at the base of the mountain in 1870. The settlement guarded by this outpost eventually grew into the town of Superior, just a few miles east of the mountain. Stoneman also commissioned the construction of a mule trail that ran from the outpost at the base of Picketpost Mountain, through the Queen Creek basin, and eventually to an area known today as "Top of the World." Although the soldiers soon abandoned the area, the mule trail remains as a reminder of the region's history.

From the end of the large trailhead parking lot, find a metal sign describing the Arizona National Scenic Trail (AZT), which stretches north from the US–Mexico border to the Arizona–Utah border. The first part of the hike follows the AZT south near and to the left of an old mining track named Alamo Canyon Road. The trail crosses a large dry creek and winds around the foothills on a gentle incline. At 0.2 mile, you'll pass an unsigned fork that angles uphill to the left. Continue straight here to remain on the AZT. Around 0.4 mile, after crossing another sizable dry wash, leave the AZT at a signed intersection for Picketpost Mountain. Turn left here onto an old mining road that heads straight for the rock fortress in front of you.

The trail begins to climb southeast toward the foothills, gently at first but more steeply at 0.7 mile. The road soon ends at a flat area next to an old, abandoned mineshaft that has since been buried to prevent injuries. A rather abused wooden sign marks the continuation of the trail, which then steeply switchbacks up a grassy slope. Typical desert plants like chollas, ocotillos, and jojobas line the trail. In late spring, however, look for the bright-orange blossoms of the desert mariposa lily, which thrives here.

Picketpost Mountain

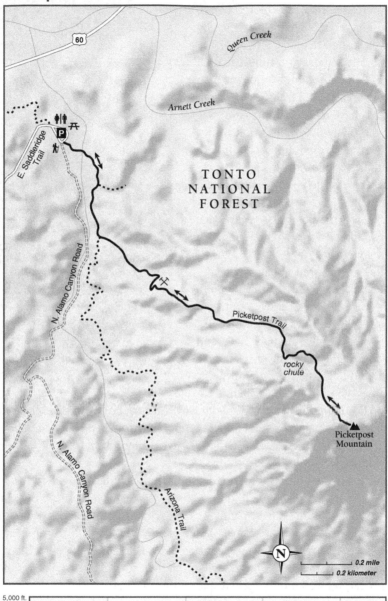

Queen Creek

Arnett Creek

60

E. Saddleridge Trail

P

N. Alamo Canyon Road

N. Alamo Canyon Road

TONTO
NATIONAL
FOREST

Picketpost Trail

rocky chule

Picketpost
Mountain

Arizona Trail

N

0.2 mile
0.2 kilometer

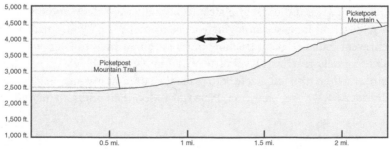

5,000 ft.
4,500 ft.
4,000 ft.
3,500 ft.
3,000 ft.
2,500 ft.
2,000 ft.
1,500 ft.
1,000 ft.

Picketpost
Mountain

Picketpost
Mountain Trail

0.5 mi.   1 mi.   1.5 mi.   2 mi.

185

Bearing three delicate and colorful petals, these flowers resemble butterflies, thereby earning their Spanish name.

One mile from the trailhead, you'll reach an open mound where you can catch your breath. At 2,800 feet elevation, you already have quite an impressive view toward the valley below, allowing you to visually retrace your approach through the foothills. US 60 lies in the distance, and the Superstition Mountains frame the horizon. The trail bends south next to a ravine and then climbs a rocky ridge where wildflowers grow in abundance after a wet winter.

A fork in the trail appears near the 1.3-mile mark—take either branch uphill, clamber over the rocks above, and then veer right. What follows is a section of incredibly steep hills, some bare rock, and slippery, rocky inclines. The trail bends to the right and hugs the base of cliff walls.

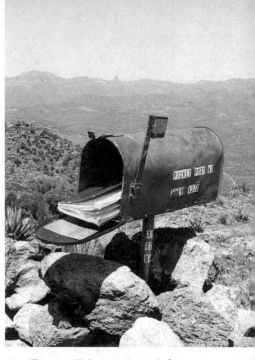

A mailbox atop Picketpost Mountain frames the view of Weaver's Needle.

At 1.5 miles, you must cross a slightly exposed ledge on the side of a gulley. It's an easy traverse, but tread carefully and don't look down. Also, make a mental note that upon returning, you need to keep far to the right after crossing this ledge. Otherwise, you might drop too low too soon and end up stranded among steep drop-offs.

Enter a narrow chute soon after crossing the scary ledge, and try to remember this spot so you know where to exit the chute later. You're not in the chute for very long, but ascending the deep gulley can be tricky in a few places where the trail goes over boulders. Leave the chute at 1.6 miles, where the trail breaks left, and then climb up a smooth bowl into the upper basin. With all the difficult parts behind you, take time to enjoy the scenery as the gulley opens wider. Agave stalks dot the hills, and a vertical cliff wall frames the left side of the gulley below.

Switchback toward the upper plateau. The trail is still steep and often slippery with loose dirt, and it passes annoyingly close to cacti; keep your guard up as you hike to prevent injury. Having trekking poles here may help to keep your balance. The trail eventually reaches a level plateau at 2 miles from the trailhead. Cross this high plain, and then turn left at a fork to reach the summit, just shy of 2.2 miles from the trailhead. At 4,375 feet elevation, Picketpost Mountain offers an incredible view of the Superstition Mountains and Weaver's Needle to the northwest. The town of Superior lies to the east, and an expansive wilderness stretches across the southern horizon as far as the eye can see.

An old mailbox stands proud on the summit, propped up by piles of rocks. The red flag on its side has been raised, and I wonder how long it takes a stamped post-card to reach its destination from here. Inside the mailbox is a summit logbook, in which you can leave words of wisdom for fellow hikers. There are also some trin-kets and mementos, but the most interesting artifact may be a story inscribed on the inside of the mailbox door. Apparently the previous owner of this tattered mailbox got tired of having it knocked down all the time, so he brought it up here for a safe retirement! It's a cute story worth reading. In recent years, someone also hauled a large metal bench up here to keep the mailbox company.

Take plenty of time to admire the panorama from the summit of Picketpost Mountain before you retrace your steps. On the way back, remember to leave the chute at the place where you entered, and stay to the right after you cross the scary ledge. If you do end up straying too low too soon, climb back up instead of trying to make an unsafe cliff traverse.

NEARBY ACTIVITIES

Boyce Thompson Arboretum State Park (see Hike 29, page 157), at the base of Picketpost Mountain, is one of the most intriguing botanical gardens in the South-west. The Superstition Wilderness northwest of Picketpost Mountain offers many more hiking opportunities.

• •

GPS TRAILHEAD COORDINATES N33° 16.310' W111° 10.588'

DIRECTIONS Drive east from Phoenix on US 60 toward Superior. After about 60 miles, past Florence Junction and beyond mile marker 221, follow the signs for Picketpost Trail and turn south (right) onto Forest Road 231/Uno Trail. Follow this dirt road 0.3 mile, and then make a sharp left onto paved Saddleridge Trail. Take this paved road 0.75 mile until it ends at the large parking area for the Picketpost Trailhead.

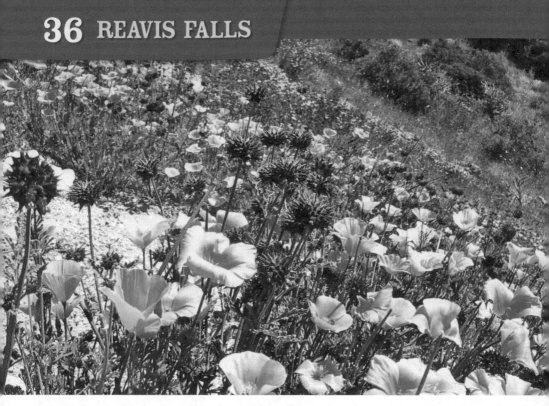

Mexican gold poppies and chia flowers flourish along Reavis Ranch Trail en route to Reavis Falls.

A 140-FOOT-TALL WATERFALL nestled deep in the Superstition Wilderness is your ultimate destination, but the journey to the falls is equally rewarding. Superb views of Apache Lake and the surrounding mountains abound.

DESCRIPTION

You may find it difficult to believe that a 140-foot-tall waterfall exists in the Arizona desert, but Reavis Falls proves doubters wrong with a spectacular cascade only miles from Phoenix. Fed by mountain springs deep within the Superstition Wilderness, Reavis Creek meanders around high plateaus and through deep valleys. At one particular spot in the shadows of Castle Dome, the creek tumbles down a sheer cliff to form a spectacular waterfall. The amount of water in the creek varies with the seasons and rainfall—sometimes it's a mere trickle, but when conditions are right, Reavis Falls sends a powerful torrent of water tumbling over the cliff.

Getting to the falls isn't easy. Your adventure begins with the drive to the Reavis Trailhead, which traces the historic Apache Trail nearly 30 tortuous miles. Upon arriving at the Reavis Trailhead, enjoy a bird's-eye view of Apache Lake while you mentally prepare for the 13-mile hike. To reach the falls, you must descend 1,625 feet into a deep valley. Hiking down first adds a degree of difficulty not normally encountered on a mountain hike, as it requires that you know your hiking ability. The bulk

DISTANCE & CONFIGURATION: 13.3-mile out-and-back

DIFFICULTY: Strenuous

SCENERY: Reavis Falls, Superstition Wilderness, Castle Dome, Apache Lake, Four Peaks, wildlife

EXPOSURE: Mostly exposed; some shade in Reavis Creek

TRAIL TRAFFIC: Light

TRAIL SURFACE: Gravel, packed dirt, loose dirt, rock; some scrambling necessary along creek

HIKING TIME: 8 hours

WATER REQUIREMENT: 4 quarts

DRIVING DISTANCE: 60 miles from Phoenix Sky Harbor Airport

ELEVATION GAIN: 3,550' at trailhead, 4,675' at highest point, 3,080' at Reavis Creek

ACCESS: Sunrise–sunset; no permits or fees required

MAPS: USGS *Pinyon Mountain;* USFS *Superstition Wilderness* (see nationalforestmap-store.com /product-p/az-18.htm)

FACILITIES: None

WHEELCHAIR ACCESS: None

CONTACT: 480-610-3300, www.fs.usda.gov /activity/tonto/recreation/hiking

COMMENTS: Also popular as a backpacking trip; dogs must leashed at all times

of the uphill toil remains for the return trip, and you can't simply turn around when you get tired: once in the canyon, you must climb out. Dire warnings aside, this hike and the falls are definitely worth the effort.

Begin by heading east on Reavis Valley Trail 109. Wide and smooth, the trail winds through rolling hills toward Reavis Ranch. Dense patches of purple chia flowers often line the trail in spring, which is also the best time to visit Reavis Falls. Patches of Mexican gold poppies add contrasting color, while delicate mariposa lilies bloom in April.

At 0.4 mile, the trail rounds a bend and opens to a northeastern view of Apache Lake and Apache Trail in the distance. To the east, rolling hills and distant mountains stretch as far as the eye can see. The trail levels and then descends slightly as it contours around a wide basin. Enjoy wide-open views as the trail traces a path over the hilltops.

The first 2 miles of the hike are relatively flat, but then you'll climb a moderately steep hill to a saddle at 2.2 miles from the trailhead. Another high basin comes into view, with the tip of Castle Dome in the distance. The trail turns left and contours around this basin at roughly 4,000 feet elevation, with expansive views of Fish Creek Mountain, Black Cross Butte, and Four Peaks on the horizon. On a clear day, you can see Camelback Mountain in the center of town. At 2.4 miles, the trail becomes notably rougher and rockier. Tall grasses blanket the hillside and sway back and forth with the slightest breeze. The entire scene looks quite out of place in Arizona.

At exactly 3.5 miles from the trailhead, with Castle Dome directly ahead, cairns mark a conspicuous spur trail that heads uphill to the left—leave Reavis Valley Trail at this point and branch onto this nameless spur. Steep and rocky, the next 0.25 mile requires significant effort. Hike up the narrow, grass-lined trail to a wide saddle at 4,675 feet—the high point of this hike—where you'll view an expansive valley with a deep ravine. Don't panic, but your destination is at the bottom of the ravine! Try not to get discouraged, and just keep going.

Reavis Falls

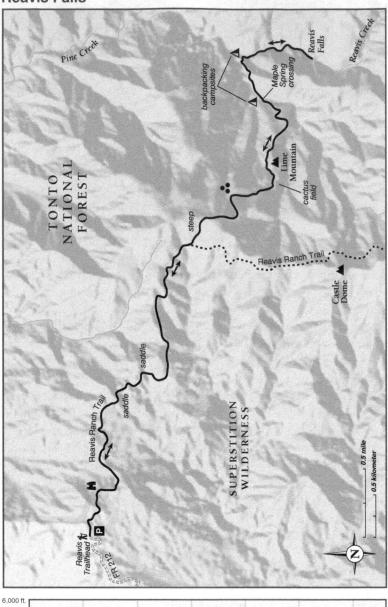

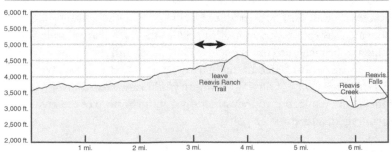

Crossing the saddle, the trail drops steeply, then eases slightly at 4 miles from the trailhead before turning south and then east. A lone juniper tree next to the trail marks a natural backpacker camp. Stone ruins just off the trail mark where the route bends south along a ridge. The trail then begins to descend. And descend. And descend. Watch your footing on loose rocks: prickly pear cacti may break your fall if you're not careful.

Turn left and hike around the northern side of Lime Mountain, where hackberry, juniper, and manzanita bushes provide some shade. Next, descend still farther on steep switchbacks to reach Cedar Basin at 5.5 miles. Some concrete slabs here, perhaps remnants of an old shelter, mark another backcountry camp. A bit farther, cross Maple Spring and continue past thick bushes and some malnourished cacti. After this, you'll pass through some hop bushes and grassy meadows to ascend a thin ridge. Cross the ridge and descend yet another steep, slippery hill to reach Reavis Creek at 6 miles from the trailhead.

Now the fun truly begins. Turn right and follow the creek upstream. The trail fades and reappears, crosses the creek several times, and goes over boulders and fallen logs. When in doubt, look for cairns, or just bushwhack up the creek. There are no established trails here, so you'll have to be creative. Watch out for poison ivy.

After 0.6 mile of bushwhacking and boulder-hopping, you'll finally see Reavis Falls over the treetops. As you get closer, the view of the falls gets more impressive. Tall cliffs and rocky slopes encircle the falls, forming a secluded alcove at the head of the canyon. It's an ideal place to picnic or just enjoy the scenery. Rest well, because climbing out of the canyon is a lot tougher than entering it was. Return the way you came.

NEARBY ACTIVITIES

Apache and **Canyon Lakes** are popular destinations for water sports. The Superstition Wilderness holds a treasure trove of trails, including **Boulder Canyon** (see Hike 28, page 151), **Reavis Ranch** (see next hike), **Rogers Canyon** (see Hike 38, page 196), and **Fish Creek** (see Hike 31, page 165), all of which are in the vicinity.

• •

GPS TRAILHEAD COORDINATES N33° 33.398' W111° 13.687'

DIRECTIONS From central Phoenix, drive east on US 60 and take Exit 196 north onto Idaho Road. After 2.25 miles, turn northeast (right) onto AZ 88/Apache Trail, and follow it 29 winding miles. Past mile marker 227, look for a sign that reads REAVIS TRAILHEAD and turn south (right), onto FR 212. Drive 2.9 miles on Forest Road 212 to the large trailhead parking lot. Note that FR 212 and portions of AZ 88 are dirt roads, which are normally passable by most cars. During the rainy season, however, deep ruts may develop, requiring a high-clearance vehicle for safe passage.

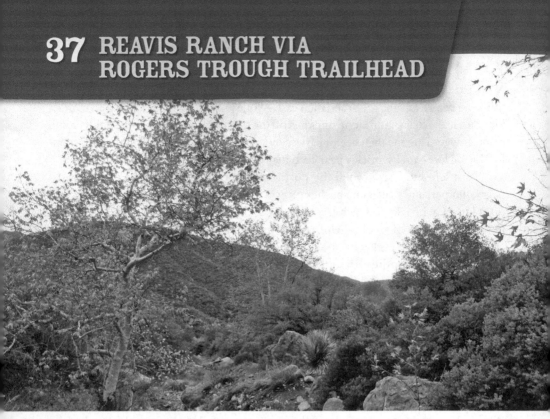

An Arizona sycamore shows its autumn colors next to Reavis Ranch Trail.

REAVIS RANCH SITS high in the remote Superstition Wilderness adjacent to a perennial creek. A popular destination for backpackers, it's reachable only via a scenic but long hike, ensuring its preservation from overuse.

DESCRIPTION

In 1874 Elisha M. Reavis, an eccentric recluse remembered as the "Hermit of Superstition Mountain," constructed his home in a mountain meadow deep in the wilderness. The first Anglo settler in the Superstitions, he established a farm next to a perennial creek that bears his name. Its waters fed a 140-acre ranch and nourished the fruits and vegetables Reavis cultivated on his property, then carted down long, winding hills to sell in nearby mining communities. In the winter of 1896, Reavis died along the trail while making one of his trips to town, and passersby buried him where they found him. His makeshift grave remains as a reminder of the trail's colorful history.

After Reavis's death, the ranch passed through many hands, getting fancier with each successive proprietor's embellishment. An apple orchard sprang up, a dirt road came in from the north, and a ranch house was built. The lush Reavis Ranch meadow became a popular place to visit. Some people had even tried to build a resort here to take advantage of cooler temperatures and trickling springs. The U.S. Department of

DISTANCE & CONFIGURATION: 15-mile out-and-back

DIFFICULTY: Moderate–strenuous

SCENERY: Pine forest, high desert, Superstition Wilderness, Reavis Ranch, Reavis Creek, wildlife

EXPOSURE: Significant shade

TRAIL TRAFFIC: Light

TRAIL SURFACE: Gravel, rock, riverbed, packed dirt, grass

HIKING TIME: 8 hours

WATER REQUIREMENT: 4–5 quarts

DRIVING DISTANCE: 65 miles from Phoenix Sky Harbor Airport

ELEVATION GAIN: 4,830' at trailhead, 5,350' at highest point (Reavis Saddle)

ACCESS: Sunrise–sunset; no permits or fees required

MAPS: USGS *Iron Mountain;* USFS *Superstition Wilderness* (see nationalforestmap-store.com /product-p/az-18.htm)

FACILITIES: None

WHEELCHAIR ACCESS: None

CONTACT: 480-610-3300, www.fs.usda.gov /activity/tonto/recreation/hiking

COMMENTS: Part of the Arizona National Scenic Trail; popular as a backpacking destination; dogs must be leashed at all times

Agriculture acquired the property in the late 1960s as part of Tonto National Forest and subsequently closed the dirt access road. The orchard, however, thrives to this day.

With cool pine forests, an apple orchard, and a flowing stream, Reavis Ranch has become a mecca for backpackers. The ranch house served as a shelter for hikers and equestrians until a fire leveled it in 1991, and the ranch is slowly but surely returning to nature—today, only the apple trees and some rusty farm tools survive. The ranch is still a pleasant place to visit, however. Retracing Reavis's footsteps on historic Reavis Valley Trail 109 transports you back in time, while trekking through the pine forest imparts an experience some might think impossible so close to Phoenix.

Begin this hike from the Rogers Trough Trailhead. A prominent sign indicates that this trail is a segment of the Arizona National Scenic Trail (AZT). The trail runs north, parallel to Rogers Creek, and soon passes a junction with West Pinto Trail 212. At 4,800 feet elevation, the trailside vegetation bears little resemblance to the desert plants near Phoenix. Alligator junipers and scrub live oaks dominate the landscape, and the air temperature is likely 15–20 degrees cooler than in town.

Pass through a gated fence at 0.3 mile from the trailhead; then follow the defined trail across Rogers Creek a few times, with Iron Mountain looming over your right shoulder. At 0.5 mile, manzanita lines the trail as it descends into the canyon. A set of switchbacks near 0.9 mile takes you farther down, and you can't help but think of the return trip and the climb it will require. Reach another manzanita patch at the nadir of your descent, nearly 1.7 miles from the trailhead. Here, Rogers Canyon Trail 110 (see next hike) forks left and eventually leads to some well-preserved Salado cliff dwellings.

Veer right at the Rogers Canyon junction to stay on Reavis Valley Trail. For the next 0.6 mile, generally follow the creekbed northeast. Riparian grasses and sugar sumacs have replaced manzanitas as the predominant plant life. At 2.3 miles, just before the trail begins to switchback, a small cairn on the left side of the trail marks an overgrown

Reavis Ranch via Rogers Trough Trailhead

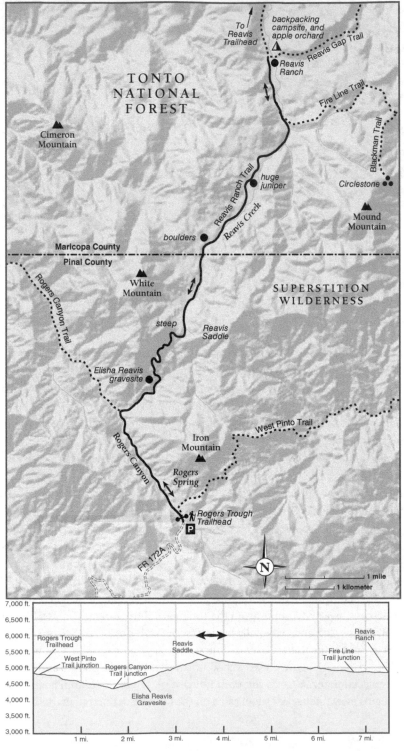

To
Reavis
Trailhead

backpacking
campsite, and
apple orchard

Reavis
Ranch

Reavis Gap Trail

Fire Line Trail

Blackman Trail

TONTO
NATIONAL
FOREST

Cimeron
Mountain

Reavis Ranch Trail

huge
juniper

Circlestone

Reavis Creek

Mound
Mountain

boulders

Maricopa County
Pinal County

Rogers Canyon Trail

White
Mountain

SUPERSTITION
WILDERNESS

steep

Reavis
Saddle

Elisha Reavis
gravesite

West Pinto Trail

Rogers Canyon

Iron
Mountain

Rogers
Spring

Rogers Trough
Trailhead
P

FR 172A

N

1 mile
1 kilometer

7,000 ft.
6,500 ft.
6,000 ft.
5,500 ft.
5,000 ft.
4,500 ft.
4,000 ft.
3,500 ft.
3,000 ft.

Rogers Trough
Trailhead

West Pinto
Trail junction

Rogers Canyon
Trail junction

Elisha Reavis
Gravesite

Reavis
Saddle

Fire Line
Trail junction

Reavis
Ranch

1 mi.   2 mi.   3 mi.   4 mi.   5 mi.   6 mi.   7 mi.

path to Reavis's grave. His unassuming makeshift memorial lies atop a small knoll with a view of surrounding hills.

Return to the main trail after paying your respects; then begin ascending switch-backs on the left side of the canyon. Dense patches of sugar sumacs line the smooth trail as you attack the steep hills. After a long ascent, the trail reaches Reavis Saddle at an elevation of 5,300 feet, where you enjoy an impressive view back down the canyon.

On the high plateau, the scenery changes abruptly from high desert to forest. A convenient fallen tree next to the trail makes a good rest spot. As you hike farther north, the trail gently descends and then enters a forest of pinyon pines and alligator junipers. You'd swear you were in Flagstaff if you hadn't just hiked up from Rogers Trough.

Reavis Valley Trail remains relatively flat for the rest of the hike, crossing a dry creek several times atop the plateau and traversing a large meadow at 5.2 miles from the trailhead. A quarter mile farther on, you'll encounter Reavis Creek, whose flow-ing water emerges from an underground spring. Tiny blue butterflies dance around the water in a wide-open meadow blanketed by tall grasses.

Hike past a gigantic alligator juniper at 5.8 miles; then cross the creek twice, at 6.3 and 6.5 miles from the trailhead. Fire Line Trail 118 merges in from the right at 6.8 miles. After you pass that trail junction, it's only a half mile or so to Reavis Ranch.

The first obvious sign of the Reavis property is an old well to the left of the trail. Some rusty remnants of farm machinery are strewn about. A large sunken meadow, home to a horse corral, sits to the right of the trail, while Reavis Creek flows east of the meadow. Allow plenty of time to explore the large property. In autumn, be sure to sample the plentiful crop of apples from the orchard on the north end of the ranch.

At 7.5 miles from the trailhead, reach the junction with Reavis Gap Trail 117, your turnaround point. The AZT follows Reavis Gap Trail east as it cuts across the meadow. If you head north on Reavis Valley Trail another 10 miles, you'll reach the Reavis Trail-head near Apache Lake. Retrace your steps to complete the 15-mile round-trip.

• •

GPS TRAILHEAD COORDINATES N33° 25.335' W111° 10.403'

DIRECTIONS From Phoenix, drive east on US 60. Past mile marker 214, turn northeast (left) onto Queen Valley Road, reset your trip odometer, and drive 1.7 miles. Bear right onto gravel Hewitt Station Road and follow it to the signed turnoff to Forest Road 172, at odometer 4.8 miles. Turn north (left) onto FR 172, cross Queen Creek, and drive to a junc-tion with FR 172A at 14.1 miles. Turn right, onto FR 172A, and follow the rough dirt road to a T-intersection at odometer 17.7 miles. Turn left and continue 0.4 mile to the Rogers Trough Trailhead. *Note:* A high-clearance vehicle or four-wheel-drive is recommended.

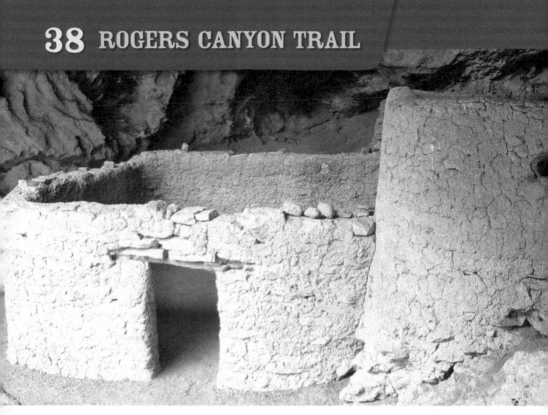

A well-preserved Salado cliff dwelling deep within Rogers Canyon in the Superstition Wilderness

SCENIC ROGERS CANYON makes the long and rough drive to the Rogers Trough Trailhead worthwhile. Shady streamside trails, beautiful deep canyons, and well-preserved Salado cliff dwellings make this hike a must for any outdoor enthusiast or history buff.

DESCRIPTION

The rugged Superstition Wilderness never ceases to amaze me, because within its confines are some of the finest hikes in Arizona. The seasonal spring and sheer cliffs in Rogers Canyon typify the natural beauty of this region, and many consider it a hidden gem within the wilderness. Add a scenic drive to the trailhead and the mystique of ancient cliff dwellings, and you have an experience you won't soon forget.

The long drive to the Rogers Trough Trailhead passes through gorgeous canyons, sandy wash crossings, and mountain vistas, setting the proper frame of mind for this excursion. When you arrive at the trailhead, the outdoor experience gets even better. At its finest, Rogers Canyon offers a winding hike through colorful fall leaves. Ample shade and the sound of trickling water along this trail make it a desirable destination regardless of season.

From the wide parking area at Rogers Trough, head north on Reavis Valley Trail 109. The 4,800-foot elevation here discourages most desert plants. Instead, junipers

DISTANCE & CONFIGURATION: 9-mile out-and-back

DIFFICULTY: Moderate

SCENERY: Rogers Canyon, Salado cliff dwellings, mountain stream, rock formations

EXPOSURE: Significant shade

TRAIL TRAFFIC: Light

TRAIL SURFACE: Rock, packed dirt, gravel, streambed

HIKING TIME: 5 hours

WATER REQUIREMENT: 3 quarts

DRIVING DISTANCE: 65 miles from Phoenix Sky Harbor Airport

ELEVATION GAIN: 4,830' at trailhead, 3,800' at Rogers Canyon cliff dwellings

ACCESS: Sunrise–sunset; no permits or fees required

MAPS: USGS *Iron Mountain;* USFS *Superstition Wilderness* (see nationalforestmap-store.com /product-p/az-18.htm)

FACILITIES: None

WHEELCHAIR ACCESS: None

CONTACT: 480-610-3300, www.fs.usda.gov /activity/tonto/recreation/hiking

COMMENTS: Well-preserved ancient cliff dwellings; dogs must be leashed at all times

and other evergreens dot the hills, and thick grasses cover the ground. The trail follows Rogers Spring, which feeds large deciduous trees such as the Arizona sycamore. At 0.1 mile, pass the junction with West Pinto Trail 212, which branches off to the east. Continue along Reavis Valley Trail, and pass through a gated fence at 0.3 mile. The trail becomes sandy here as it crosses the spring.

A half mile into the hike, you'll descend a steep, slippery slope. Thickets of manzanita bushes line the trail, their silky-smooth red bark contrasting with silver-green leaves. Cross the spring again, and then climb out of the canyon to a high ledge where an expansive view opens before you. Iron Mountain towers above you to the right. The trail drops off steeply again and returns to the streambed at 0.9 mile.

Hike the next 0.5 mile near the spring and among giant sycamore trees with their signature white bark. Pass a bend in the trail where there's a rocky drop-off on the left; then dive into another patch of manzanita providing cool shade. At 1.7 miles veer left onto Rogers Canyon Trail 110, which begins in a thick forest of manzanitas and live oaks.

As you enter Rogers Canyon, crisscrossing the spring and passing sycamores and sugar sumacs, the scenery steadily improves. Thick brush surrounds the trail, and rocky ridges top both sides of the canyon. In the rainy season, many stream crossings take you past small cascades where water tumbles a few feet into shallow pools. When hiking next to the spring, you are often walking in the shade of tall trees, enjoying views of oddly shaped hoodoos along the ridgetops. Near 2.7 miles, you'll reach a flat section parallel to the spring, where you face a massive jagged mountaintop.

Roughly 3.3 miles into the hike, cross the spring again at a rocky spot, and then climb up its right bank. Soon a clearing opens to reveal views of yellowish volcanic tuff on the hills framing the canyon. The trail can be a little hard to find here, but it runs along the right side of the spring. Streamside rocks and clearings along

Rogers Canyon Trail

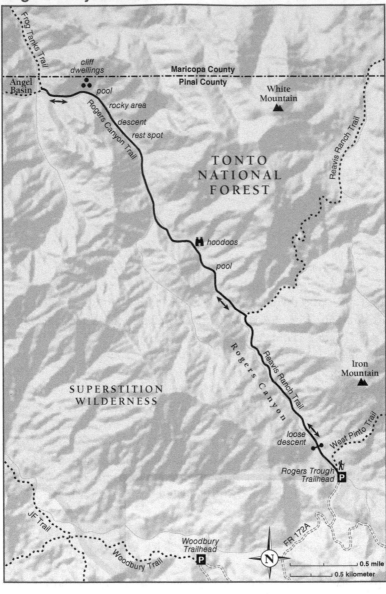

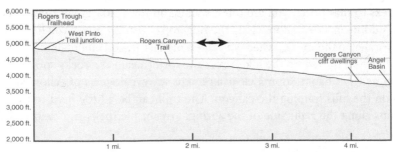

this stretch make great rest stops. The trail then descends through rougher terrain. Watch out for thorny catclaw acacias tearing at your clothing.

Entering the depths of Rogers Canyon, the trail undulates, passing over rocky areas that require a bit more effort and attention. Thankfully, the scenery continues to improve. At 3.7 miles, you'll cross a rocky mound where you have an open view straight into the canyon. Continuing beside the spring and seasonal pools, look for the cliff dwellings ahead; they're on the right bank about 100 feet above the canyon floor.

At 4.1 miles, a cairned turnoff takes you across the spring and up a steep slope to the cliff dwellings. In the 1300s, the Salado people built many such dwellings in canyon walls and caves throughout the region. Judging by the location of this particular settlement, they picked a beautiful and strategic place to live. Taking advantage of the natural shelter provided by the canyon walls, the Salado built several multistory homes and common living quarters within deep caves. From these ruins, you command a gorgeous view up and down the canyon, making this spot an ideal picnic setting. Note the large plaque reminding hikers to keep off the walls and to protect the fragile buildings. The most important structure in this cliff-dwelling complex is located high up in the rocks and requires a little light scrambling to visit. Please leave everything as you found it.

Most people turn back after reaching the ruins, but it's worthwhile to hike another 5–10 minutes to visit Angel Basin. Backtrack to the main trail and continue west along Rogers Canyon Trail. Hike through thick thorny brush to a clearing approximately 4.3 miles from the trailhead. Head toward the large, open basin directly in front of you to reach the signed junction with Frog Tanks Trail 112 at 4.5 miles. This is Angel Basin, a favorite destination of backpackers and campers. A ring of mountains surrounds the wide-open plain, which is covered in deep, soft grass. In front of you looms a mound topped by massive boulders, perched like a castle overlooking a kingdom. A narrow vertical gap serves as the doorway to the castle, and there's even a rock in the shape of a dog guarding its entrance.

Rogers Canyon Trail continues west and terminates at JF Trail 106. If you have a shuttle vehicle, you can take JF Trail to the Woodbury Trailhead, at the end of Forest Road 172; most hikers are content with seeing Angel Basin and the cliff dwellings, though. Rest here before returning the way you came. Remember that the hike out of Rogers Canyon gains over 1,000 feet in elevation, with the toughest climb near the end, so save some strength for that last mile.

NEARBY ACTIVITIES

Rogers Canyon lies in the heart of the Superstition Wilderness, the site of many hikes in this book, including **Siphon Draw** (see next hike), **Boulder Canyon** (see Hike 28, page 151), **Peralta Canyon** (see Hike 34, page 179), and **Lost Goldmine** (see Hike 33, page 174). Farther out on US 60, **Picketpost Mountain** (see Hike 35, page 183) and **Boyce Thompson Arboretum State Park** (see Hike 29, page 157) offer additional hiking opportunities.

• •

GPS TRAILHEAD COORDINATES N33° 25.335' W111° 10.403'

DIRECTIONS From central Phoenix, drive east on US 60 past mile marker 214. Turn northeast (left) onto Queen Valley Road, reset your odometer, and drive 1.7 miles. Bear right onto gravel Hewitt Station Road and follow it to the signed turnoff to Forest Road 172, at odometer 4.8 miles. Turn north (left) onto FR 172, cross Queen Creek, and drive through the desert foothills to a junction with FR 172A at 14.1 miles. Turn right, onto FR 172A, and follow the rough dirt road to a T-intersection, at odometer 17.7 miles. Turn left and continue 0.4 mile to the Rogers Trough Trailhead.

Note: This drive is very scenic but requires a high-clearance vehicle. A four-wheel-drive vehicle may be necessary after storms.

Desert globemallow flowers adorn the Rogers Canyon cliff dwellings.

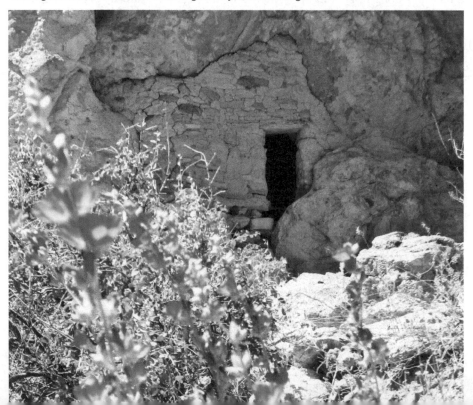

39 SIPHON DRAW TRAIL

The Flatiron and surrounding cliffs tower above Siphon Draw Trail.

SIPHON DRAW TRAIL and The Flatiron capture the rugged beauty of the Superstition Mountains and package the essence of this wondrous wilderness into a short but very challenging hike.

DESCRIPTION

The Superstition Wilderness area offers arguably the best hikes near Phoenix. With a rich and storied history and hundreds of miles of trails running through a land of stark contrasts, the Superstitions draw visitors of all types. Hikers especially enjoy its diverse scenery and challenging trails. Siphon Draw Trail 53 ranks high on most people's list because it is readily accessible and packs so much scenery into just a 6-mile hike.

Along Siphon Draw Trail, fields of wildflowers cover gentle foothills in spring. Fantastic rock formations frame the canyon and The Flatiron, a massive yet smooth protrusion of rock, looms over the trail. A seasonal waterfall delights visitors. Views from Siphon Draw, and especially atop The Flatiron, are unparalleled. The upper half of the canyon, however, remains raw and rugged, requiring much scrambling and plenty of sweat and toil to explore fully. If you like switchbacks, this hike is not for you: there are no switchbacks at all, and the elevation profile rises dramatically.

DISTANCE & CONFIGURATION: 6-mile out-and-back

DIFFICULTY: Strenuous

SCENERY: Superstition Mountains, The Flatiron, seasonal waterfall, city panoramas

EXPOSURE: Early-morning shade; otherwise exposed

TRAIL TRAFFIC: Moderate–heavy

TRAIL SURFACE: Rock, gravel, boulders, scrambling, climbing

HIKING TIME: 5 hours

WATER REQUIREMENT: 3 quarts

DRIVING DISTANCE: 33 miles from Phoenix Sky Harbor Airport

ELEVATION GAIN: 2,080' at trailhead, 5,024' at unnamed summit above The Flatiron

ACCESS: Sunrise–10 p.m.; $7/vehicle entry fee

MAPS: USGS *Goldfield;* map available at park entrance; USFS *Superstition Wilderness* (see nationalforestmap-store.com/product-p /az-18.htm)

FACILITIES: Restrooms, water, picnic area, campground, shower, ranger station

WHEELCHAIR ACCESS: None

CONTACT: 480-982-4485, azstateparks.com /lost-dutchman

COMMENTS: Spectacular climb to a spectacular viewpoint; dogs permitted on leash but may have trouble getting to The Flatiron due to scrambling

Perhaps the challenge of conquering Siphon Draw, though, is part of its mystique, and those who succeed are duly rewarded.

The trailhead for Siphon Draw lies inside Lost Dutchman State Park—the state park closest to Phoenix—although most of the trail stretches beyond park boundaries into Tonto National Forest. The park is named after the legend of the Lost Dutchman, actually a German prospector named Jacob Waltz, who purportedly stashed gold in these mountains in the late 1800s. He left a legacy of maps and fantasies of treasures, but no one has ever found gold here.

Begin this hike from the western end of the Saguaro Day-Use Area at a signed trailhead. The first part of the hike follows Discovery Trail, which takes you on a gentle stroll among desert plants along a path with interpretive signs. Turn left at a signed junction to access Siphon Draw Trail, and you'll soon pass the campground restroom and showers. If you find yourself at the restrooms, then you've missed the turn—veer left and you'll rejoin the trail. At 0.5 mile turn left again and head toward the mountains on a bed of crushed rock.

Siphon Draw Trail heads southeast into the Superstition Mountains, passing a fence and equestrian guard as it enters Tonto National Forest. Climbing a wide, gentle path, cross the intersections with Prospector's View Trail and Jacob's Crosscut Trail. Note the trailside remnants of a bunker, which was part of the nearby Palmer Mine. During certain springs, when there has been sufficient winter rain, these foothills display a gorgeous blanket of golden brittlebush flowers. Poppies, lupine, and globemallows also add a dash of vibrant color. This area is one of the most photographed landscapes in Arizona.

As the trail enters the Superstition Wilderness and approaches the canyon, it gets progressively steeper. At 1.6 miles from the trailhead, look to your right for a large protruding boulder in the shape of a thumb; some call this formation Thumb

Siphon Draw Trail

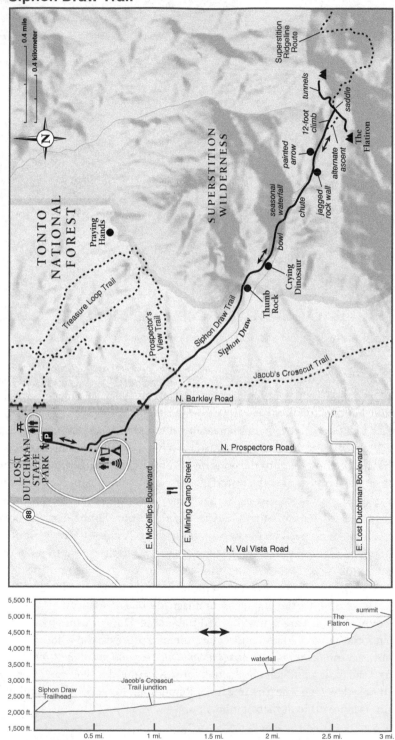

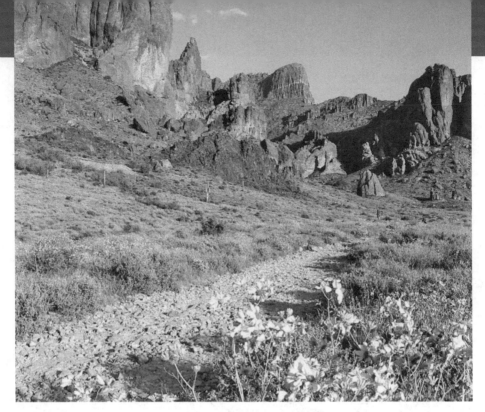
Golden brittlebush flowers blanket the foothills below The Flatiron during spring.

Rock. The trail continues to rise as you enter the mouth of the canyon. Notice a tall spire named the Crying Dinosaur across the canyon. Near 1.8 miles, the trail makes a surprise left turn uphill toward the canyon wall and hooks around a large boulder. Deeper into Siphon Draw, the trail dives into a wooded wash but soon emerges into a large bowl of smooth rock. After seasonal rains, a small waterfall cascades down the cliff face and empties into the bowl, providing an ideal backdrop for a picnic.

The official trail ends at the waterfall, but there's so much more to Siphon Draw. Who can resist? Just be aware that the next mile covers very rocky terrain on insanely steep slopes and gains more than 1,500 feet of elevation. Climb out of the bowl right of the waterfall, and head up the narrow chute directly ahead. After a bit of slipping and sliding on a gravelly hill, you'll reach a narrow saddle with a tremendous view of The Flatiron directly above. Take time to admire the view behind you and to survey the route ahead. The correct path drops from the saddle and heads straight up Siphon Draw, which is the first major drainage left of The Flatiron.

Scrambling skills are a must beyond the saddle. Dots of white paint guide your way, but forest rangers sometimes remove them to preserve the wilderness, so when in doubt, *stay inside the main drainage of Siphon Draw and avoid the temptation to drift right.* If faced with a difficult climb, look for ways around it; you can often bypass it altogether or leverage a nearby tree limb. Remember, however, that climbing down to return is more difficult than climbing up.

Three especially tricky spots deserve mention. The first is a jagged wall of granite not far from the saddle. When you reach this wall, simply climb over it. The rock surface has plenty of good footholds. The second tricky area is about halfway up the canyon. Look for a painted white arrow telling you to climb up and turn left around a large boulder. If you turn right here, you end up on a slope of loose scree. It is possible to get to the top that way, but it's fairly miserable. The final tricky spot is a 12-foot wall that you'll encounter just before you reach the high plateau. Tackle this climb by using the stepping-stones in the crevice to the right.

Beyond the final climb, you'll emerge from Siphon Draw to reach a ledge level with the top of The Flatiron. Strangely eroded rock formations called hoodoos cap the mountaintops. Head right 0.25 mile to visit The Flatiron, a large and incredibly flat area covered with strawberry hedgehogs that display bright-purple flowers in April and May. Leave the trail and walk west to the cliff's edge, where you can admire dizzying views of the valley below.

If you're not too tired yet, consider taking a 15-minute detour to visit the unnamed summit above The Flatiron. Backtrack to the point where the trail emerges from Siphon Draw. Continue straight uphill to a saddle point, where you can access the Superstition Ridgeline route (see next hike). From the saddle, turn left to head uphill toward the hoodoos, and look for a smooth slope on the right side of the small basin—ascend this slope, and follow a narrow brushy track to an angled slab of rock wedged between boulders. Climb over the slab and then duck through the first rock arch. Turn left and then right to reach the second rock tunnel. Crawl through the opening and immediately climb up the boulder on the left. Follow the faint trail all the way to the summit.

This unnamed 5,024-foot summit is the highest point on the western end of the Superstitions. From its peak, you can gaze into the heart of the Superstition Wilderness and see Weaver's Needle, view the distant Four Peaks, and survey the ridgeline all the way to Superstition Peak, the highest point on the eastern end. You can spend hours up here exploring the nooks and crannies among the hoodoos. When satisfied, return by descending Siphon Draw. Be careful not to dislodge loose rocks onto hikers below as you climb down the steep gulley.

• •

GPS TRAILHEAD COORDINATES N33° 27.558' W111° 28.801'

DIRECTIONS From central Phoenix, drive east on US 60 and take Exit 196 north onto Idaho Road. After 2.25 miles, turn northeast (right) onto AZ 88/Apache Trail, and continue 5 miles to the entrance of Lost Dutchman State Park. Pay the entrance fee and follow the signs to the Siphon Draw Trailhead in the Saguaro Day-Use Area.

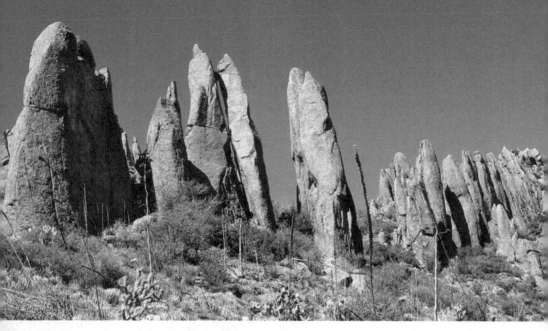

A picket fence of hoodoos high atop the Superstition Ridgeline

CROSSING THE SUPERSTITION Ridgeline is one of those feats that you brag about for a long time. This combination hike and scramble challenges even the hardiest of outdoor aficionados.

DESCRIPTION

With a nickname like "Superstitions Death March," this grueling endurance test has attained legendary status. Despite the ridgeline's well-deserved reputation as the toughest hike near Phoenix, most hikers who tackle it can't wait to try it again—after a period of recovery, of course. With open views of Weaver's Needle, the Superstition Wilderness, and Four Peaks, the scenery along this high ridge is nothing short of stunning.

There is no official trail across the ridgeline, but years of use have carved an established route marked by cairns. *Route-finding and scrambling skills are required for this rigorous hike; therefore, only experienced hikers should attempt it, preferably with someone already familiar with the route.* Because of its difficulty, crossing Superstition Ridgeline is not recommended in summer. Always tell someone where you're going, and remember to bring plenty of water. Also, leave your four-legged friends at home, because they'll have trouble in several spots that require climbing.

You can hike the ridgeline in either direction, though I find going from east to west somewhat easier. Stash a vehicle at Lost Dutchman State Park and then drive to the Lost

DISTANCE & CONFIGURATION: 12.2-mile point-to-point with shuttle

DIFFICULTY: Very strenuous

SCENERY: Superstition Mountains, Flatiron, Weaver's Needle, canyons, seasonal waterfalls

EXPOSURE: Mostly exposed, some canyon shade

TRAIL TRAFFIC: Light

TRAIL SURFACE: Rock, gravel, boulders

HIKING TIME: 8–10 hours

WATER REQUIREMENT: 4 quarts

DRIVING DISTANCE: 33 miles from Phoenix Sky Harbor Airport

ELEVATION GAIN: 2,080' at trailhead, 5,057' at Superstition Peak

ACCESS: Sunrise–10 p.m., $7/vehicle entry fee at Lost Dutchman State Park; sunrise–sunset at Lost Goldmine Trailhead, no permits or fees required

MAPS: USGS *Goldfield* and *Weavers Needle;* USFS *Superstition Wilderness* (see nationalforest mapstore.com/product-p/az-18.htm)

FACILITIES: *Lost Dutchman:* restrooms, water, picnic area, campground, shower, ranger station; *Lost Goldmine Trailhead:* none

WHEELCHAIR ACCESS: None

CONTACT: 480-982-4485, azstateparks.com /lost-dutchman

COMMENTS: Most difficult hike near Phoenix; not a good hike for dogs due to scrambling

Goldmine Trailhead on Peralta Road. Avoid starting from the Carney Springs parking area—that approach, though 0.5 mile shorter, requires a paid state-land permit. Instead, follow Lost Goldmine Trail (see Hike 33, page 174) 1.1 miles to find a small gate and equestrian guard in the Superstition Wilderness boundary fence. This gate lies opposite a fairly open area, an old dirt track called Carney Springs Road that approaches from your left. Your epic Superstitions adventure begins at this wilderness access point. Cross the boundary fence here, and head north on a narrow path.

The trail begins as a gentle stroll through desert foothills. Keep right and pass an unsigned turn for Wave Cave (see next hike) about 800 feet after the fence. The slope soon turns steeply uphill. Look for a seasonal waterfall on a mountainside crevice in the distance. Climb ridiculously steep and rocky slopes beginning at 1.8 miles, using cairns to guide your ascent. Take a breather at an open intermediate saddle 2 miles from the trailhead. In the spring, you'll see many wildflowers along the way. One particularly interesting succulent indigenous to this region is the rock echeveria, or "live-forever." Look for its candy corn–shaped red and orange flowers clinging to rocky crags.

Resume the torturous climb to reach the higher West Boulder Saddle (3,680'), 2.35 miles from the trailhead. You've now gained 1,350 feet, most of it in only 0.5 mile. Turn around to survey your ascent of the canyon below. Notice the trapezoidal Picket-post Mountain (see Hike 35, page 183) in the distance.

Turn left at West Boulder Saddle and hike west toward Superstition Peak. The trail mercifully flattens awhile as you snake around boulders and thick patches of vegetation. Descend slightly into upper West Boulder Canyon, and cross seasonal Willow Spring at 2.9 miles. Next, turn left uphill where the trail flattens out again with a view of Weaver's Needle jutting out above the opposite ridge.

Superstition Ridgeline

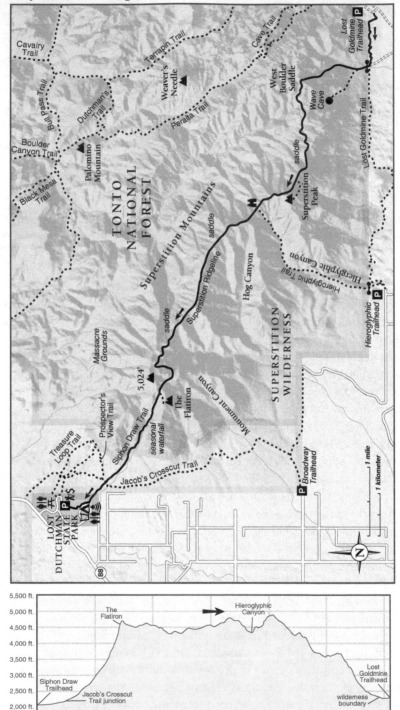

At 3.3 miles, cross a small, dry wash and begin another steep climb through thick grasses. Turn left up a rocky chute with a small cairn on top, and hike up a rocky ridge with views to the south. The trail begins yet another steep, slippery ascent here. At these considerably higher elevations, the plants are noticeably different from those lower in the canyon. Sotols and agaves thrive, and banana yuccas display stalks of delicate white flowers in April and May. The climb culminates at a saddle with views of Gold Canyon and Apache Junction to the south. Weaver's Needle stands distinct in the northeast.

Continue up the ridge and down to another saddle. Watch out for the shin dagger, a small, sharp, agave-like plant. At 4.1 miles from the trailhead, make your way up a slope of loose shale to find the trail bending north toward Weaver's Needle. The trail then contours around the mountain and takes aim at Superstition Peak. The path can be hard to find here, so look carefully for cairns; when in doubt, head for the tallest peak you see, which upon closer inspection comprises a tight grouping of hoodoos.

From the southeastern end of the summit ridge, at the base of the hoodoos that form the summit, a spur trail visits Superstition Peak. Look for a cairned path that heads left into the hoodoos, flanks them on the left, and leads to the 5,057-foot summit. Some light scrambling is required near the top. Now atop the highest point in the Superstitions, admire the sweeping views of the city and the expansive wilderness below.

Retrace your steps to the southeast corner of the summit ridge and resume your hike. Ridgeline Trail skirts the summit hoodoos on the right this time. Reach a wide saddle 4.7 miles (not counting the summit spur) from the trailhead.

Cross the saddle toward the west; then go north around the left side of the hoodoos to a large flat area with sheer drop-offs. Look for a cairn near the northern cliff, marking your first scary Class 3 scramble down a rocky chute. Next, head for the southwestern (left) side of the boulders straight ahead. The trail descends about 50 feet along a steep slope, then turns north across the base of the boulders. This section also requires some scrambling and bushwhacking; again, cairns guide you along a faint path.

Past the scrambling section, a saddle greets you nearly 5.1 miles from the trailhead. Notice scenic Hieroglyphic Canyon (see Hike 32, page 169) to the south. Tackle the uphill to the south of the ridge, and then cross to the northern side as you bob up and down across several saddles. One of the most challenging aspects of this hike is enduring the undulations along the ridge. Near 5.6 miles, the trail fades once more. You can either veer right and climb to the ridgetop, or you can take a climbing traverse along the southern side of the hill. Look for a lone pine tree on the ridgeline at 6.1 miles—if you lose the trail, head for this tree, because the trail runs right next to it.

You'll reach a high point on the ridgeline just past the pine tree. From this vantage point, gaze down at Weaver's Needle to the northeast and Hog Canyon to the southwest. You can see Superstition Peak behind you, and the unnamed peak above Siphon Draw Trail (see Hike 39, page 201), your destination for the day. Descend from this pinnacle toward a confusing forest of boulders. The trail veers slightly left and squeezes through a crevice before dumping you out on the ridgeline again.

Route-finding becomes much easier now as you pick up the pace along the chiseled ridgeline. The trail tackles the ridge head-on and ducks to the north when it seems impassible, only to return to the ridgeline later. The next mile is a classic ridge walk, where you literally walk the spine of the Superstitions. Admire grand views to either side of the trail, and look for bright-purple blossoms on spiny hedgehog cacti in April.

Near 7.6 miles, the trail comes to a flat outcropping, a scenic overlook into Monument Canyon and a great place to take a quick break. A quarter mile farther, another steep descent awaits. This is the second steep scramble down a rocky, loose chute, but it's less technical than the first. Dropping to 4,200 feet, you'll reach the final low saddle on the ridge. Climbing again feels tough, but the worst is behind you.

You'll regain most of the lost elevation and draw level with the ridge again. The trail takes a long, flat traverse around the top of Monument Canyon and across the level ledge ahead. At 9.2 miles you'll begin your final ascent, which leads to a high saddle overlooking the famous Flatiron. Those familiar with Siphon Draw Trail now breathe a sigh of relief because this is the end of the ridgeline. However, more challenges lurk around the corner. Descending Siphon Draw is no easy task.

Refer to Siphon Draw (see previous hike) for how to return to Lost Dutchman State Park, where you should have a shuttle vehicle or a ride waiting.

NEARBY ACTIVITIES

The Superstition Mountains are home to many hikes detailed in this book, including the **Peralta, Lost Goldmine**, and **Siphon Draw Trails** (see pages 179, 174, and 201). The Usery Mountains to the west offer additional hiking opportunities.

• •

GPS TRAILHEAD COORDINATES
N33° 27.558' W111° 28.801' (Siphon Draw Trailhead)
N33° 23.589' W111° 21.242' (Lost Goldmine Trailhead)

DIRECTIONS *Siphon Draw Trailhead:* From central Phoenix, drive east on US 60 and exit at Idaho Road. Drive 2.25 miles north on Idaho Road to AZ 88, Apache Trail. Turn northeast (right) onto AZ 88, and continue 5 miles to the entrance of Lost Dutchman State Park. Pay the entrance fee and follow the signs to the Siphon Draw Trailhead, in the Day-Use Area.

Lost Goldmine Trailhead: From the Siphon Draw Trailhead, retrace your route to US 60, turn east (lef), and drive 7.5 miles. At mile marker 204, turn northeast (left) onto Peralta Road, and reset your odometer. Follow Peralta Road, which becomes a graded dirt road, to a fork at 5.5 miles. Bear left at the fork to continue to the Lost Goldmine Trailhead (see Hike 33, page 174) at 7.1 miles—if you've reached the Peralta Trailhead, you've gone too far.

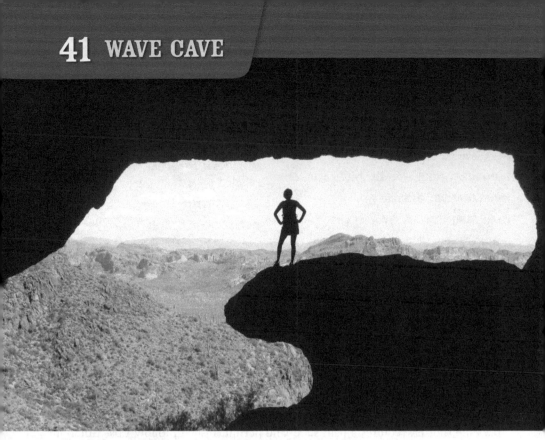

A hiker rides the wave at the mouth of Wave Cave

THOUGH NOT ACCESSIBLE via an official trail, the Wave Cave has neverthe-less become a popular destination over the years. Its unique rock formation draws many hikers to visit and to take silhouette photographs of themselves posing like they're surfing in the desert.

DESCRIPTION

Arguably, the best hiking near Phoenix lies within the expansive 160,200-acre Super-stition Wilderness. Its mysterious rugged mountain ranges and deep forests host hundreds of miles of remote trails and hold hidden gems such as waterfalls, swim-ming holes, abandoned mines, and unique rock formations. Some of these treasures are reachable by trail, while others require a bit more bushwhacking. One hidden gem is actually easily reached: a shallow cave on the south side of Superstition Mountain known as the Wave Cave, so named because a tonguelike rock protrusion near its entrance resembles a crashing wave.

To reach the Wave Cave, one must travel along a popular use trail, or unmain-tained trail made accessible by frequent foot traffic. The arid landscape of the South-west makes such trails possible: there is a lack of vegetation that may overgrow and obscure unmaintained trails over time. The drawback is that these unofficial trails

DISTANCE & CONFIGURATION: 4.1-mile out-and-back

DIFFICULTY: Moderate

SCENERY: Superstition Mountain, Wave Cave, desert

EXPOSURE: Mostly exposed, shaded at the cave

TRAIL TRAFFIC: Moderate

TRAIL SURFACE: Gravel, packed dirt

HIKING TIME: 1.5 hours

WATER REQUIREMENT: 1 quart

DRIVING DISTANCE: 43 miles from Phoenix Sky Harbor Airport

ELEVATION GAIN: 2,300' at trailhead, 3,070' at Wave Cave

ACCESS: Sunrise–sunset at Lost Goldmine Trailhead, no permits or fees required

MAPS: USGS *Weavers Needle;* USFS *Superstition Wilderness* (see nationalforestmap-store.com /product-p/az-18.htm)

FACILITIES: None

WHEELCHAIR ACCESS: None

CONTACT: 480-610-3300

COMMENTS: Secluded cave with a tonguelike rock formation that resembles a crashing wave, dogs leashed at all times

may erode the natural desert landscape. (South Mountain in Phoenix is an example where use trails have become rampant.) Fortunately, the trail to Wave Cave is well defined, and there are few, if any, spur trails to confuse hikers.

Begin this hike from the Lost Goldmine Trailhead (see Hike 33, page 174). Avoid starting from the traditional Carney Springs parking area—that approach, though 0.5 mile shorter, requires a paid state-land permit. Instead, follow Lost Goldmine Trail 1.1 miles to find a small gate and equestrian guard in the Superstition Wilderness boundary fence. Pass through this angled opening in the fence, which keeps out wildlife and pack animals but grants hikers access.

Hike north toward Superstition Mountain, with the cliffs of Three Sisters to your left and the Swiss-cheesy Dacite Cliffs to your right. Look toward Three Sisters from here, and you can actually see the Wave Cave, nestled at its base along a chartreuse-colored band of volcanic tuff. Follow the trail toward the mountain, but make a mental note of the distance from the fence. You'll leave the main trail in about 800 feet.

Cross a dry wash about 500 feet after the fence as the trail narrows and becomes rocky. Look for a sizable rock in the middle of the trail; then find a use trail branching left, often marked with a cairn. There are no major landmarks here, except for a couple ironwood trees, some chain fruit cholla, and a saguaro. Leave the main trail and turn left onto a conspicuous use trail under the ironwood tree.

Once on the use trail, hike along the left edge of a dry wash, amid brittlebush and mesquite trees. About 1.3 miles from the Lost Goldmine Trailhead, follow the use trail as it turns left and crosses the dry wash in a patch of canyon ragweed. Note that some smaller paths are blocked by a line of rocks, so don't step over them. Occasional cairns mark the proper route as you work your way through the underbrush, heading in the general direction of Three Sisters.

Wave Cave

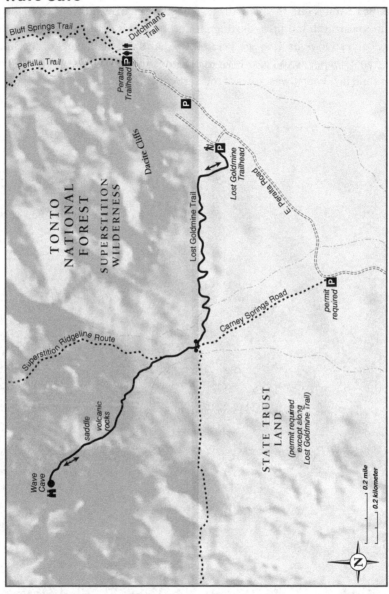

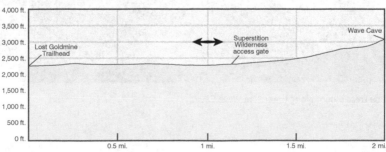

About 1.5 miles into the hike, the trail becomes narrow and rocky. Begin a gentle climb toward the foothills, darting around saguaros and jojoba bushes. Higher up now, you can look back to see Peralta Road and the plains of Apache Junction. The trail gets steeper as you get closer to your destination. You'll pass a couple giant boulders and head northwest toward the vertical cliff in front of you.

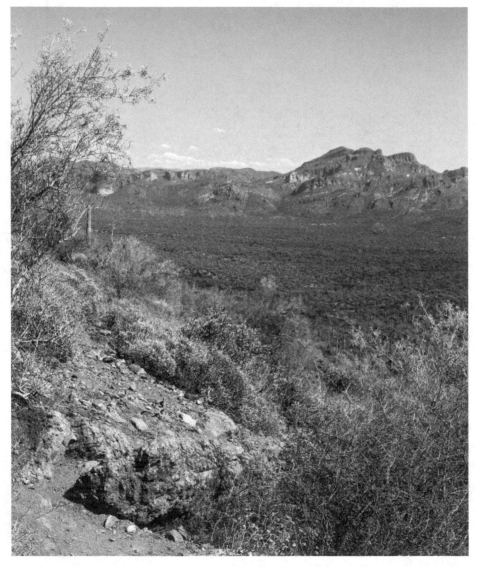

Palo verde trees bloom along the trail to Wave Cave.

A large volcanic rock presents a "threshold" in the trail. Step up and over it to peer into a dry wash. Atop this drainage and to the left, Wave Cave, carved out of giant boulders by eons of erosion, lies at the base of a cliff. Continue following the trail up until you arrive at a little saddle point next to two sizable boulders on the left. Here, the trail dips to cross the ravine. Make sure to turn and memorize this spot. Upon your return, you'll need to climb out of this drainage instead of following it downstream.

Continue making your way across the drainage and follow the defined trail and cairns up the opposite side. There are spots where the footing becomes loose and the slope fairly steep. Take your time here to avoid a slip. The trail winds around jojoba bushes, gaining elevation quickly. The last part of this hike is the steepest. At 1.8 miles from the trailhead, you'll pass a vertical rock wall on your left. Follow the trail as it passes some palo verde trees. The remainder of the ascent is obvious.

When you arrive at Wave Cave, the first thing to notice is the large rock formation at its mouth. A hollowed-out shady cave lies behind it. It is not very deep, but it provides ample shelter from the elements and a cool place to rest. As you look out from within the cave, the tonguelike rock resembles a dark wave against the bright desert landscape beyond. Take time to enjoy the view and take some silhouette pictures. Return to the trailhead the same way you came.

NEARBY ACTIVITIES

Superstition Ridgeline (see previous hike), a beautiful but difficult traverse along the spine of Superstition Mountain, begins from the same wilderness-boundary gate. **Lost Goldmine Trail** (see Hike 33, page 174) runs along the wilderness border and connects to **Hieroglyphic Canyon** (see Hike 32, page 169). The nearby **Peralta Trail** (see Hike 34, 179) is the most popular trail in the Superstitions. Many other trails crisscross the Superstition Wilderness, affording endless possibilities for hiking and backpacking.

• •

GPS TRAILHEAD COORDINATES N33° 23.589' W111° 21.242'

DIRECTIONS From central Phoenix, drive east 42.5 miles on US 60. At mile marker 204, turn northeast (left) onto Peralta Road, and reset your odometer. Follow Peralta Road, which eventually becomes a graded dirt road, to a fork at 5.5 miles. Bear left at the fork and continue to the Lost Goldmine Trailhead (see Hike 33, page 174) at 7.1 miles—if you've reached the Peralta Trailhead, you've gone too far.

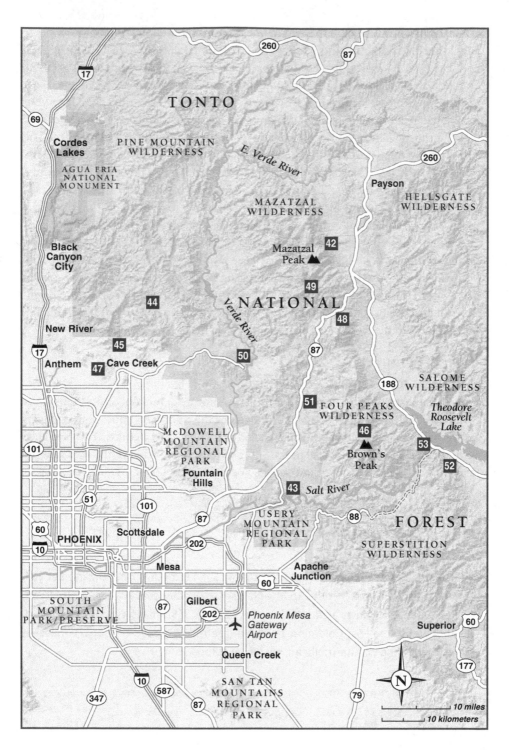

NORTHEAST
(Including Cave Creek and Mazatzal Mountains)

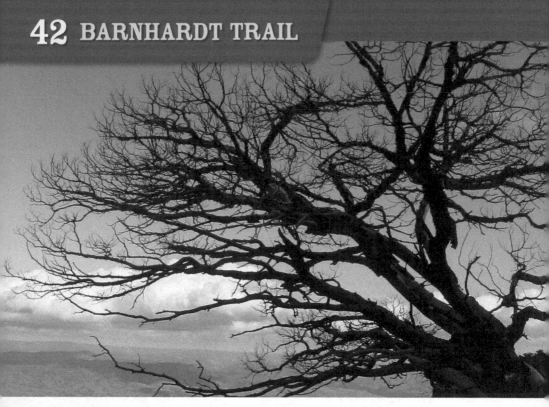

A barren tree silhouetted against the sky along Barnhardt Trail in Mazatzal Wilderness

BARNHARDT TRAIL TAKES you on a tour into the heart of the Mazatzal Wilderness, offering thrilling views into deep gorges, up rugged mountains, and across picturesque hills. Rocky cliffs and spectacular waterfalls accentuate an already dramatic landscape.

DESCRIPTION

The massive Mazatzal mountain range lies within Tonto National Forest and stretches from the Salt River Valley all the way north to Payson. Characterized by a line of rocky summits well in excess of 7,000 feet in elevation, most of which are within 60 miles of Phoenix, the Mazatzals offer desert dwellers a convenient escape from the summer heat. The Mazatzal Divide, a north–south watershed along its major axis, separates the Verde River and Tonto Creek Valleys and delineates Gila County from Maricopa County.

Many trails crisscross these rugged mountains, but perhaps none offers a better overall hiking experience than Barnhardt Trail 43. In spite of this trail being the most popular trail into the Mazatzal Wilderness, many Phoenix hikers have yet to discover its charm. The Barnhardt trailhead-access road intersects AZ 87, a major transportation vein connecting Phoenix and Payson, but most people who pass the

DISTANCE & CONFIGURATION: 14-mile out-and-back, 6 miles to waterfall only

DIFFICULTY: Moderate–strenuous

SCENERY: Barnhardt Canyon, waterfalls, Mazatzal Wilderness, Horseshoe Reservoir

EXPOSURE: Partial shade in Barnhardt Canyon; exposed on the plateau above

TRAIL TRAFFIC: Moderate

TRAIL SURFACE: Rock, gravel, packed dirt

HIKING TIME: 7 hours, 3.5 hours for waterfall portion only

WATER REQUIREMENT: 4 quarts, 2.5 quarts for waterfall portion only

DRIVING DISTANCE: 70 miles from Phoenix Sky Harbor Airport

ELEVATION GAIN: 4,190' at trailhead, 5,800' at waterfall, 6,100' at highest point

ACCESS: Sunrise–sunset; no permits or fees required

MAPS: USGS *Mazatzal Peak;* USFS *Mazatzal Wilderness* (see nationalforestmapstore.com /product-p/az-15.htm)

FACILITIES: None

WHEELCHAIR ACCESS: None

CONTACT: 928-474-7900, www.fs.usda.gov /activity/tonto/recreation/hiking

COMMENTS: Dogs must be leashed at all times

unremarkable trail sign think it's just another desert trail like so many others near town. They couldn't be more wrong!

Barnhardt Trail begins on the plateau east of the mountain, climbs Barnhardt Canyon to a high basin, and terminates at roughly the midpoint of the 29-mile-long Mazatzal Divide Trail, which is also a segment of the Arizona Trail. Along the way, Barnhardt Trail cuts through arguably the most beautiful canyon in the Mazatzals, passes near several seasonal waterfalls, and provides plenty of overlooks from which to admire the surrounding landscape. I should note that the lightning-induced Willow Fire of 2004 devastated more than 100,000 acres of forest in these mountains. Barnhardt Canyon escaped fairly unscathed, but the high plateaus suffered significant damage. Recent new growth and regrowth above Barnhardt Canyon, however, is starting to show remarkable progress toward recovery.

From the large trailhead parking area, which also serves Y Bar Trail 44 and Half Moon Trail 288, begin by hiking west toward the mountain, staying right at the junction where Y Bar Trail forks south. Initially, large rocks covering the trail challenge your balance, but trail conditions steadily improve once you pass through the forest boundary fence at 0.1 mile. The trail soon enters shady groves of alligator juniper and live oak. A few cacti and agaves lie hidden under the trees, signifying the transition zone between desert and forest.

The trail bends around the hills and begins a moderate but steady ascent of many miles. The slope is mostly moderate, but seemingly unrelenting uphills keep your pulse high and legs burning. As you enter Barnhardt Canyon, the trail carves a path along the steep left hillside, forming a natural ledge at certain bends from which to survey the canyon below. Garden Spring, at the bottom of the deep canyon, gurgles among enticing pools and inaccessible narrow passages, sending the sound of refreshing water reverberating high up into the hills. Twisted and gnarled layers of

Barnhardt Trail

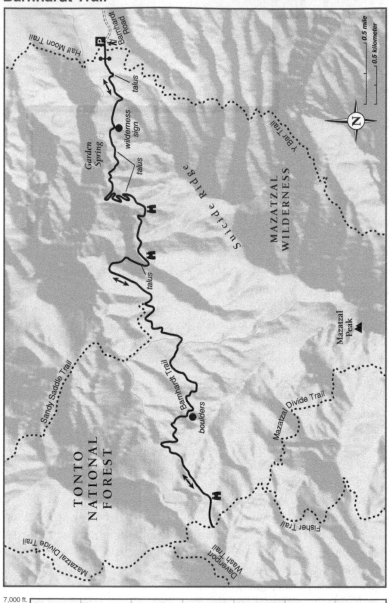

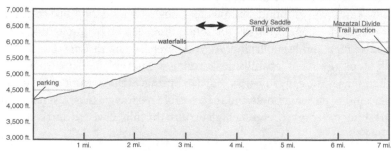

sedimentary rock lie exposed across the canyon, a testament to the violent geologic forces that created this rocky wonderland.

Near 1.5 miles from the trailhead, Barnhardt Trail makes a sharp bend and begins to ascend switchbacks that take you into a smaller but steeper side canyon. These switchbacks offer amazing views at every outer turn; dense tree cover engulfs the inner bends. Pass a talus at 2.3 miles, and dive deeper into the rocky canyon walled by sheer cliffs. Another quarter mile along, look for a rock outcropping from which you command a dizzying view straight down into the canyon.

At 2.7 miles, the trail passes a stunning wall of layered sedimentary rock. Just when you think the scenery couldn't possibly improve, some seasonal waterfalls prove you wrong. In winter, spring, and even early summer, cascading falls tumble over the cliffs that line the trail. Depending on the amount of snowmelt, you may see quite a few of them. The biggest one is near a sharp bend in the trail 3 miles from the trailhead. You'll likely hear rushing water as you walk by. To visit the waterfall, scramble up large boulders to find a secluded and shady rocky alcove where the waterfall tumbles over the cliff from an upper pool. Though reflected sunlight from the upper pool may tempt you, do not try to climb the vertical rock face to investigate. Be satisfied with admiring the waterfall from below and return to the trail.

Beyond the waterfall, Barnhardt Trail takes on a completely different character, and understandably, many hikers go no farther. A short ascent beyond the waterfall takes you to an expansive upper basin, where, from an elevation of 5,870 feet, views of the valley below are stunning. You can look back down Barnhardt Canyon to see the town of Rye in the distance. Manzanita forests that once stood here were devastated by the Willow Fire. Although this high plateau has made a steady recovery, some eerie stands of manzanita skeletons remain, serving as reminders of the fire damage.

Continue hiking west on Barnhardt Trail, which skirts the upper basin at 6,000 feet. The interior of the Mazatzal Wilderness appears almost tame compared with the rugged cliffs in Barnhardt Canyon. The trail intersects Sandy Saddle Trail 231 at 4 miles from the trailhead. Stay left and continue following Barnhardt Trail as it crosses a series of dry washes in the wide upper basin.

Near 4.6 miles, the trail briefly follows a large, dry wash. Look for cairns to guide you across. On the other side, enter the remnants of a thick ponderosa pine forest and hike on fallen pine needles and recovering undergrowth. More signs of regrowth appear in the forest at 5.2 miles in the form of lush grasses and shrubs.

Reach the crest of Mazatzal Divide at 6.1 miles from the trailhead. This saddle point straddles the county line and affords an excellent view of surrounding mountains. A small trail leads to the right—make a sharp left turn to stay on Barnhardt Trail. Over the next hill, begin a gradual descent with a distant view of Horseshoe Reservoir in the Verde River valley. Barnhardt Trail terminates at the junction with Mazatzal Divide Trail, 7 miles from the Barnhardt Trailhead. You can either backtrack from there or turn south onto Mazatzal Divide Trail and then return via the

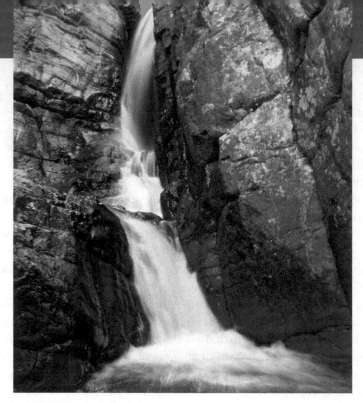

A spectacular waterfall along Barnhardt Trail

Y Bar Trail. However, be aware that hiking the Y Bar loop adds 4 miles on rougher trails and 1,000 feet of elevation gain to your trip.

NEARBY ACTIVITIES

The Barnhardt Trailhead also serves **Y Bar Trail** and **Half Moon Trail.** Nearby **Payson** is a popular summertime retreat for Phoenix residents and provides access to many hiking destinations on the Mogollon Rim. Farther south on AZ 87, many trails lead to other summits in the Mazatzal range, including **Mount Peeley** (see Hike 49, page 251), **Mount Ord** (see Hike 48, page 246), and the 7,657-foot **Brown's Peak** (see Hike 46, page 237). AZ 188, which intersects AZ 87 just south of the Barnhardt trailhead-access road, leads to **Roosevelt Lake,** the largest of the Salt River reservoirs.

• •

GPS TRAILHEAD COORDINATES N34° 05.576' W111° 25.330'

DIRECTIONS From Loop 202, exit onto Country Club Drive, which is also AZ 87/Beeline Highway. Drive north 60 miles on AZ 87 to the signed Barnhardt Trailhead turnoff, north of mile marker 239. Turn west (left) onto FR 419, a dirt road that is passable by most passenger cars. Follow it 5 miles to the wide trailhead parking area.

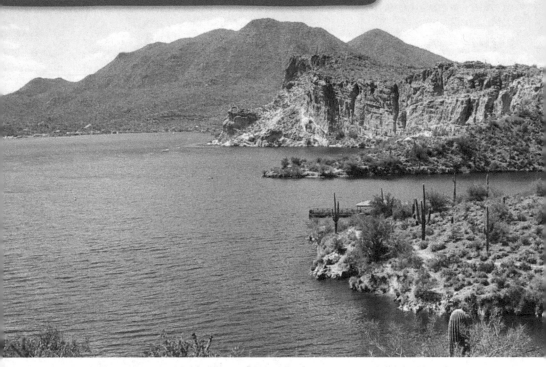

Butcher Jones Trail overlooks Saguaro Lake and Peregrine Point.

BUTCHER JONES TRAIL runs along a section of Saguaro Lake's northern shore, offering overlooks of the lake and surrounding mountains. Burro Cove, this hike's destination, commands an impressive view of Four Peaks across the lake.

DESCRIPTION

As the reservoir closest to Phoenix, Saguaro Lake draws plenty of visitors seeking summer fun in the sun. While most people come here for water sports, hikers can enjoy a scenic trail along Saguaro Lake's shoreline, especially during the cooler winter months. Butcher Jones Trail 463 provides access to some choice vantage points from which to catch a bird's-eye view of the lake.

Easy and well marked, Butcher Jones Trail makes an excellent hike for beginners. The trail's name recalls a 19th-century doctor and rancher whose nickname was "Butcher." (I wonder which of his occupations earned him that gruesome moniker.) Snaking along a portion of Saguaro Lake's 22-mile shoreline, this trail passes through alcoves, rocky slopes, shady riparian zones, and Sonoran Desert landscape as it cuts across a peninsula in the lake. Many spurs branch out to provide waterfront access for fishing, camping, or swimming. With impressive overlooks of the lake and reflections of distant mountains, views along this trail are nothing short of stunning.

DISTANCE & CONFIGURATION: 5-mile out-and-back

DIFFICULTY: Easy

SCENERY: Saguaro Lake, riparian zone, desert, Goldfield Mountains, Four Peaks

EXPOSURE: Mostly exposed, some shade in riparian areas

TRAIL TRAFFIC: Moderate

TRAIL SURFACE: Gravel, packed dirt

HIKING TIME: 2.5 hours

WATER REQUIREMENT: 1.5 quarts

DRIVING DISTANCE: 36 miles from Phoenix Sky Harbor Airport

ELEVATION GAIN: 1,525' at trailhead, with no significant rise

ACCESS: Sunrise–sunset; a Tonto Pass ($8/vehicle) is required but not sold on-site; buy it from a nearby store, or display your National Forest Pass (see www.fs.usda.gov/detail/tonto/passes-permits for more information)

MAPS: USGS *Stewart Mountain*

FACILITIES: Restrooms, picnic areas, beach, fishing dock

WHEELCHAIR ACCESS: One short section only

CONTACT: 480-610-3300, www.fs.usda.gov/activity/tonto/recreation/hiking

COMMENTS: Dogs must be leashed at all times

Begin the hike from a signed trailhead near Butcher Jones Beach. Though the sign reads SAGUARO LAKE NATURE TRAIL, it marks the correct starting point for Butcher Jones Trail. Diving right into some shady trees, the initial trail segment is paved and has a handrail. Turn right when the first handrail ends. As you head south on the paved Nature Trail next to the water, a few pullouts and benches provide excuses to stop and read the interpretive signs. The paved trail, which is wheelchair-accessible, ends at Peregrine Point, where a floating fishing dock protrudes into the lake.

Peregrine Point sits at the tip of a scenic peninsula. The Arizona Game and Fish Department stocks the lake with many species of fish, and this fishing dock is a popular destination for anglers seeking walleye, trout, bass, and catfish. It's worth walking out onto the fishing dock for a view from the lake.

From Peregrine Point, pass through a gate and onto a narrow dirt path that hugs the water's edge and follows the contour of Peregrine Cove inland. At the tip of the cove, under shady cover of thick brush, a spur runs north while the main trail curves right and heads back out toward the lake. If you feel adventurous, take a small detour up this faint spur 0.1 mile to find a 7-foot-high dry waterfall. If you climb this rock crevice and continue up the dry creekbed for another 0.1 mile, you'll find a small but charming slot canyon carved through large boulders by eons of occasional runoff. After visiting the slot canyon, return to the main trail and resume your hike on Butcher Jones Trail.

As you hike out toward the lake again, the trail begins to climb a moderate hill. In the spring, look for wildflowers such as owl clover, lupine, and buckwheat along this hilly section. About a mile from the trailhead is a small mound with an excellent view of the lake and Butcher Jones Beach. The view gets even better at another vista 0.3 mile farther down the trail. Situated 175 feet above the water, this overlook is the highest point on the entire hike. You can see the marina across the lake. Lakeside cliffs to your left frame the distant Superstition Mountains and The Flatiron.

Butcher Jones Trail

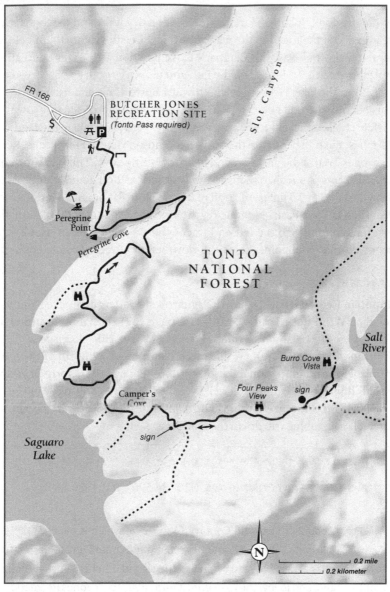

TONTO
NATIONAL
FOREST

FR 166

BUTCHER JONES
RECREATION SITE
(Tonto Pass required)

Peregrine
Point

Peregrine Cove

Slot Canyon

*Salt
River*

Burro Cove
Vista

Four Peaks
View

sign

Camper's
Cove

sign

*Saguaro
Lake*

N

0.2 mile
0.2 kilometer

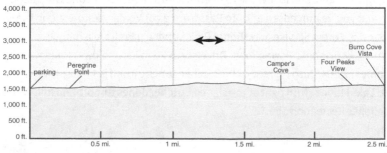

After the overlook, follow the trail as it crosses a dry wash and descends toward the lake. Several side trails lead to the waterfront; feel free to explore them before returning to the main trail. Pass the Camper's Cove junction at 1.7 miles and another signed trail junction at 1.9 miles. Then dip into and cross a large dry wash as you begin to pull away from the lake. Heading inland toward Burro Cove and leaving the noisy motorboats behind, the trail enters a peaceful desert landscape. Saguaros tower over the trail, while chollas, triangle-leaf bursage, and palo verdes dominate the landscape.

At 2.2 miles, the trail bends north to reveal a head-on view of Four Peaks. Remain on Butcher Jones Trail at the next fork and head for Burro Cove. The lake soon comes into view again, and you realize that the trail's desert section actually cuts across a peninsula in the lake. At 2.5 miles, the trail reaches a large flat mound overlooking the lake, with majestic Four Peaks looming on the horizon. Though a faint, sometimes overgrown trail continues to the left and traces the shoreline, the overlook is your recommended turnaround point. Enjoy the view before retracing your steps.

NEARBY ACTIVITIES

Usery Mountain Regional Park, south of Saguaro Lake, offers many excellent hiking trails, including **Wind Cave Trail** (see Hike 26, page 139) and **Pass Mountain Trail** (see Hike 19, page 108). **Brown's Trail** to Four Peaks (see Hike 46, page 237), **Pine Creek Trail,** and **Ballantine Trail** are all accessible from AZ 87 north of Bush Highway. **McDowell Mountain Regional Park** (see Hike 18, page 104), north of Fountain Hills, presents hiking opportunities as well. Nearby **Salt River Tubing** (9200 N. Bush Highway; 480-984-3305, saltrivertubing.com) provides a shuttle service and tube rentals for a relaxing tubing trip down the Salt River.

· ·

GPS TRAILHEAD COORDINATES N33° 34.525' W111° 30.869'

DIRECTIONS *From Loop 202:* Exit onto Country Club Drive, which is also AZ 87/Beeline Highway. Drive 22 miles north on AZ 87, and turn east (right) onto Forest Road 204/Bush Highway toward Saguaro Lake. Proceed 3 miles to the signed Butcher Jones turnoff. Turn north (left) onto FR 166, and follow the road until it ends at Butcher Jones Recreation Site. Make sure that you've purchased a Tonto Pass from a convenience store along the way, or display your U.S. Forest Service or National Park Service pass from a hang tag.

From US 60: Exit onto Power Road. Drive north 20 miles on Power Road, which eventually becomes FR 204/Bush Highway. The Butcher Jones turnoff is 1 mile past the entrance to Saguaro Lake Marina. Turn right at the signed Butcher Jones turnoff, and follow the road to Butcher Jones Recreation Site.

44 CAVE CREEK TRAIL AND SKUNK TANK TRAIL

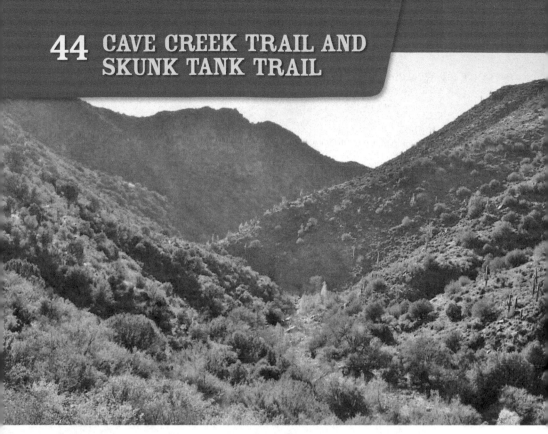

Cave Creek runs through rugged mountains north of Phoenix.

CAVE CREEK TRAIL provides a pleasantly shaded and mild hike along the banks of the perennial Cave Creek. Enjoy the classic riparian flora and the trickling water. Then hike the hilly Skunk Tank Trail for a good workout as you loop back to the trailhead.

DESCRIPTION

Perennial Cave Creek flows through part of Tonto National Forest northeast of Phoenix. Because it supplies water year-round, Cave Creek feeds a riparian oasis and sustains a wide variety of plant and animal life normally not found in the desert. Largely shaded, this area attracts summer hikers aiming to escape the harsh desert environment, and its proximity to town also draws visitors. Hiking Cave Creek Trail 4 is an exercise in serenity—and an experience the whole family can enjoy.

If you crave a more challenging hike and prefer not to backtrack, looping back via Skunk Tank Trail 246 satisfies both fancies. Skunk Tank Trail touts a 1,125-foot elevation gain and takes visitors high above the canyon, where they can admire sweeping views of the surrounding mountains and plateaus. This moderately strenuous trail adds variety and a cardio workout to your day hike.

DISTANCE & CONFIGURATION:
10.4-mile balloon

DIFFICULTY: Cave Creek Trail, easy; Skunk Tank Trail, moderate

SCENERY: Cave Creek, riparian zone, desert, wildlife, Quien Sabe Mine

EXPOSURE: Considerable shade on Cave Creek Trail; Skunk Tank Trail exposed

TRAIL TRAFFIC: Light

TRAIL SURFACE: Packed dirt, creek crossings, gravel, crushed rock

HIKING TIME: 5.5 hours

WATER REQUIREMENT: 3 quarts

DRIVING DISTANCE: 49 miles from Phoenix Sky Harbor Airport

ELEVATION GAIN: 3,365' at trailhead, 4,075' at highest point, 2,960' at lowest point

ACCESS: Sunrise–sunset; no permits or fees required

MAPS: USGS *New River Mesa* and *Humboldt Mountain*

FACILITIES: Toilet, campground, picnic area, but no water

WHEELCHAIR ACCESS: Only near campground and picnic area

CONTACT: 480-595-3300, www.fs.usda.gov /activity/tonto/recreation/hiking

COMMENTS: Dogs must be leashed at all times

Access Cave Creek Trail 4 from a parking lot just past the campground, 0.6 mile inside the entrance to Seven Springs Recreation Area. A large trailhead plaque maps out trails in the area. Begin by following the trail south behind the campground. You'll immediately notice that this hike differs from other desert hikes. Shady shrubs shroud the trail as you walk along junipers, Fremont barberry, and lush grasses. The trail runs parallel to the creek, where white-barked sycamores display golden leaves in November.

At 0.7 mile, the trail crosses Forest Road 24B and dives into a thicket of trees. Look for a marker for Trail 4, and keep right. Climb over a metal stepstool straddling the fence, and then head down toward the creek, where the trail soon intersects Cottonwood Creek Trail 247. At this junction, you can choose to hike this large loop in either direction—I prefer the counterclockwise route, so take the right fork to continue along Trail 4.

Cave Creek Trail parallels the creek and provides plenty of shade under live oaks. Sycamores trees and even a few quaking aspens stand closer to the water. Hoof prints in the dirt trail indicate significant equestrian traffic, but this trail is only lightly used. At 1.8 miles, pass through a gated fence, remembering to secure the gate behind you. Then make the first of three crossings over Cave Creek by hopping carefully across stepping-stones.

The trail meanders up and down the hills on the creek's left bank, where vegetation is recovering from a recent wildfire. As you hike farther downstream, look for a forest of saguaros on opposing slopes that escaped the fire. These giant cacti prefer the warmer and drier environment on sun-drenched southern hillsides. At 2.5 miles, the trail follows Cave Creek southwest and enters a narrow canyon flanked by

Cave Creek Trail and Skunk Tank Trail

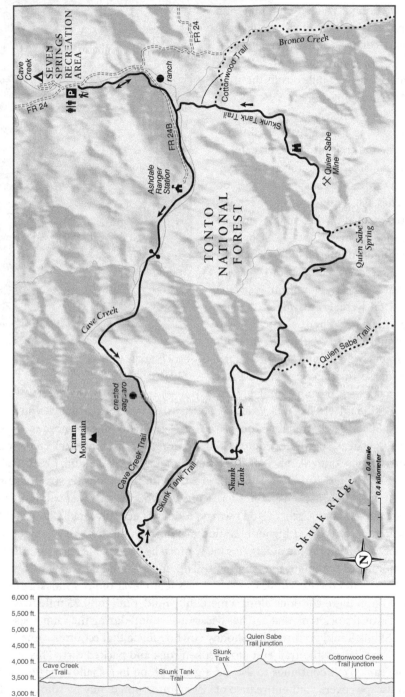

Cramm Mountain. Watch the shimmering water in the creek flicker in the sunlight as the trail descends back to the creekbed.

Cross the creek a second time at a wide, rocky area 2.9 miles from the trailhead. After crossing the creek, climb up the right side of the canyon and continue west, paralleling Cave Creek. Look carefully beside the trail for a rare cristate, or crested, saguaro, which for reasons yet unknown grows fan-shaped crowns on its branches. This stretch of the creek lies in a narrow canyon, where a lush riparian habitat shelters many animals. Don't be surprised to encounter families of javelina grunting and racing along next to you. Follow the undulating trail until you reach the third and final creek crossing at 4 miles from the trailhead. There, the trail leaves the creek and enters a vastly different landscape. Grass-covered open slopes take the place of dense riparian vegetation. Evergreens such as sugar sumac and juniper

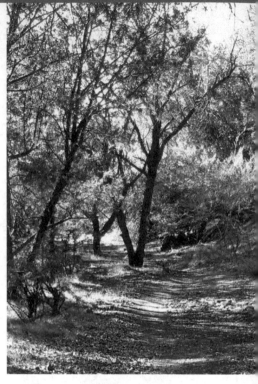

Cave Creek Trail offers a shaded hike from Seven Springs Recreation Area.

replace deciduous trees like the sycamore. Shortly past the creek crossing, you'll find the signed Skunk Tank Trail junction. Cave Creek Trail continues 6 more miles and ends on FR 48 near Spur Cross Ranch Conservation Area. To loop back to the trailhead, turn left here onto Skunk Tank Trail, sometimes also called Skunk Creek Trail.

The hilly Skunk Tank Trail contrasts greatly with the creekside stroll. It turns east and immediately ascends a long series of switchbacks and steep straights to a ridgeline next to Skunk Creek. (Don't worry; it doesn't actually smell like a skunk.) The resultant visibility and higher elevation maximize your views in all directions. New River Mesa's flat profile dominates the western horizon, while various hills and distant mountains complete the panorama. The upward gradient remains punishing until the trail crosses Skunk Creek at 3,665 feet elevation, 5.3 miles from the trailhead. From there continue along a mercifully milder hill for 0.25 mile to Skunk Tank, a seasonal stock tank that catches occasional runoff during the rainy season.

Past Skunk Tank, go through a shoddy cowboy fence that requires some effort to close. Next, follow the trail east atop broken rock and packed dirt. This section of Skunk Tank Trail continues to ascend a gentle slope in a shallow basin. Wide-open landscape covers your entire field of vision, interrupted only by some trailside shrubs recovering from the Cave Creek Complex fire. A moderately challenging trail segment remains at 5.9 miles, where you tackle some loose crushed rock. The trail bends south and then tops out at a clearing where it meets Quien Sabe Trail 250, which takes off south toward who-knows-where, as its Spanish name suggests. This trail junction marks the highest point on the entire loop, at 4,075 feet elevation.

Stay left at the junction and hike east along Skunk Tank Trail, which wanders around the side of Quien Sabe Peak, skirts drainages, drops gently in elevation, and then ascends. At 7.7 miles the trail opens up into what looks like a wide dirt road and descends a slope packed with loose rock. Pass Quien Sabe Spring at the bottom of the hill, and then forge your way east on a high plateau. From here, you can see a distant ranch house near FR 24. A 0.2-mile-long spur trail leads uphill to Quien Sabe Mine at 8.2 miles from the trailhead. Past the mine, the trail finally begins to descend in earnest. Notice an old miner's camp next to the trail, where hundreds of rusted tin cans lie strewn under a tree.

Skunk Tank Trail 246 eventually meets Cottonwood Creek Trail 247 at a flat spot 9.3 miles along the loop. Turn left onto the rough Cottonwood Creek Trail toward Cave Creek. Near the creek crossing, Cottonwood Creek Trail is deeply rutted and bends west before crossing the creek to join Cave Creek Trail at 9.6 miles. Complete the hike by turning east (right) here, and then retrace your steps across FR 24B and back to the Cave Creek Trailhead.

NEARBY ACTIVITIES

Seven Springs Recreation Area offers creekside camping and picnic areas. **Bronco Trail** and the historic **Sears Kay Ruins** are also accessible from FR 24. **Elephant Mountain** (see Hike 45, page 232), in Spur Cross Ranch Conservation Area, lies downstream from Cave Creek. The nearby **Bartlett** and **Horseshoe Reservoirs** provide scenic hikes and opportunities for water sports.

• •

GPS TRAILHEAD COORDINATES N33° 58.344' W111° 52.000'

DIRECTIONS From Loop 101, exit onto Princess Drive and turn east. The road soon becomes Pima Road. Drive north on Pima Road for 12 miles, and then turn east (right) onto Cave Creek Road. Follow Cave Creek Road for 6 miles to the Tonto National Forest boundary. Cave Creek Road extends into Forest Road 24 and eventually becomes a dirt road (suitable for most passenger cars). Drive 10 more miles along FR 24 to Seven Springs Recreation Area, and then continue a final 0.6 mile to the Cave Creek Trailhead.

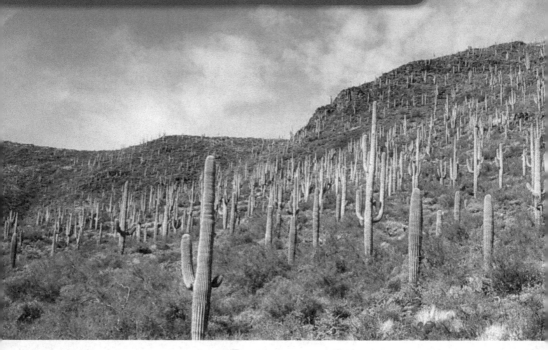

Giant saguaros thrive on the south-facing slopes of Elephant Mountain.

THE RELATIVELY NEW Spur Cross Ranch Conservation Area is the scene of a beautiful hike through undisturbed desert in the shadow of Elephant Mountain. Hiking this trail might make you think you're the first to discover the scenery—and that wouldn't be too far from the truth.

DESCRIPTION

One of the newer additions to Maricopa County's park system, Spur Cross Ranch Conservation Area clearly shows its raw charm. Upon arrival, you immediately get the sense that this hike is going to be a rugged adventure. Crossing the park boundary on foot, using a self-pay drop box, and seeing portable toilets and a portable office all add to that perception. However, volunteer rangers may staff the entrance to welcome visitors. The facilities may be minimal, but they foretell a hike through a pristine desert teeming with abundant plant and animal life yet unmarred by frequent traffic.

As suggested by its name, the Spur Cross Ranch area has a rich history of ranching and even mining. Early settlers of the region found a thriving ecosystem along the banks of perennial Cave Creek on which to build their livelihoods. Today there are still many ranches, but the Town of Cave Creek and the State of Arizona set aside 2,154 acres of desert wilderness bordering Tonto National Forest to create Spur Cross Ranch Conservation Area.

DISTANCE & CONFIGURATION: 9-mile out-and-back

DIFFICULTY: Moderate–strenuous

SCENERY: Pristine desert, Cave Creek, Elephant Mountain

EXPOSURE: Mostly exposed

TRAIL TRAFFIC: Light

TRAIL SURFACE: Packed dirt, gravel, sandy wash, broken rock

HIKING TIME: 4.5 hours

WATER REQUIREMENT: 3.5 quarts

DRIVING DISTANCE: 35 miles from Phoenix Sky Harbor Airport

ELEVATION GAIN: 2,345' at trailhead, 3,150' at highest point

ACCESS: Park open 6 a.m.–8 p.m. (until 10 p.m. Friday–Saturday); trails close at sunset; $3/person entry fee

MAPS: USGS *New River Mesa;* maricopacounty parks.net/maps

FACILITIES: Toilets but no water

WHEELCHAIR ACCESS: None

CONTACT: maricopacountyparks.net/park -locator/spur-cross-ranch-conservation-area (no phone)

COMMENTS: One of the newest Maricopa County preserves; dogs leashed at all times

Elephant Mountain is the most prominent feature in the conservation area. A large, monolithic hill, this mountain resembles its namesake pachyderm roughly in shape and certainly in stature. Elephant Mountain Trail carves an S-shaped track around the base of the mountain, offering outstanding vistas from many angles. The trail also crosses a high saddle near the elephant's head, giving you an up-close look.

Begin the trek at an information kiosk just inside the park entrance. Head northwest on Spur Cross Trail, which is really a wide dirt road and serves as a good warm-up for the hike. Sharing a segment of Maricopa Trail, this trail begins on level ground and gradually increases in slope. The first trail segment passes through a grove of palo verde and mesquite trees that provide limited shade. Then, at 0.3 mile, the trail crosses Cave Creek just downstream from the Cottonwood Creek confluence and turns up a mildly sloped hill. The foundations of an old ranch building lie in ruins next to the trail.

At 0.7 mile you'll continue straight, onto Tortuga Trail, which soon levels out and reveals a head-on view of Elephant Mountain. A bit farther, the trail crosses an arroyo before resuming its climb. At this point, the dirt road deteriorates into a steep, rough pile of rocks. Huff and puff your way to the top of this hill, where you will find an obvious trail junction. Elephant Mountain Trail begins here. Veer right and hike along a service road toward the national forest boundary another 250 yards to find the continuation of Elephant Mountain Trail, 1.5 miles from the park entrance.

Leave the service road and turn west (left) onto Elephant Mountain Trail, a narrow footpath that at times passes dangerously close to some prickly chollas. Soon, a giant basin opens up in front of you, and the trail descends steeply into it. Watch your step on the slippery gravel while descending 150 feet. At 1.75 miles from the park entrance, the trail intersects a sandy, rocky dry wash at the bottom of the basin. Follow cairns and footprints 0.3 mile as the trail zigzags through the dry wash.

233

Elephant Mountain Trail

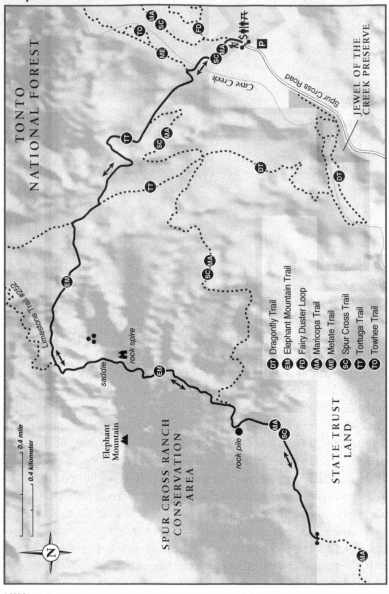

Dragonfly Trail
Elephant Mountain Trail
Fairy Duster Loop
Maricopa Trail
Metate Trail
Spur Cross Trail
Tortuga Trail
Towhee Trail

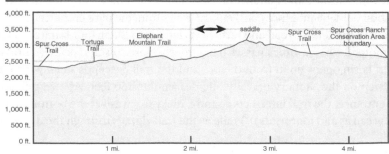

Eventually, the trail leaves the dry wash at a signed point of egress. Follow the steep trail uphill on loose dirt as you draw near a fence demarcating the edge of Tonto National Forest. Continue west, parallel to the fence, in shadows of the huge rock spire that forms Elephant Mountain's imaginary trunk. The flat plateaus of Black Mesa and New River Mesa can be seen to the north across the fence. At 2.3 miles, you'll pass a small trail junction. This spur trail cuts across the fence into Tonto National Forest, where it joins Limestone Trail 252. Stay to the left here to remain on Elephant Mountain Trail.

After the trail junction, follow the path southward and aim straight for the saddle between the rock spire and the "head" of Elephant Mountain. This ascent gets increasingly steep. Even the plants notice the elevation change—you begin to see some yuccas, hop bush, and ocotillos in lieu of dense palo verde trees down by the dry wash. Continue fighting your way up the punishing hill beside the rock spire's sheer northern face. This climb is the most strenuous part of the entire hike, but it's reasonably short.

Located 2.7 miles from the park entrance, the 3,150-foot saddle commands a splendid view toward the town of Cave Creek and Black Mountain (see Hike 18, page 96) to the southeast. Take a well-deserved break here to enjoy the scenery and cool breezes rushing through the saddle. Notice a series of small rock walls constructed of piled stones atop the spire to the east of the saddle. There are many mysterious ruins like this in central Arizona. Table Top Mountain (see Hike 59, page 298), for example, holds a nearly identical wall on its summit; you may be tempted to climb up for a closer look, but a sign prohibits entry into the area.

Many hikers feel content with getting this far and turning back at the saddle. Should you choose to press on, the remainder of the trail rewards your efforts with impressive profiles of Elephant Mountain from its photogenic southern side and a tour through a variety of desert microclimates, each with characteristic geology and flora. Follow the trail south over the saddle as it quickly descends through a layer of chalky, loose dirt. As is the case with typical desert hills, the sunny southern slopes host many species of warmth-loving cacti. The teddy bear cholla fare especially well here. Watch for clusters of prickly branches littered about the trail.

Continue hiking along the slope to a ridgecrest at 2.9 miles where, on a clear day, you can see the Superstition Mountains and Weaver's Needle to the southeast. Turn around and look closely at the head of Elephant Mountain. Notice the strangely striated sedimentary rock that decorates its rugged cliffs like wallpaper. A quarter mile farther, you'll pass a relatively flat landing covered with teddy bear chollas. Turn southwest here onto rough igneous rock indicative of ancient volcanic activity. The trail is a bit overgrown from infrequent use, but the path remains fairly obvious. Few hikers venture this far along the trail, but their absence is your gain because the desert environment remains pristine and unspoiled. It's hard to believe that the Spur

Cross Ranch area nearly became home to condos and golf courses before state and municipal governments stepped in to preserve it in 2001.

The trail continues mostly south as it gently descends the hillside. Soon, Elephant Mountain Trail ends and you are hiking along the continuation of Spur Cross Trail. At 3.5 miles you'll cross a dry wash littered with large boulders. There's nothing but mountains and saguaros as far as the eye can see. Walk a bit farther and pass the remnants of an old fence. As the trail flattens out on a high basin, it bends west and traverses the drainage south of Elephant Mountain. The flora changes dramatically here. An eerie field of dead grasses, dead mesquite branches, and dead cacti surrounds you. You might even find some skeletons of unfortunate dead critters next to the trail. Follow the trail as it runs parallel to the park boundary, marked by a barely visible fence to the south. At 4.3 miles small trees and brush seem to be thriving again. Mesquites, acacias, and palo verdes line the trail, which is littered with large volcanic rocks.

Spur Cross Trail officially ends at the park boundary, 4.5 miles from the entrance. A sign and a loosely gated fence mark the transition between the park and Maricopa Trail. To explore further, obtain an Arizona State Land Department Recreational Permit from land.az.gov/recreational-permit-portal before you cross the fence. Otherwise, simply enjoy the solitude and the view of Elephant Mountain before returning via the same route.

NEARBY ACTIVITIES

Cave Creek Trail (see previous hike) runs along its namesake creek just north of Spur Cross Ranch Conservation Area. **Black Mountain** (see Hike 16, page 96) offers a good hike in the town of Cave Creek. Nearby **Cave Creek Regional Park** hosts many hiking trails, including **Go John Trail** (see Hike 47, page 241) and **Overton Trail.**

• •

GPS TRAILHEAD COORDINATES N33° 53.310' W111° 57.043'

DIRECTIONS Exit Loop 101 onto Scottsdale Road. Drive north on Scottsdale 11.8 miles until it meets Cave Creek Road at a T-intersection. Turn west (left) on Cave Creek Road and follow the winding road 2 miles. Turn north (right) on Spur Cross Road, and take the signed left turn to remain on Spur Cross Road. Next, drive 4.1 miles to Spur Cross Ranch Conservation Area parking lot. The last mile is unpaved but suitable for passenger cars.

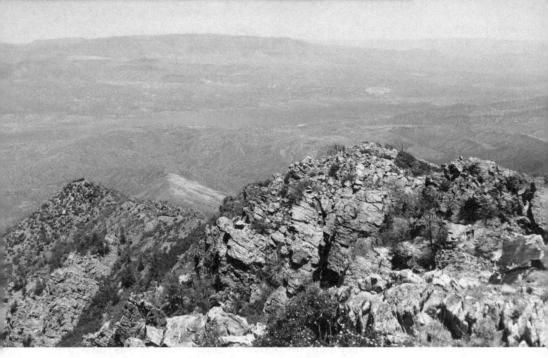

Brown's Peak commands an impressive view of Roosevelt Lake.

BROWN'S PEAK, the tallest of the Four Peaks, is the highest point in Maricopa County. Hike through its oaks and pines in summer for a cool escape from the desert heat. The thrilling scramble to the summit is an exhilarating adventure.

DESCRIPTION

Phoenix hikers often escape to Flagstaff or the Mogollon Rim to hike in cool pine forests during summer. Such hikes can be found much closer to home, however, in the Four Peaks Wilderness. The serrated outline of Four Peaks guards the eastern skyline of Phoenix. Often after winter rains in the Valley of the Sun, fresh snow caps the four summits like alpine glaciers, contrasting with the desert scenery. At 7,657 feet, Brown's Peak is the highest point in Maricopa County, is the northernmost and tallest of the four summits, and is easily doable as a day hike from Phoenix.

To reach the summit of Brown's Peak, hike forested, tranquil Brown's Trail from the Lone Pine Trailhead to Brown's Saddle; then scramble up a gulley of scree and boulders for a stunning panoramic view. The first adventure of the day, however, is getting to the Lone Pine Trailhead, hidden deep within the Mazatzal mountain range.

The most direct route from Phoenix is via Four Peaks Road, a 20-mile twisty, mountainous suspension-durability test. I have tried, and some have even succeeded

DISTANCE & CONFIGURATION: 5-mile out-and-back

DIFFICULTY: Moderate to Brown's Saddle; strenuous scramble to summit

SCENERY: Roosevelt Lake, Four Peaks Wilderness, forest, mountain vistas

EXPOSURE: Significant shade within the forest

TRAIL TRAFFIC: Light

TRAIL SURFACE: Packed dirt, gravel, scree, and exposed scramble near summit

HIKING TIME: 4 hours

WATER REQUIREMENT: 2 quarts

DRIVING DISTANCE: 55 miles from Phoenix Sky Harbor Airport

ELEVATION GAIN: 5,690' at trailhead, 6,850' at Brown's Saddle, 7,657' on Brown's Peak

ACCESS: Sunrise–sunset; no permits or fees required

MAPS: USGS *Four Peaks*

FACILITIES: None

WHEELCHAIR ACCESS: None

CONTACT: 480-610-3300, www.fs.usda.gov /activity/tonto/recreation/hiking

COMMENTS: Exposed Class 4 scramble near summit. Dogs are permitted on leash, but this hike is not recommended for them due to the scrambling.

in, negotiating this road in a passenger car—a rental is best—but it's not advisable. Although four-wheel drive isn't necessary, having a high-clearance vehicle would certainly help. If you don't have an off-road vehicle or a friend who owns one, take the smoother El Oso Road from the eastern side of the mountain (see Directions).

At 5,690 feet elevation, the Lone Pine Trailhead sees temperatures 20 degrees cooler than those on the valley floor. You notice the difference as soon as you step out of the car: the air is crisper and more fragrant, and it seems easier to breathe. Look for a sign that reads BROWN'S TR. 133 near the end of the parking lot, and begin hiking up the well-maintained trail. Live oaks and ponderosa pines provide ample shade as you begin the climb. A quarter mile from the trailhead, use your imagination and look for a large rock that resembles Woodstock, Snoopy's tiny friend from the Charlie Brown cartoons, or perhaps a profile of Barney the purple dinosaur's head.

Continue up the switchbacks. Notice the trailside manzanita bushes, with their distinctive red, silky-smooth bark. Blooming in April and May, their delicate pink flowers resemble decorative lightbulbs hanging upside down. At 0.7 mile, the trail crests a ridge where you can see Roosevelt Lake and the Sierra Ancha Mountains to the east.

Brown's Trail ascends more switchbacks, then turns toward the eastern side of the mountain. The slope is never unreasonably steep, but its consistent grade quickens the pulse. Once the trail straightens a bit, it also levels considerably. Hike a gentle traverse along the eastern slope through Gambel oaks. At 2 miles from the trailhead, Brown's Trail merges into Amethyst Trail at a signed junction. Follow the continuation of Amethyst Trail a short distance to Brown's Saddle, where you can rest and take in extensive views. You can see Saguaro Lake to the southwest and metro Phoenix in the distance. The Superstition Mountains loom on the southern horizon. From Brown's Saddle, Amethyst Trail continues south along the western flank of Four Peaks and eventually ends at Amethyst Mine, a privately owned (but inaccessible) mine where amethyst was once extracted for fine jewelry.

Four Peaks: Brown's Peak

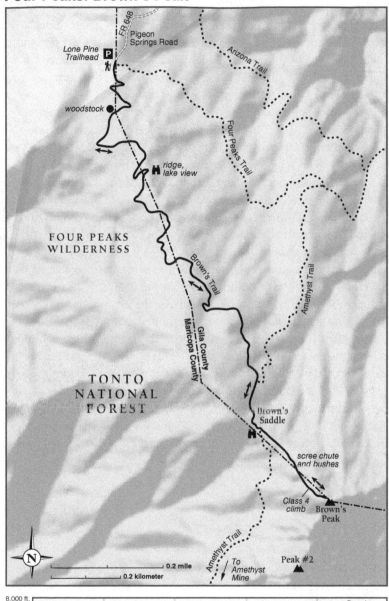

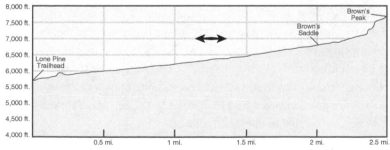

The hike to Brown's Saddle has so far been moderate and nontechnical. Though Brown's Peak beckons from above, the scramble to its summit is for experienced hikers only. In addition to steep inclines and loose scree, you have an exposed Class 4 scramble up a rock wall. The summit route can also be packed with snow in winter and early spring and should *not* be attempted under icy conditions.

To scale Brown's Peak, break from Amethyst Trail at the saddle and start climbing southeast along a faint trail. Look up to find a long, vertical crevice on the western side of the rocky mountaintop—that's the scree chute you'll need to scale. The faint trail eventually peters out, and you must scramble over large boulders. Find your way into the chute by picking a route over the boulders and through some shrubs. Once atop the scree, slog your way straight up the chute. At one point, you'll have to scoot to the right along a thicket of bushes next to the cliff to continue. Look back at these bushes from which you emerge, and remember this spot—when descending, you may find cairns unreliable, and you don't want to overshoot this exit point. When you reach a 15-foot rock wall, climb carefully. The hand and foot holds are solid, but there is considerable exposure—a fall would certainly ruin your day. Continue climbing until you come to a spot where it seems you can no longer continue. Look for a cairn on the ledge above your head and to the left. Scramble up the final few boulders to the summit of Brown's Peak.

Once your heart has stopped racing, soak in the breathtaking panorama from your perch atop the Everest of Maricopa County. On a clear day, you can see for 100 miles. Phoenix looks almost small from up here. Your view also includes the Superstitions, Roosevelt Lake, and Mogollon Rim. Descend the way you came, taking care while descending the scree chute. For a little variety, you can return on Amethyst Trail at the junction just below Brown's Saddle. Amethyst Trail eventually dead-ends into Four Peaks Trail. Turning left onto Four Peaks Trail takes you back to the Lone Pine Trailhead.

• •

GPS TRAILHEAD COORDINATES N33° 42.321' W111° 20.273'

DIRECTIONS *High-clearance vehicles:* From Loop 202, exit onto AZ 87/Country Club Drive, and drive north about 25 miles to mile marker 204. Turn east (right) onto Four Peaks Road/Forest Road 143. Proceed cautiously 18 miles on the rough dirt road to the junction with FR 648. Turn sharply south (right) and go 1.8 miles down FR 648 to reach the Lone Pine Trailhead. Keep left at a final fork in the road near your destination.

Passenger cars: Continue 30 miles on AZ 87. Turn southeast (right) onto AZ 188 and drive 20 miles to El Oso Road, at the other end of FR 143. Turn west (right) onto El Oso Road, continuing 9 miles. Turn southeast (left) on Pigeon Spring Road toward Lone Pine Trailhead at a signed junction, and drive 1 mile to the FR 648 junction. Turn south (left) and follow FR 648 for 1.8 miles to the Lone Pine Trailhead.

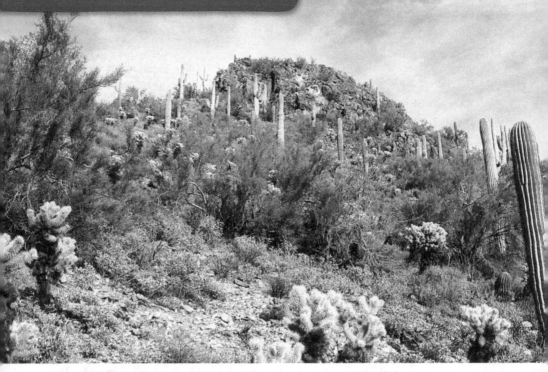

A typical Sonoran Desert scene along Go John Trail in Cave Creek Regional Park

GO JOHN TRAIL is one of the best moderate loop trails you can hope for. Scenic hills surround Cave Creek Regional Park, and the undulating hike has just enough ups and downs to keep you on your toes.

DESCRIPTION

Part of the Maricopa County park system, Cave Creek Regional Park spans nearly 3,000 acres of mountain preserves north of Phoenix and west of the town of Cave Creek. Go John Trail, the most popular trail in the park, encircles its most prominent feature: a 3,060-foot-tall mountain. Contrary to popular belief, however, the mountain at the trail's center is not Go John Mountain; that mountain is outside the park to the east.

Go John Trail offers an excellent loop hike through landscape typical of the mountains near Cave Creek. This trail touches hills, plains, dry washes, and unique rock formations, and, of course, showcases plenty of desert flora. Be prepared, though, to share the trail with other hikers, equestrians, and mountain bikers.

Unlike many loop hikes, where the lay of the land makes one route preferable over another, hiking in either direction works equally well on Go John—here, I've arbitrarily chosen to describe the clockwise hike. Begin by heading north from the

241

DISTANCE & CONFIGURATION: 5.8-mile loop

DIFFICULTY: Easy–moderate

SCENERY: Desert, Elephant Mountain, Black Mesa, city views

EXPOSURE: Mostly exposed

TRAIL TRAFFIC: Heavy

TRAIL SURFACE: Packed dirt, gravel, rock

HIKING TIME: 3 hours

WATER REQUIREMENT: 2 quarts

DRIVING DISTANCE: 34 miles from Phoenix Sky Harbor Airport

ELEVATION GAIN: 2,130' at trailhead, 2,545' at highest point

ACCESS: Gates open 6 a.m.–8 p.m. (until 10 p.m. Friday–Saturday); trails close at sunset; $6/vehicle entry fee

MAPS: USGS *Cave Creek*; park map available at entrance and at maricopacountyparks .net/maps

FACILITIES: Picnic areas, water, restrooms, riding stables, campground, playground

WHEELCHAIR ACCESS: Near trailhead

CONTACT: 623-465-0431, maricopacountyparks .net/park-locator/cave-creek-regional-park

COMMENTS: Dogs must be leashed at all times

trailhead parking lot on a wide, level dirt track lined with chollas, palo verdes, and mesquites. This section of Go John Trail is shared with Maricopa Trail, a cross-county system of trails connecting 10 regional parks and spanning 315 miles. Cross a dry wash at 0.1 mile, and begin a gentle ascent as the trail heads toward a series of switchbacks. The trail bends to the east and then turns northwest with an open view of the city behind you. The climb remains gradual on this smooth, well-maintained trail, which was recently rerouted. The original path can be seen to the left and below the current route. Nearly 1 mile from the trailhead, you'll catch your first glimpse of the mountains and desert wilderness to the north from a 2,450-foot saddle. You'll spot Elephant Mountain (see Hike 45, page 232), with its distinctive shape, straight ahead; you can see the tip of Black Mesa just behind it. Skull Mesa looms on the right. The trail veers to the west and begins a long hillside traverse. If you are already winded, there's a stone bench here where you can rest.

Pleasant and wide, the smooth, packed-dirt trail north of the saddle winds its way through gorgeous desert scenery. Jojoba and staghorn cholla line the trail, while majestic saguaros adorn the slopes. As the trail follows the hillside contour around the first drainage, look back up at the saddle and you'll see a fenced-in area protecting an old abandoned mineshaft. The Overton Trail connects from the west at 1.3 miles, but continue following Go John Trail northeast, overlooking Apache Wash to your right. The trail meanders in and out of hillside drainages but remains relatively level. You'll reach the northern park boundary at 2.2 miles from the trailhead, where Maricopa Trail continues north. Hiking beyond the park and onto state trust land requires an annual recreation permit, so Go John Trail makes a hairpin turn back toward the south.

Go John Trail enters Apache Wash shortly after turning back from the park boundary. Seasonal rains collect in the dry wash bed and feed a different variety of desert plant life, a shady biome of taller brush and small trees. Enjoy a moment

Go John Trail

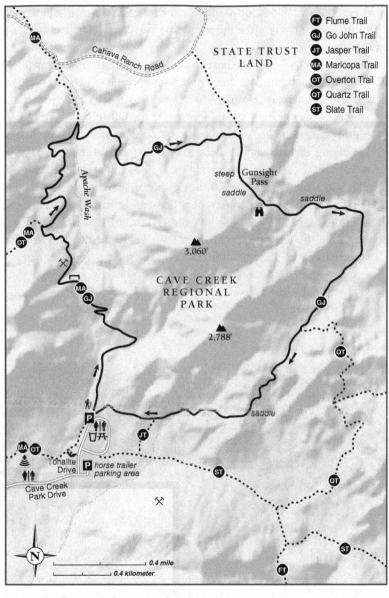

STATE TRUST LAND

FT	Flume Trail
GJ	Go John Trail
JT	Jasper Trail
MA	Maricopa Trail
OT	Overton Trail
QT	Quartz Trail
ST	Slate Trail

Cahava Ranch Road

Apache Wash

steep Gunsight Pass

saddle

saddle

3,060'

CAVE CREEK REGIONAL PARK

2,788'

saddle

Tonalite Drive

horse trailer parking area

Cave Creek Park Drive

N

0.4 mile

0.4 kilometer

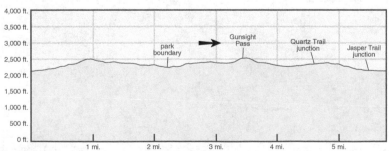

4,000 ft.						
3,500 ft.						
3,000 ft.				Gunsight Pass	Quartz Trail junction	Jasper Trail junction
2,500 ft.		park boundary	→			
2,000 ft.						
1,500 ft.						
1,000 ft.						
500 ft.						
0 ft.	1 mi.	2 mi.	3 mi.	4 mi.	5 mi.	

in the shade here, but watch out for prickly cat-claw acacias, which will tug at your clothing. Almost immediately after entering Apache Wash, you'll climb out and ascend toward the east.

The gently rolling hills of the northern leg of Go John Trail offer open views as it roughly traverses the park boundary. Trail conditions become noticeably rockier, narrower, and more rugged here. At 2.4 miles, survey the expansive views from the top of a mound. A variety of dense desert vegetation covers the hillside. In the distance, the prominent landmarks Apache Peak and Elephant Mountain provide a frame of reference. Continue hiking east through shallow basins, dry washes, and fields of jojoba bushes. Fewer folks share the path here, giving the impression of relative seclusion.

At 3.2 miles, Go John Trail meets another spur trail leaving the park boundary. Turn south (right) here to remain on Go John Trail, and climb a moderately steep, chalky hill 0.25 mile to a 2,515-foot saddle called Gunsight Pass, the highest point on this loop. Admire the view of magnificent Four Peaks on the horizon and the town of Cave Creek below. Shortly after reaching the saddle, look left for a small track leading to a cluster of sharply protruding rocks. This is a good place to take a quick break and enjoy the quiet basin.

Go John Trail winds along an arid hillside.

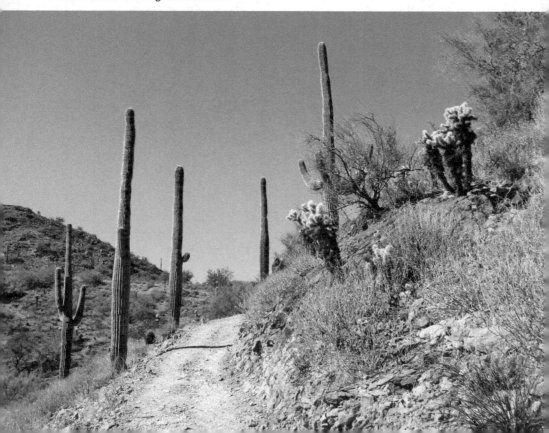

Continue southeast, with Black Mountain (see Hike 16, page 96) directly ahead, until you descend into the basin. The trail bends east here and follows a brushy, dry creekbed. Jojobas, mesquites, and canyon ragweed encroach on the trail, and a forest of saguaros covers the hill before you. Climb out of the creekbed at 3.8 miles from the trailhead. A quarter mile on, turn south for a stretch next to the remnants of a fence, and follow the trail as it bends southwest.

The next mile or so is rather unremarkable as you hike near encroaching housing developments and scrub brush, passing a few dry washes and the Quartz Trail junction along the way. Some striated layers of flaky sedimentary rock provide a little amusement about halfway through this mile. You'll pass an open basin covered in teddy bear cholla and white quartz rocks at approximately 5 miles, then skirt the side of a hill with the McDowell Mountains to the southeast. The trail reaches a ridgeline at 5.1 miles and crosses a saddle. From here, break west to head back toward the trailhead.

Go John Trail slowly descends, crossing a dry wash at 5.5 miles. After that, it meets Jasper Trail, named for the colored quartz that fooled many prospectors into thinking, "There's gold in them hills!" Notice the mine and slag heap on the hill to the south. After the Jasper Trail junction, continue west 0.25 mile to complete the loop hike.

NEARBY ACTIVITIES

Cave Creek Regional Park offers horseback riding, camping, and other popular hikes, such as **Overton Trail. Spur Cross Ranch Conservation Area,** which lies to the north, presents other hiking opportunities at the base of Elephant Mountain (see Hike 45, page 232). Even farther north, **Cave Creek Trail** (see Hike 44, page 227) runs along the perennial spring for which it is named.

• •

GPS TRAILHEAD COORDINATES N33° 49.969' W112° 0.071'

DIRECTIONS Drive north on I-17 and exit onto AZ 74/Carefree Highway. Drive east for 6 miles on AZ 74; then turn north (left) onto 32nd Street and continue 1.5 miles to the Cave Creek Regional Park entrance. Pay the entrance fee at the gate, and then proceed 1.3 miles to Go John Trailhead.

A view of snowy Four Peaks from Mount Ord

MOUNT ORD IS one of several summits in the Mazatzal Mountains more than 7,000 feet in elevation, and the only Mazatzal peak with road access to a fire lookout on the summit. This hike covers 15 miles round-trip and 4,000 feet of elevation gain, a popular endurance hike among locals, who use it to train for even tougher challenges.

DESCRIPTION

Stretching from Payson down to the outskirts of Phoenix, the majestic Mazatzal mountain range boasts a string of five named peaks more than 7,000 feet in elevation along its spine, defining the boundary between Gila and Maricopa Counties. Most of these high peaks are inaccessible by trail or road, but Mount Ord is the exception. Forest Road 626 runs to its summit, allowing easy access to a fire lookout tower and telecommunications equipment perched on top.

There are actually two converging Forest Roads that provide access to Mount Ord from AZ 87 Beeline Highway. FR 626, the main road, is drivable by passenger cars and begins from the top of a mountain pass near Sunflower, at 4,565 feet elevation. The other, FR 27, is a four-wheel-drive road that starts from Slate Creek, at 3,190 feet elevation, and eventually meets the main road 5 miles up the mountain. Both routes are roughly the same length, but the four-wheel-drive road rarely sees

DISTANCE & CONFIGURATION: 15.1-mile out-and-back

DIFFICULTY: Strenuous

SCENERY: Mount Ord, Mazatzal Mountains, Mogollon Rim, high desert chaparral, pine forest

EXPOSURE: Partial shade in upper elevations

TRAIL TRAFFIC: Light

TRAIL SURFACE: Gravel, packed dirt

HIKING TIME: 6–7 hours

WATER REQUIREMENT: 5 quarts

DRIVING DISTANCE: 59 miles from Phoenix Sky Harbor Airport

ELEVATION GAIN: 3,190' at trailhead, 7,129' on Mount Ord summit

ACCESS: Sunrise–sunset; no permits or fees required

MAPS: USGS *Reno Pass;* USFS *Tonto National Forest* (see nationalforestmapstore.com/product-p /az-19.htm)

FACILITIES: None

WHEELCHAIR ACCESS: None

CONTACT: 480-610-3300, www.fs.usda.gov /activity/tonto/recreation/hiking

COMMENTS: Hike travels along FR 27 and FR 626; dogs must be leashed at all times

any vehicle traffic and serves as a nice wide hiking trail. In the interest of maximizing your workout and minimizing potential encounters with passing vehicles, I describe a route from the lower Slate Creek access point to the summit of Mount Ord.

This strenuous hike isn't for everyone. The forest road is not a formal trail, and there are no facilities at the "trailhead." But for intrepid adventurers who seek a lengthy, rigorous, but nontechnical route with ample elevation gain, Mount Ord may be the ideal hike. Many locals use this route to train for tougher challenges, such as hiking the Grand Canyon. The higher summit elevation of this hike, however, means cooler temperatures and shady subalpine forests. Midway up the mountain is a montane zone where juniper, pinyon, and manzanita flourish. At the base, desert chaparral shrubs and woodlands dominate the landscape. Open views are unparalleled both along this winding mountain road and from the summit. You'll likely encounter some snow cover during winter and early spring, ideal if you wish to try out traction devices on a snowy hike.

Begin this hike from a small pullout along AZ 87 where it meets Slate Creek. There are no facilities here, so be sure to pack extra food, water, and emergency supplies. Enter through a gated fence, and then cross Slate Creek, a large dry creekbed, to access the four-wheel-drive forest road. The gravelly path first runs parallel to AZ 87 but then quickly turns away from the highway. Road noise steadily diminishes as you hike among desert chaparral brush, such as Fremont barberry, jojoba bushes, and catclaw acacia. A half mile into your hike, the road noise has completely subsided, and you've climbed 200 feet along the old forest road. Notice the subtle transition from chaparral into montane zones as you begin to see some sugar sumacs and junipers when the road crosses a drainage.

Roughly 0.8 mile into the hike, the road makes a U-turn and presents a stunning view down into Slate Creek Canyon where AZ 87 snakes its way north. Notice some large concrete anchors, remnants of an old mining structure, on a hillock to

Mount Ord

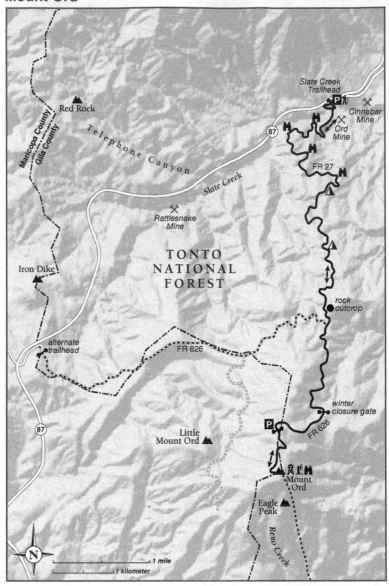

Red Rock

Maricopa County / Gila County

Telephone Canyon

Slate Creek

Slate Creek Trailhead

Cinnabar Mine

Ord Mine

FR 27

Rattlesnake Mine

TONTO NATIONAL FOREST

Iron Dike

rock outcrop

alternate trailhead

FR 626

winter closure gate

FR 626

87

Little Mount Ord

Mount Ord

Eagle Peak

Reno Creek

N

1 mile
1 kilometer

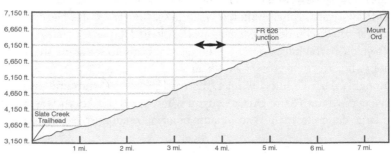

your left. Over the next mile, the dirt road makes several turns and yields impressive views around each corner. You can look back at the trail, AZ 87 winding below, and the Mogollon Rim toward the north and northeast. As you climb higher, views get more expansive. The trail alternates between a moderate climb and some fairly flat straight sections, so it's not overly taxing. Pass a survey marker on the left side of the road at 1.8 miles on a gentle ascent.

At 2.3 miles, you've gained 1,000 feet in elevation and are now hiking among more broad-leaf evergreens like sugar sumacs and manzanita bushes, with their signature smooth red bark. Look to the north and notice a cleared swath where power lines seem to climb the Mogollon Rim and stretch toward the horizon. The road becomes rocky and steep in spots as you pass several clearings on your left, where it's apparent that people camp. The next section of this forest road would put some four-wheel-drive vehicles to the test. Thankfully, navigating these obstacles on foot presents little challenge beyond the steep incline. Your second 1,000 feet of elevation gain are achieved at 3.8 miles from the trailhead.

Continue following the seemingly endless forest road upward. Notice the change in flora as you now hike through a forest of live oaks. At 4.8 miles from the trailhead, there is a unique rock outcrop that was formed by geological forces pressing and kneading layered sedimentary rock. Next, you'll pass a few more makeshift campsites before reaching the end of the old forest road and joining the main road (FR 626). Though it's difficult to miss this intersection, take a mental picture of this area for your return hike. Though not much of a landmark, there is a small personal memorial on a tree on the left side of the road.

Turn left onto the main road to continue hiking up toward Mount Ord. Far smoother than the old forest road, the trail here is much more comfortable for walking. You're now hiking among pines and oaks, and if you're lucky, in the company of passing deer. Taller trees provide ample shade, and it is noticeably cooler. Somewhere within the next mile, you'll have gained another 1,000 feet of elevation.

Pass through a winter-closure gate at 6.2 miles from the trailhead to catch your first sight of Roosevelt Lake. A small dirt road branches off to the right—stay on the wide main road, which ends at a fence and a parking area 6.8 miles from the trailhead. You could arrange a car shuttle to avoid retracing your steps to return, but because it takes almost an hour to drive the road each way, you wouldn't save much time.

To visit the summit of Mount Ord, pass the fence and continue up the service road. You'll follow it another 0.7 mile to the top, staying right at a fork in the road. Once on the 7,129-foot summit, you're duly rewarded with panoramic views of Central Arizona: Tonto Basin and Roosevelt Lake to the east, Mogollon Rim to the north, Saddle Mountain and Mazatzal Peak to the west, and Red Mountain and the Superstitions to the south. The fire lookout tower on Mount Ord is off-limits to hikers, unfortunately. Once satisfied with the view, embark on your 7.6-mile return hike along the same route, making sure that you turn onto the four-wheel-drive road at the intersection.

NEARBY ACTIVITIES

Along AZ 87/Beeline Highway are many notable hiking trails: **Barnhardt Trail** (see Hike 42, page 218) and **Ballantine Trail** (see Hike 51, page 259) are easily accessible, while **Mount Peeley** (see next hike) and **Brown's Peak** (see Hike 46, page 237) are a longer drive. Many Phoenicians escape to the **Mogollon Rim** in summer for its cooler temperatures and superb hiking and camping opportunities.

• •

GPS TRAILHEAD COORDINATES N33° 57.603' W111° 23.898'

DIRECTIONS Drive north on AZ 87/Beeline Highway toward Payson, about 35 miles past Fountain Hills. Pass the signed Mount Ord access road (FR 626), and descend a long, steep hill. After mile marker 228, you'll find a small pullout and a dirt parking area at the bottom of the hill. Slow down to avoid missing the turnoff. Upon departure, drive north 7 miles to make the legal U-turn to return to Phoenix.

Hikers descend the forest road on Mount Ord.

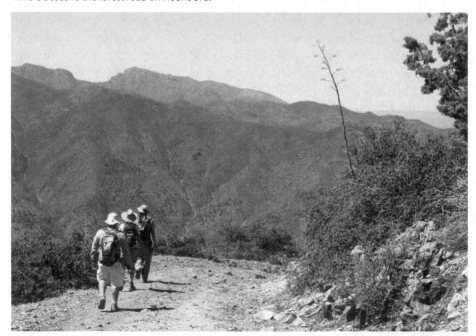

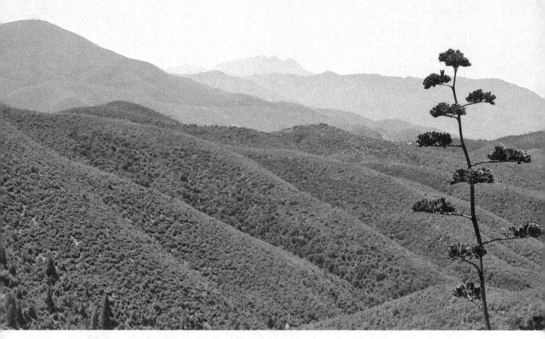

An agave along Mazatzal Divide Trail accentuates forested hillsides and distant Four Peaks.

FOLLOW A SECTION of the Arizona National Scenic Trail (AZT) to the top of Mount Peeley, a 7,034-foot peak in the Mazatzal Mountains. Superb scenery from the summit and along the trail rewards hikers, while the high elevation keeps temperatures relatively mild on hot summer days.

DESCRIPTION

The Mazatzal Mountains form a line of rugged peaks and deep valleys in the geographic center of Arizona. This extensive mountain range stretches from the Goldfield Mountains east of Phoenix north to the Mogollon Rim near Payson. Pronounced "**MAH**-zah-tsal" but often misspoken as "**MAT**-a-zal," the odd-sounding name was taken from an Aztec word meaning "land of the deer." No doubt many deer roam the forests that cover these mountainsides.

Rising to elevations well in excess of 7,000 feet, a string of tall Mazatzal summits forms a spine along the mountain range and provides a natural boundary for Maricopa, Yavapai, and Gila Counties. The most well known of these giants is, of course, Four Peaks (see Hike 46, page 237), a series of serrated summits that form a unique silhouette on Phoenix's eastern horizon. Hiking Four Peaks requires a long drive on rough roads and some scary scrambling. At 7,903 feet, Mazatzal Peak towers above all others, but there are no established trails near its summit. Mount Ord

DISTANCE & CONFIGURATION: 5-mile out-and-back

DIFFICULTY: Moderate

SCENERY: Mount Peeley, Mazatzal Mountains, forest, panoramic vistas

EXPOSURE: Mostly exposed

TRAIL TRAFFIC: Light

TRAIL SURFACE: Gravel, packed dirt, rock; some off-trail travel required

HIKING TIME: 3 hours

WATER REQUIREMENT: 2.5 quarts

DRIVING DISTANCE: 65 miles from Phoenix Sky Harbor Airport

ELEVATION GAIN: 5,570' at trailhead, 7,030' on Mount Peeley summit

ACCESS: Sunrise–sunset; no permits or fees required

MAPS: USGS *Mazatzal Peak;* USFS *Tonto National Forest* (see nationalforestmapstore.com/product-p /az-19.htm)

FACILITIES: None

WHEELCHAIR ACCESS: None

CONTACT: 480-610-3300, www.fs.usda.gov /activity/tonto/recreation/hiking

COMMENTS: Hike follows part of Arizona National Scenic Trail; dogs must be leashed at all times

(see previous hike) presents a long walk up an old mining road to the top, where there's a fire lookout tower. Mount Peeley, on the other hand, provides a reasonable compromise between difficulty and accessibility and allows hikers to pierce the 7,000-foot barrier with just the right amount of effort.

Start your adventure with the scenic drive on narrow Forest Road 201, which crawls up and down the foothills leading to the Peeley Trailhead. Already, at 5,600 feet, you've left behind the desert heat and entered a cooler climate. Find a large ARIZONA TRAIL (AZT) sign, and begin by hiking west on Cornucopia Trail 86. Similar to several other hikes in this book, Mount Peeley requires hiking a section of the AZT, a system of trails that runs from the Mexican border to Utah.

Cornucopia Trail begins in a nicely shaded forest of manzanitas, pines, and live oaks dotting the hillsides. After a few bends, the trail settles into a mild but steady incline heading southwest. At this elevation, colorful wildflowers, such as Palmer's penstemon, bloom well into June. The trail turns west again and unveils an open view toward Mount Ord and Four Peaks to the south. At 0.6 mile from the trailhead, you reach a signed trail junction and the southern end of Mazatzal Divide Trail 23.

Mazatzal Divide Trail traces the spine of its namesake mountain range for 29 miles, intersecting nearly every other trail in Mazatzal Wilderness. Thankfully, you don't have to hike the whole thing to access Mount Peeley! Veer right at the trail junction and turn onto Mazatzal Divide Trail, whose switchbacks demand significantly more from your muscles than Cornucopia Trail. Lined with sugar sumacs and manzanitas, these switchbacks offer ever-grander vistas with each turn. Soon the tip of Weaver's Needle and the Superstition Ridgeline come into view. To the north, two unnamed peaks of more than 7,500 feet rise from the horizon, while Mazatzal Peak remains hidden for the time being.

At 1.75 miles from the trailhead, the trail crosses a dry wash and turns away from the canyon through which you have been hiking. The slope lessens somewhat

Mount Peeley

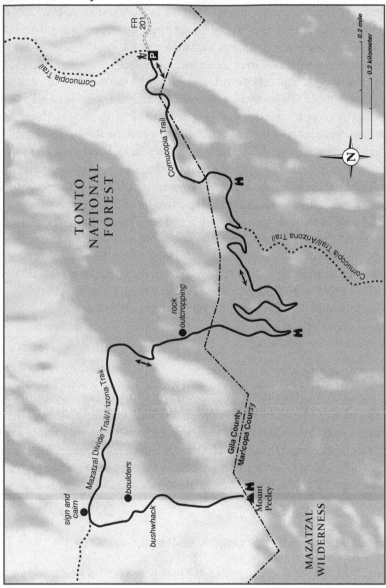

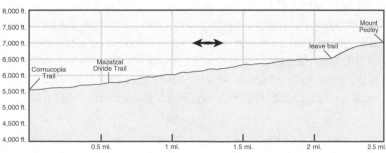

as you contour around the north slope of Mount Peeley. You'll see evidence of the 2004 Willow Fire here. That lightning-sparked blaze destroyed more than 100,000 acres of forest and many pristine trails in the Mazatzals. Fortunately, much of the wilderness has recovered nicely over the years.

Along a relatively straight section of trail, look for a cairn and a burnt sign at 2.1 miles from the trailhead. To your left, a dense forest covers a very steep hill. To make the ascent slightly more tolerable, pass the sign about 50 yards ahead to leave Mazatzal Divide Trail. Turn left and bushwhack uphill through the thick trees. Despite the lack of a trail, finding a route through the forest should be fairly easy. Climbing the nearly 40-degree incline is anything but easy, however. Take your time as you slog up the steep slope, and make a mental note of your surroundings for the return trip. A handheld GPS unit with a topographical map could be of help here.

After 0.2 mile of arduous ascent, you'll reach a rocky overlook where the forest clears and the hill flattens considerably. Notice the intricate gridlike patterns of reddish mineral deposits on the rocks. Finish your climb with relative ease, reaching the wide-open rocky summit of Mount Peeley at 2.5 miles from the trailhead. You can trace the scenic drive along FR 201, admire Saddle Mountain to the southwest, look down upon Horseshoe Reservoir on the Verde River, and sneak a peek at Mazatzal Peak to the north. When satisfied with the view, return to Mazatzal Divide Trail and backtrack to the Peeley Trailhead.

NEARBY ACTIVITIES

The Peeley Trailhead also serves **Deer Creek Trail.** Many **abandoned mines** sprinkled throughout the hills near Sunflower provide a look into the history of the area. Other excellent trails in the Mazatzal Mountains include **Barnhardt Trail** (see Hike 42, page 218), and **Mazatzal Divide Trail.** Other hikes accessible from AZ 87 include **Ballantine Trail** via **Pine Creek Loop** (see Hike 51, page 259) and **Brown's Peak** (see Hike 46, page 237), which takes you to the highest of the Four Peaks.

• •

GPS TRAILHEAD COORDINATES N34° 0.289' W111° 28.275'

DIRECTIONS Take Loop 202 to Country Club Drive, which is also AZ 87/Beeline Highway. Drive northeast on AZ 87 to the Sycamore Creek/Mount Ord turnoff, just past mile marker 222. Turn west (left) onto Sycamore Creek Road and drive 1.2 miles to Forest Road 25. Turn right to cross a cattle guard; then proceed another 1.2 miles to the junction with FR 201. Take the right fork and begin driving uphill on FR 201. Follow FR 201 until it ends at the Peeley Trailhead parking lot, 8.3 miles farther. *Note:* FR 201, a narrow dirt road, has a few rough spots that may require a high-clearance vehicle.

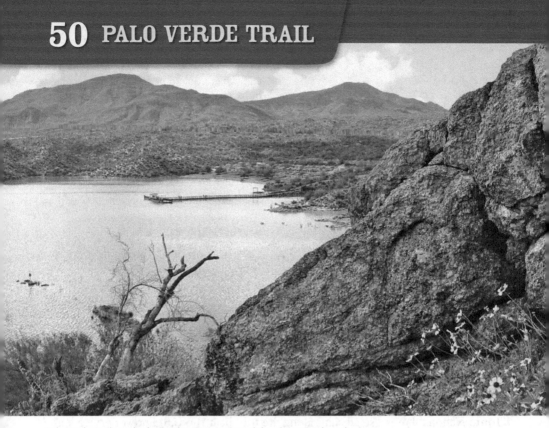

Palo Verde Trail overlooks Bartlett Reservoir and the pier at Rattlesnake Cove.

PALO VERDE TRAIL winds along the shoreline of Bartlett Reservoir, giving hikers an up-close view of the lake and surrounding mountains. Plenty of ups and downs along this trail give your legs and lungs a workout.

DESCRIPTION

Hiking near water is a treat for desert dwellers. Fortunately, Arizona has plenty of artificial lakes, many of which are close to Phoenix. A series of dams on the Salt and Verde Rivers provides the necessary water to sustain the fifth-largest US city, which is in the middle of a desert. These reservoirs also offer valley residents a place to enjoy water sports. A popular urban myth ascribes to Arizona the highest-per-capita boat ownership of any state in the country; though that's not accurate, Arizona does have a relatively high percentage of boat owners.

Bartlett Reservoir, near Cave Creek, is the backdrop for this lakeside hike. Palo Verde Trail 512 links Rattlesnake Cove and SB Cove, two recreational areas on the lake's western shore. Along this trail, hikers enjoy views of Bartlett Reservoir, surrounding mountains, and desert foothills. Though the hike is described as an out-and-back, you could also do it one-way with a shuttle car or boat. A shortcut near the trail's northern end shaves off a mile along the shore, giving you the option to create

DISTANCE & CONFIGURATION: 8.2-mile out-and-back

DIFFICULTY: Easy–moderate

SCENERY: Bartlett Reservoir, mountain views, desert

EXPOSURE: Completely exposed

TRAIL TRAFFIC: Light

TRAIL SURFACE: Gravel, sand

HIKING TIME: 4 hours

WATER REQUIREMENT: 2.5 quarts

DRIVING DISTANCE: 51 miles from Phoenix Sky Harbor Airport

ELEVATION GAIN: 1,800' at trailhead, 1,960' at highest point, with numerous ups and downs

ACCESS: Sunrise–sunset; a Tonto Pass ($8/vehicle) is required but not sold on-site; buy it from a nearby store, or display your National Forest Pass (see www.fs.usda.gov/detail/tonto/passes-permits for more information)

MAPS: USGS *Bartlett Dam;* USFS *Tonto National Forest* (see nationalforestmapstore.com/product-p/az-19.htm)

FACILITIES: Restrooms, picnic area, drinking water, outdoor shower

WHEELCHAIR ACCESS: None

CONTACT: 480-595-3300, www.fs.usda.gov/activity/tonto/recreation/hiking

COMMENTS: Dogs must be leashed at all times

a balloon-shaped hike and enjoy a change of scenery. Though the trail never gains more than 100 feet at any one stretch, it undulates with the wavy terrain and satisfies those who crave a workout on their hikes.

From the parking lot at Rattlesnake Cove, walk down to a line of ramadas and picnic sites to find the signed trailhead at the northeastern end. The lake sits inside Tonto National Forest, so all signs along the trail bear the U.S. Forest Service logo. Hike toward the boardwalk jutting out into the lake. At the base of the boardwalk, turn sharply uphill to embark on a gravel trail. At 0.25 mile, you'll pass a short peninsula that projects into the lake; continue on the trail as it traces the shoreline.

This lakeside trail is surprisingly rugged, with several steep climbs and descents. A good variety of flora lines the trail; some conspicuous flowers you might encounter include tubular chuparosas, pink fairy dusters, fragrant desert lavender, odd-looking chias, and Mexican gold poppies. Plenty of palo verde trees, for which this trail is named, jojoba bushes, brittlebush, and various cacti also inhabit these sandy hills.

Cross a dry wash at 0.6 mile, and then climb a hefty slope to a rocky hilltop. The trail gradually rounds the tip of the hill, affording views of Maverick Mountain and SB Mountain across the lake. At 1.1 miles, the trail turns west atop a mound overlooking the lake. The next 1.5-mile section heads up and down hills, and in and out of coves. The trail also crosses several dry washes that feed the lake and follows a high ridge with open views of the mountains and surrounding desert.

Near 2.9 miles from the trailhead, you descend into a wide, sandy wash with a tall saguaro guarding the opposite bank. The trail forks here. Turning left up the wash shortens the hike by 1 mile, while crossing the wash takes you along the lakeshore. You can go either way, but if you wish to make a loop out of the hike, you should take the scenic route first because it's easier to find your way when you're coming down the wash.

Palo Verde Trail

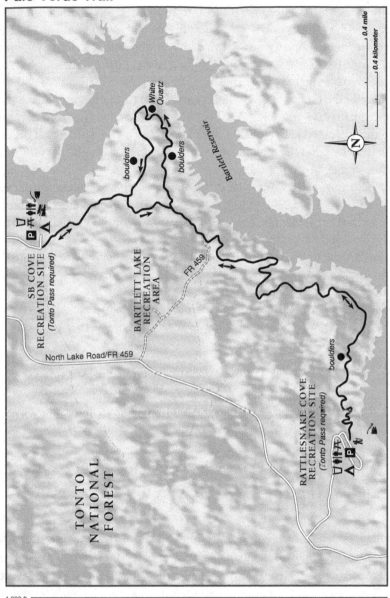

White Quartz

boulders

boulders

Bartlett Reservoir

N

SB COVE
RECREATION SITE
(Tonto Pass required)

BARTLETT LAKE
RECREATION
AREA

FR 459

North Lake Road/FR 459

boulders

RATTLESNAKE COVE
RECREATION SITE
(Tonto Pass required)

TONTO
NATIONAL
FOREST

0.4 mile

0.4 kilometer

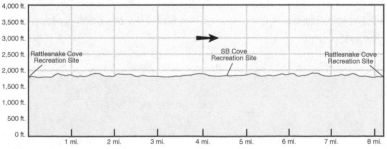

4,000 ft.	
3,500 ft.	
3,000 ft.	
2,500 ft.	Rattlesnake Cove Recreation Site / SB Cove Recreation Site / Rattlesnake Cove Recreation Site
2,000 ft.	
1,500 ft.	
1,000 ft.	
500 ft.	
0 ft.	

1 mi. 2 mi. 3 mi. 4 mi. 5 mi. 6 mi. 7 mi. 8 mi.

Past this fork, the trail becomes difficult to follow at times, so look carefully for trail markers in the form of cairns or plastic ribbons tied to tree limbs. At 3.4 miles, the trail crosses another wash and passes a patch of white quartz. Here, you'll round the end of a wide peninsula near an elbow in the lake and turn uphill toward the west. As you hike across a ridge with the lake on either side, look for a large boulder that oddly resembles the profile of a face. This route rejoins the shortcut trail at a saddle point approximately 0.5 mile from SB Cove, which was named after Sam Bartlett.

From this intersection, turn right to head downhill if you wish to visit SB Cove. The trail descends a gravelly section and then follows the shoreline toward the recreation area, ending at a point on the beach about 0.2 mile shy of the parking lot. Upon your return from SB Cove, take the shortcut at this trail junction by heading southwest. One-tenth of a mile farther, the trail bends south and enters a wide, dry wash. Follow this wash 0.2 mile toward the lake, where it meets the scenic route again at the base of the tall saguaro.

Turn right at the trail junction and follow the common section of Palo Verde Trail back to Rattlesnake Cove. The distance from Rattlesnake Cove to SB Cove along the scenic route is 4.6 miles, while returning via the shortcut is only 3.6 miles, forming an 8.2-mile circuit. One good thing about hiking next to a lake is having the option to jump in to cool off. You can also use the outdoor showers beside the restrooms.

NEARBY ACTIVITIES

Bartlett Reservoir has a shorter lakeside trail called **Jojoba Trail,** which also starts at Rattlesnake Cove Recreation Site but heads in the opposite direction from Palo Verde Trail. The scenic **Cave Creek Trail** (see Hike 44, page 227), on Cave Creek Road, is 10 miles past the Bartlett Dam Road turnoff.

• •

GPS TRAILHEAD COORDINATES N33° 50.919' W111° 37.975'

DIRECTIONS From Loop 101, exit onto Princess Drive and turn east. The road soon becomes Pima Road. Follow Pima Road north for 12 miles; then turn east (right) onto Cave Creek Road. Go 6 miles, and turn right onto Bartlett Dam Road. Follow Bartlett Dam Road for 14 miles to the Bartlett Reservoir entrance. Turn left onto AZ 459; then follow the signs to Rattlesnake Cove Recreation Site. Take the one-way loop drive and park near the last restroom.

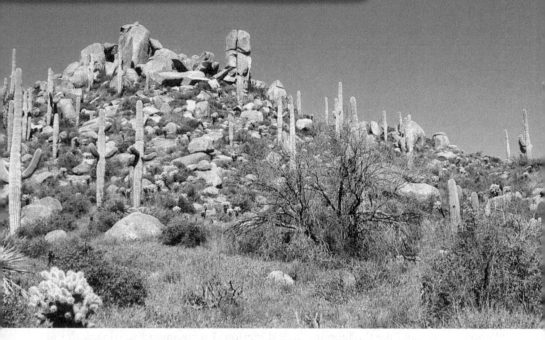

Craggy boulders and a forest of giant saguaros dot the landscape along Ballantine Trail.

THOUGH PINE CREEK LOOP and Ballantine Trail offer easy access to a scenic hike, relatively few people bother to explore these trails. Those who do visit this area enjoy stunning boulder-strewn canyons, views of mountains near Four Peaks, and some delightful seasonal springs.

DESCRIPTION

A major transportation artery between Phoenix and Payson, AZ 87 (aka the Beeline Highway) runs from the low-lying valleys of Phoenix through the rugged Mazatzal Mountains to the pine-covered Mogollon Rim. In recent years, this route has grown quickly from a two-lane twisty mountain road into a busy divided highway. Many Mazatzal trails can be accessed via this road, and the Ballantine Trailhead is perhaps the most obvious.

Situated on AZ 87 and prominently signed, the Ballantine Trailhead sees thousands of vehicles speed by every day. Despite easy access, Ballantine Trail 283 and Pine Creek Loop 280 remain relatively unknown to Phoenix hikers. Those who hike Ballantine for the first time often express their surprise at how pleasant the trail is and their regret for not having explored it sooner. Pine Creek Loop, named for a large seasonal stream north of the trailhead, loops over a hill next to AZ 87. Ballantine Trail begins

DISTANCE & CONFIGURATION: 8.8-mile inverse balloon

DIFFICULTY: Moderate

SCENERY: Desert, Four Peaks Wilderness, rock formations, mountain vistas, seasonal streams

EXPOSURE: Mostly exposed

TRAIL TRAFFIC: Light

TRAIL SURFACE: Gravel, rock, packed dirt

HIKING TIME: 4.5 hours

WATER REQUIREMENT: 3 quarts

DRIVING DISTANCE: 43 miles from Phoenix Sky Harbor Airport

ELEVATION GAIN: 2,240' at trailhead, 3,650' at highest point

ACCESS: Sunrise–sunset; no permits or fees required

MAPS: USGS *Boulder Mountain;* USFS *Superstition Wilderness* (see nationalforestmapstore.com /product-p/az-18.htm)

FACILITIES: None

WHEELCHAIR ACCESS: None

CONTACT: 480-610-3300, www.fs.usda.gov /activity/tonto/recreation/hiking

COMMENTS: Dogs must be leashed at all times

at the farthest point on the loop and extends east into Ballantine Canyon, parallel to many other canyons that channel rainfall from mountains near Four Peaks. The continuation of Ballantine Trail eventually wraps around Pine Mountain and ends at the Cline Trailhead about 11 miles from its start on Pine Creek Loop.

The hike described follows a scenic route through Pine Creek Loop, takes in a portion of Ballantine Trail, and makes a detour to Rock Creek before returning. Although you can hike the loop in either direction, I recommend starting with the southern half: it's more visually interesting, and you also save all the downhill parts for the end. From a signed trailhead at the end of the large parking area, begin by turning right, onto Pine Creek Loop South. The trail circles the hill's southern tip and turns northeast up its main ridge. Plentiful desert plants, such as palo verdes and chollas, cover the slopes. When in season, a variety of wildflowers also graces the landscape. Bluedicks, popcorn flowers, phacelias, goldfields, fairy dusters, brittle-bush, and many others bloom in a kaleidoscope of colors.

At 0.4 mile from the trailhead and about halfway up the hill, pause to survey the landscape. Behind you, AZ 87 swoops across the valley, broadcasting loud tire noise from passing vehicles deep into the hills. Toward the east, a basin opens where seasonal Camp Creek flows from the high hills. Continue following the ridge among chollas and brittlebushes. At 0.8 mile from the trailhead, you'll reach the highest point on Pine Creek Loop. This 2,785-foot vantage point offers a superb panorama of the surrounding mountains and valleys. The trail then proceeds northeast along a flat ridge, with Boulder Mountain towering over the horizon. A quarter mile farther, you'll descend to a saddle where the Ballantine Trail begins.

At 1.4 miles from the trailhead, Ballantine Trail meets Pine Creek Loop at a well-marked three-way intersection. The northern half of Pine Creek Loop turns back sharply toward the west. Save that trail for the return trip, and start hiking northeast on Ballantine Trail. A plaque says it is 3 miles to Boulder Flat, but the true

Pine Creek Loop and Ballantine Trail

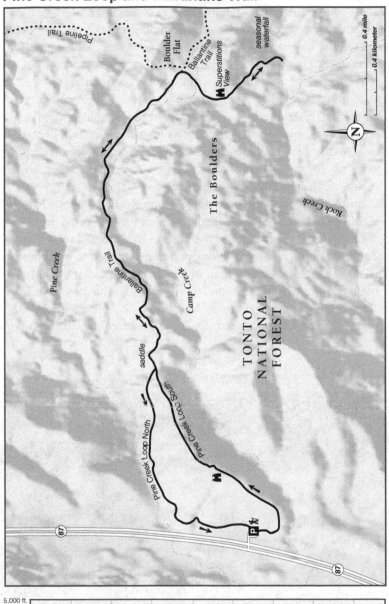

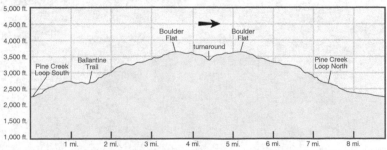

distance is just over 2 miles. The trail first passes some hop bushes and sotols on level ground but soon begins to climb. More charming and noticeably quieter than Pine Creek Loop, Ballantine Trail is also more rugged and challenging. It quickly surpasses Pine Creek Loop's highest elevation and then steadily gains more. An old camp at 1.9 miles from the trailhead offers a convenient rest stop if you need one.

As you climb higher and farther east, you'll see a hilly landscape dotted with large boulders. The farther you go along the trail, the more boulders you'll see. If you use a little imagination, some misshapen boulders look like animals or perhaps Easter Island statues. At 2.3 miles, you'll reach a clearing where a variety of cacti flourish. Giant saguaros tower over their smaller siblings, chollas and prickly pears. Stringy ocotillos, though not technically cacti, also thrive here.

Farther into the hike, the trail draws near Camp Creek. In the spring, the gurgling of trailside Camp Creek replaces road noise from AZ 87, providing a soothing ambience for the hike; at other times of year, you're likely to find total silence here. Follow Ballantine Trail as it enters a large open basin studded with stunning boulders and tall saguaros. Near 3.2 miles, you'll cross a small oasis fed by a Camp Creek tributary and then resume your eastbound traversal of the wide basin. Notice a large reddish hill to your right seemingly comprised of crumbly piles of rocks. On topographical maps of the area, this hill is labeled "The Boulders," for obvious reasons.

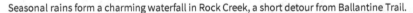

Seasonal rains form a charming waterfall in Rock Creek, a short detour from Ballantine Trail.

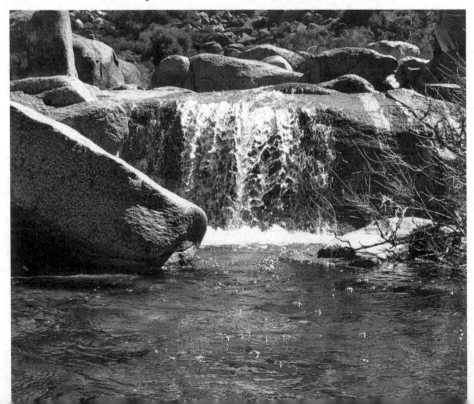

At 3.6 miles from the trailhead, Ballantine Trail climbs to a 3,700-foot saddle guarded by a huge stack of boulders on the left and a lone pine tree on the right. This point is essentially the entry into Boulder Flat, and many hikers make this their turn-around spot. Should you choose to explore further, be aware that several confusing and unmarked trail junctions await just beyond this saddle. (A trail sign explaining your options would be most welcome, should the Forest Service see fit to install one here.) Ballantine Trail proper goes straight through a wide valley and then continues several more miles before bending south toward the Cline Trailhead. A left fork heading uphill eventually becomes the northbound Pipeline Trail. When seasonal streams are flowing, however, I suggest that you visit Rock Creek by turning right and hiking around The Boulders.

The detour to Rock Creek travels south 0.8 mile from the aforementioned saddle. Though unmarked, the narrow trail is easy to follow. Along the way, capture a splendid southern view encompassing The Flatiron in the Superstitions, AZ 87, and the McDowell Mountains. This view is worth the extra effort, even if Rock Creek is out of season. When there is water in the mountains, proceed farther and head downhill to where the unmarked trail intersects Rock Creek. There you will find a slick-rock area in the stream, ideally suited for a picnic.

Return via Ballantine Trail to the three-way intersection with both branches of Pine Creek Loop. Take the gentle northern route back to the trailhead. This flat 1.4-mile section of trail hugs the hillside above Pine Creek until it reaches AZ 87. Though the trail doesn't actually meet Pine Creek, some people bushwhack down to the stream to explore the creekbed. Finally, head south, parallel to the road, to complete the loop.

NEARBY ACTIVITIES

The nearby **Four Peaks Wilderness** contains many miles of rugged and remote hiking trails. **Brown's Peak,** the tallest point in Maricopa County, can be reached via **Brown's Trail** (see Hike 46, page 237). Trails such as **Barnhardt** (see Hike 42, page 218), **Mazatzal Divide** (see Hike 49, page 251), and **Deer Creek** in the Mazatzal Mountains are also accessible from AZ 87.

• •

GPS TRAILHEAD COORDINATES N33° 45.862' W111° 29.601'

DIRECTIONS Exit Loop 202 onto AZ 87/Country Club Drive, also known as Beeline Highway. Follow AZ 87 north 33 miles to the signed Ballantine Trailhead beyond mile marker 210.

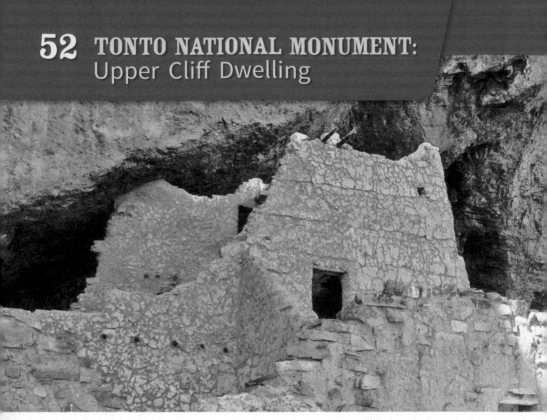

The Upper Cliff Dwelling in Tonto National Monument is accessible only by guided tour.

A LESSON IN desert ecology featuring several microclimates, a history lesson on the Salado people, and an archaeology lesson, this educational trip to the Upper Cliff Dwelling at Tonto National Monument has it all. The hike and views aren't bad either.

DESCRIPTION

Tonto National Monument is small by national park standards, but it has plenty to offer visitors in the way of history, scenery, and a memorable hike for the entire family. For an educational outdoor experience, make a reservation for the Upper Cliff Dwelling tour, pack a picnic lunch, and spend a day learning about the lives of the Salado people who inhabited the area 700 years ago.

Leave extra early for this trip, because it requires a considerable amount of time to navigate the twisting mountain roads of the very scenic Apache Trail. Arriving at the Tonto National Monument visitor center, check in with the rangers to make sure you can get on this exclusive tour. They allow only 15 people per day to visit the Upper Cliff Dwelling, and the tour is available only three days a week between November and April. The extremely low traffic on the trail to the ruins makes this trip a pleasant experience every time. Knowledgeable park rangers guide you up the canyon at an easy pace, stopping often to explain various desert features along the way.

DISTANCE & CONFIGURATION: 2.4-mile out-and-back

DIFFICULTY: Easy

SCENERY: Cliff dwellings, Roosevelt Lake, high-desert panorama, riparian habitat

EXPOSURE: Partially shaded, open areas can be windy

TRAIL TRAFFIC: Very light; by reservation only

TRAIL SURFACE: Packed dirt, creek bed, gravel

HIKING TIME: 3.5 hours for guided tour

WATER REQUIREMENT: 1 quart

DRIVING DISTANCE: 70 miles from Phoenix Sky Harbor Airport

ELEVATION GAIN: 2,838' at trailhead, 3,600' at Upper Cliff Dwelling

ACCESS: Friday–Monday, November–April; $10/person fee, or show your National Park Pass

MAPS: USGS *Boulder Mountain;* USFS *Tonto National Forest* (see nationalforestmapstore.com /product-p/az-19.htm)

FACILITIES: None

WHEELCHAIR ACCESS: None

CONTACT: 928-467-2241, nps.gov/tont

COMMENTS: By guided tour only (15-person limit, reservations required); no dogs allowed

The tour begins at the southern end of the parking lot. After some quick, obligatory safety reminders, the group heads out on the lightly used but well-maintained trail. The rangers unlock a gate and lead the group into Cave Canyon, a delightful and pristine desert canyon that sees very little foot traffic. The first lesson in ecology begins here at a riparian habitat next to the creekbed. Standing in the shade of large walnuts and sycamores, you learn about how this surprisingly moist desert environment provides precious water to feed the plants and animals living here.

Knowledge of plants and their uses helped the Salado people thrive in this seemingly harsh environment. As the hike progresses, you tour several microclimates. Each of these tiny ecosystems is distinct and supports a specific kind of plant. The colonies of hackberries and dewberries supplied tasty fruits. Clusters of mesquite provided firewood, and their seedpods are an important source of nutrition.

Hike farther up the canyon as the trail zigzags across the creekbed several times. The upper Cave Canyon is drier; the presence of more cacti, agaves, and yuccas indicates a dearth of water. The Salado people made ample use of these important plants. The giant saguaro leaves behind a column of tough spines when it dies, and the Salado used them extensively as construction material for their cliff dwellings. Yucca root can be used to create soap as well as to sooth arthritis, and its fibrous leaves make great weaving material. The juices from agaves can be fermented into an alcoholic drink. Indeed, we still drink it today in the form of tequila.

Approximately a half mile into the hike, the trail leaves the canyon and makes a switchbacking ascent of the western slopes. Even though you're climbing 600 feet to reach the Upper Cliff Dwelling, the rangers go at a sufficiently slow pace to make the hike an easy stroll. (On cold, windy days, you might even be itching to go faster to keep warm.) The switchbacks eventually give way to a long straight traverse toward the cave where the cliff dwelling is located. As you climb higher, Roosevelt Lake comes into view in the distance. The Sierra Ancha Wilderness lies beyond the lake.

Tonto National Monument: Upper Cliff Dwelling

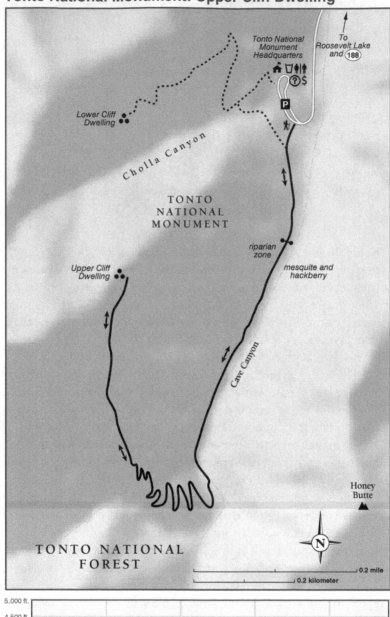

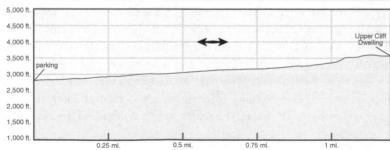

The final segment of the hike skims the base of an imposing, overhanging cliff. When the Upper Cliff Dwelling comes into view, you realize how well protected these ancient homes really are. The inhabitants can see for many miles, and the cave shielded their adobe-style homes from the elements. Break out the picnic lunch here, and listen to the park ranger's lesson in archaeology. Admire the Salado people's engineering feat in constructing these elaborate multilevel homes from the raw materials at hand. Explore the ruins to get a sense of how they lived. Close your eyes. Try to imagine being among the ancients nearly a millennium ago, and wonder what kind of legacy we will leave 1,000 years from now.

After the informative tour, take a moment to relish the views from the Upper Cliff Dwelling. Roosevelt Lake is even more beautiful when framed by one of the cliff dwelling's windows. Once satisfied that you have learned all you can, descend the mountain at your own pace along the same trail.

• •

GPS TRAILHEAD COORDINATES N33° 38.656' W111° 06.760'

DIRECTIONS From central Phoenix, drive east on US 60 and take Exit 196 north onto Idaho Road. After 2.25 miles, turn northeast (right) onto AZ 88, and follow it 41 miles until the road ends at Roosevelt Dam. From the dam, turn southeast (right) onto AZ 188, and drive 4.5 miles to the signed entrance of Tonto National Monument. *Note:* Half of AZ 88 is a gravel road but still suitable for passenger cars.

For a paved alternative, continue east on US 60 past the Idaho Road exit, traveling 50 miles past Miami, Arizona. Turn northwest (left) onto AZ 188, and drive 27 miles to Tonto National Monument.

Enjoy this view of Roosevelt Lake framed by Cholla Canyon as you descend from the Upper Cliff Dwelling.

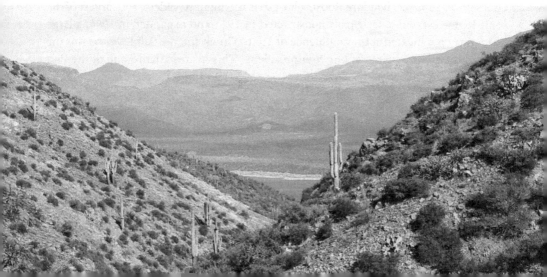

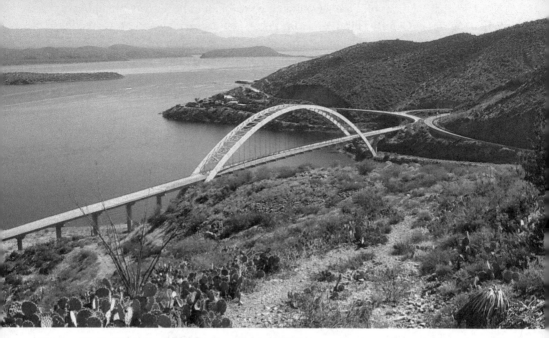

Vineyard Trail offers a stunning view of Roosevelt Lake Bridge.

STRIKING VIEWS OF Roosevelt Lake, Apache Lake, and Four Peaks grace this secluded and scenic hike in Tonto National Forest. Vineyard Trail, a segment of the Arizona National Scenic Trail (AZT), passes the site of historic Camp O'Rourke, where Roosevelt Dam construction workers lived in the early 1900s.

DESCRIPTION

A system of dams and reservoirs along the Salt River Valley manages most of Phoenix's water supply. Theodore Roosevelt Lake is the highest, oldest, and largest of the Salt River reservoirs. Originally constructed in 1911 and expanded in 1996, a large concrete dam located at the confluence of Tonto Creek and the Salt River retains the lake that bears the name of our 26th president. This historic dam—one of the first reclamation projects in the West—provides the backdrop for a picturesque hike in Tonto National Forest.

Vineyard Trail 131 connects Roosevelt Lake with mountains in the Four Peaks Wilderness. The trail begins next to Roosevelt Lake Bridge and ends at the Mills Ridge Trailhead high above Tonto Basin. Along this 6-mile trek, expansive views abound. Hikers can expect dramatic panoramas overlooking two major reservoirs on the Salt River watershed, one of the prettiest bridges in the Southwest, historic Roosevelt Dam, the rugged Four Peaks, and the Superstition Wilderness. With so

DISTANCE & CONFIGURATION: 6.1-mile point-to-point

DIFFICULTY: Moderate

SCENERY: Roosevelt Lake, Apache Lake, Four Peaks, Superstition Wilderness, pristine desert

EXPOSURE: Completely exposed

TRAIL TRAFFIC: Very light

TRAIL SURFACE: Crushed rock, grass, packed dirt

HIKING TIME: 3 hours

WATER REQUIREMENT: 2.5 quarts

DRIVING DISTANCE: 68 miles from Phoenix Sky Harbor Airport

ELEVATION GAIN: 2,200' at Roosevelt Lake Bridge, 3,675' at Mills Ridge Trailhead

ACCESS: Sunrise–sunset; no permits or fees required

MAPS: USGS *Theodore Roosevelt Dam;* USFS *Tonto National Forest* (see nationalforestmap store.com/product-p/az-19.htm)

FACILITIES: None on trail; nearest facilities at Roosevelt Lake Marina

WHEELCHAIR ACCESS: None

CONTACT: 602-225-5395, www.fs.usda.gov /activity/tonto/recreation/hiking

COMMENTS: Secluded trail can be overgrown in places; dogs must be leashed at all times

many nearby attractions, and despite being part of the AZT, Vineyard Trail receives surprisingly few visitors. You'll likely enjoy complete solitude while hiking this trail.

With a shuttle vehicle, you can hike Vineyard Trail in either direction. Starting from Roosevelt Lake Bridge and climbing uphill toward Mills Ridge Trailhead is obviously the more challenging route. The first 1.5 miles yields a heart-pounding workout as you ascend 1,100 feet to Inspiration Point and Vineyard Mountain. The remainder of the trail undulates over rolling hills and winds its way toward Four Peaks. If you don't have a shuttle, just start from the bridge and hike out as far as you like before turning around. Even if you traverse the entire trail in both directions for a 12.2-mile round-trip, the endless vistas will make it worth your while.

From the pullout immediately north of Roosevelt Lake Bridge, walk across the road to find a trail marker behind the guard rail. Begin by hiking into a small canyon and away from the lake. An interpretive sign at 0.2 mile marks the site of Camp O'Rourke, where dam workers and their families lived in the early 1900s. The population reached 400 near this location, although remnants of the camp are barely visible today.

Continue up the trail and climb switchbacks to a large flat area offering overhead views of the dam. Before the construction of Roosevelt Lake Bridge in the early 1990s, the dam itself carried AZ 188 traffic. An interesting bit of trivia is that the original width of the dam barely accommodated two Ford Model Ts traveling abreast. It's easy to see why a new bridge had to be constructed in preparation for the expansion of Roosevelt Lake.

From the dam overlook, backtrack 200 feet and follow the trail as it resumes a steep ascent. At 0.7 mile, you'll reach a saddle where the slope tapers off for a short stretch and the trail parallels Roosevelt Lake's shoreline. Sotols, yuccas, and hop bushes frame an open view of the lake's northern half. Much of the lake you see is

Vineyard Trail

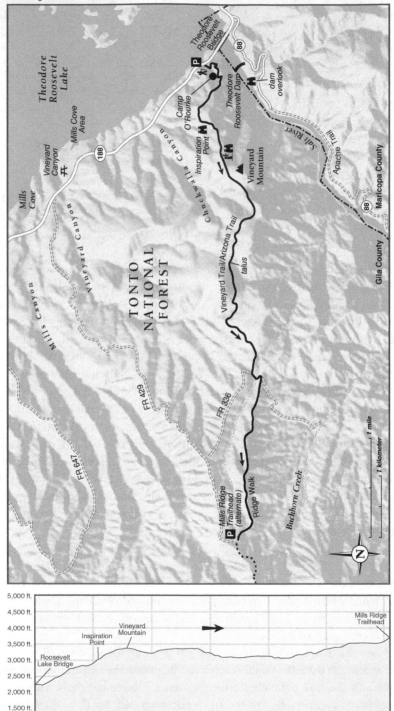

part of the 1996 expansion, which remained dry for nearly a decade until heavy rainfall in 2005 finally filled the lake to capacity.

Vineyard Trail soon bends away from the lake and again climbs steeply up to Inspiration Point. Follow a wide ridge toward an abandoned reflector on Vineyard Mountain. The Roosevelt Lake area hosts a wide range of birds and wildlife. Herons, migrating ducks, and other waterfowl flock near the water while hawks and even bald eagles cruise the higher elevations. Birds of prey often perch on the metal framework of the reflector while scouting their next meal.

Past the reflector, the trail skirts Vineyard Mountain and the surrounding hills. With most of the hard work behind you, you can now savor open views of Four Peaks straight ahead and the Superstition Wilderness to the left. Around a bend in the trail at 1.75 miles, the long, narrow Apache Lake comes into view, with Apache Trail winding along its banks. Though still fairly obvious, the trail becomes somewhat overgrown with tall grasses here. Watch out for hidden cacti and prickly catclaw acacia.

The trail descends slightly while traversing the side of a steep hill. To your left, the Salt River flows through Alchesay Canyon on its way down to Apache Lake. Across the canyon, you can make out the tips of Castle Dome and Mound Mountain in the Superstition Wilderness. This canyon was named after an Apache chief who earned the Congressional Medal of Honor while serving as a scout for the U.S. Army. He also reportedly convinced Geronimo to surrender in 1886.

The trail continues to bend around the hills and remains relatively level. Near 3 miles from the trailhead, descend toward a dense stand of saguaros on a rocky hill, and then cut across a steep talus overgrown with brittlebush and chia. In the spring, when wildflowers bloom in unison, this area is especially beautiful. Beyond the talus, Vineyard Trail dips into a shallow basin and approaches Forest Road 336. The trail becomes somewhat faint and difficult to follow here. Look for cairns to guide you.

Reach the FR 336 junction at 4.2 miles from the trailhead. Turn left and follow FR 336 as it crosses a dry wash and crests a small hillock. Atop the hill, you'll find an open parking area where a prominent sign directs you to leave the road and head up a gentle ridge. The trail again becomes very faint. When in doubt, continue straight up the ridge crest. Follow the ridge 1.5 miles with wide-open views to either side. Vineyard Trail terminates at Mills Ridge Trailhead, at the end of FR 429.

NEARBY ACTIVITIES

Four Peaks Trail 130 (see Hike 46, page 237) connects the Mills Ridge and Lone Pine Trailheads in the shadow of Four Peaks. **Tonto National Monument** (see previous hike), south of Roosevelt Lake Bridge, showcases prehistoric Salado cliff dwellings. Many hikes in the **Superstition Wilderness** begin from trailheads on or near AZ 88. The **Inspiration Point** and **Roosevelt Dam Interpretive Overlooks**

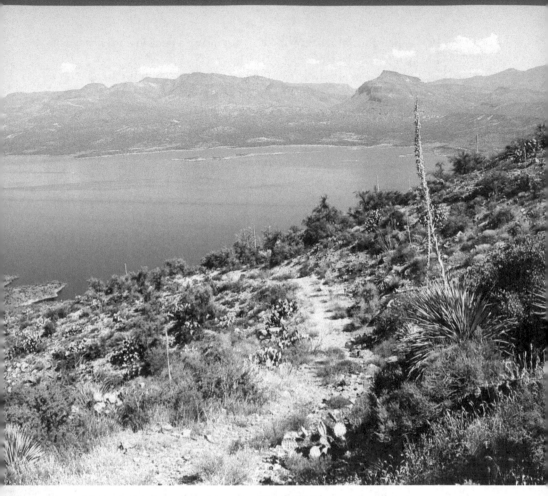

Roosevelt Lake provides a scenic backdrop along Vineyard Trail.

on AZ 88 provide fascinating facts and up-close views of the dam. Behind the dam, **Roosevelt Lake** offers ample opportunities for camping, fishing, water-skiing, and boating.

• •

GPS TRAILHEAD COORDINATES
N33° 40.305' W111° 14.460' (Mills Ridge Trailhead)
N33° 40.609' W111° 09.668' (Roosevelt Lake Bridge)

DIRECTIONS *Mills Ridge Trailhead:* From central Phoenix, drive east on US 60 and take Exit 196 north onto Idaho Road. After 2.25 miles, turn northeast (right) onto AZ 88/Apache

Trail, and then follow this scenic but twisty road 44 miles until it ends at the Roosevelt Lake Bridge. Turn left onto AZ 188 to cross the bridge, and drive northwest for 2 miles. Turn west (left) onto Forest Road 429 just north of Vineyard Canyon Picnic Area; note that there is a subtle left turn on FR 429 shortly after you leave AZ 188. Drive 4.8 miles along FR 429 until it ends at the Mills Ridge Trailhead. *Note:* FR 429 is a rough dirt road but should be navigable by most passenger cars.

Part of AZ 88 is a graded dirt road suitable for most passenger cars. Two alternate routes exist, however, if you prefer smoother and straighter roads. You can continue east on US 60 through the town of Miami and then turn north (left) onto AZ 188—a distance of about 50 miles past the Idaho Road exit. About 32 miles farther, turn west (left) onto FR 429 to reach the Mills Ridge Trailhead. Or, from US 60 in Mesa, you can take Exit 179 north onto AZ 87, drive about 62 miles, and then turn southeast (right) onto AZ 188. About 35 miles farther, turn west (right) onto FR 429 to reach the Mills Ridge Trailhead. While both alternate routes add significant mileage to the approach, traveling at highway speeds should shave a few minutes off your total commute time.

Roosevelt Lake Bridge: From the Mills Ridge Trailhead, retrace your route to AZ 188, turn right, and drive 2 miles southeast. Look for a parking pullout on the north (opposite) side of the road just before the bridge crossing.

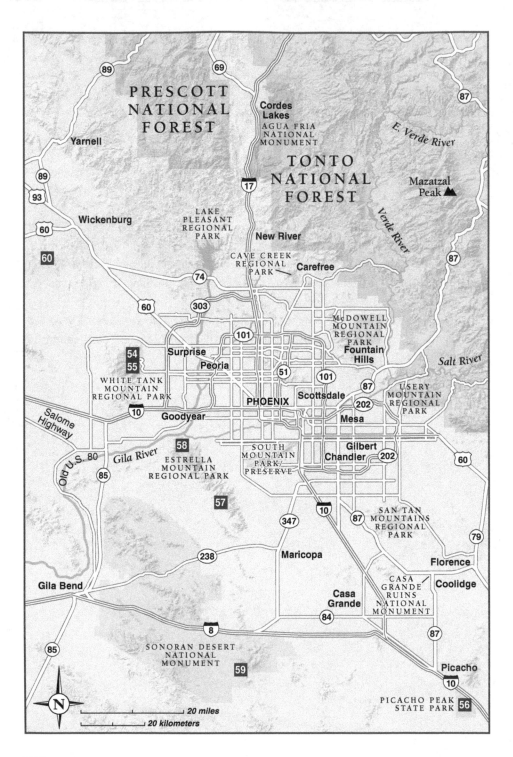

PRESCOTT
NATIONAL
FOREST

Yarnell

Cordes
Lakes

AGUA FRIA
NATIONAL
MONUMENT

E. Verde River

TONTO
NATIONAL
FOREST

Mazatzal
Peak ▲

Wickenburg

LAKE
PLEASANT
REGIONAL
PARK

New River

Verde River

CAVE CREEK
REGIONAL
PARK

Carefree

Surprise

Peoria

WHITE TANK
MOUNTAIN
REGIONAL PARK

McDOWELL
MOUNTAIN
REGIONAL
PARK

Fountain
Hills

Salt River

PHOENIX

Scottsdale

USERY
MOUNTAIN
REGIONAL
PARK

Goodyear

Salome
Highway

Old U.S. 80

Gila River

ESTRELLA
MOUNTAIN
REGIONAL
PARK

Mesa

SOUTH
MOUNTAIN
PARK/
PRESERVE

Gilbert
Chandler

SAN TAN
MOUNTAINS
REGIONAL
PARK

Maricopa

Florence

Gila Bend

CASA
GRANDE
RUINS
NATIONAL
MONUMENT

Coolidge

Casa
Grande

SONORAN DESERT
NATIONAL
MONUMENT

Picacho

PICACHO PEAK
STATE PARK

N

20 miles

20 kilometers

274

WEST AND SOUTH
(Including White Tank and Sierra Estrella Mountains)

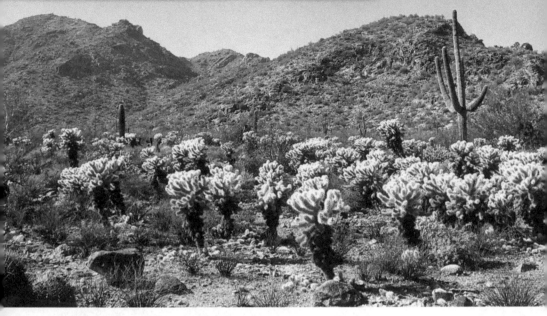

A stand of teddy bear cholla nestled in the foothills along Ford Canyon Trail

FORD CANYON AND MESQUITE CANYON TRAILS showcase the best features of White Tank Mountain Regional Park west of Phoenix. This 10-mile loop takes you through beautiful rocky canyons, sandy washes, and grassy hillsides.

DESCRIPTION

The White Tank Mountains form a massive wall northwest of Phoenix. Seemingly a single mountain running north–south when viewed from town, the White Tanks are actually a complex network of mostly east–west ridges and scenic canyons. White Tank Mountain Regional Park encompasses 30,000 acres on the mountains' eastern flank, which faces metro Phoenix. Within the park, 25 miles of hiking trails tempt visitors with sculpted canyons, sweeping views, seasonal waterfalls, and rugged desert scenery.

Ford Canyon Trail takes hikers up through a canyon carved from white granite. Turquoise-colored water from drenching desert storms pools in deep pockets, or "tanks," eroded into the white bedrock, giving the mountains their name. Even in this desert environment, some pools of water remain year-round. Ford Canyon Trail then climbs out of the canyon and intersects Willow Canyon, Mesquite Canyon, and Goat Camp Trails. Returning on Mesquite Canyon Trail makes a reasonable 10-mile loop.

The official trailhead is at the Trailhead Staging Area, but our hike starts from the trailhead opposite Picnic Area 9 to save a long, flat approach. Follow a short

DISTANCE & CONFIGURATION: 10.3-mile loop

DIFFICULTY: Moderate

SCENERY: Pristine desert, mountain vistas, rock formations, white-granite creekbed

EXPOSURE: Shady in creekbed, otherwise exposed

TRAIL TRAFFIC: Light

TRAIL SURFACE: Packed dirt, sand, gravel, rock

HIKING TIME: 4.5 hours

WATER REQUIREMENT: 3 quarts, 4 quarts during summer

DRIVING DISTANCE: 37 miles from Phoenix Sky Harbor Airport

ELEVATION GAIN: 1,565' at trailhead, 2,950' at highest point

ACCESS: Gates open 6 a.m.–8 p.m. (until 10 p.m. Friday–Saturday); $6/vehicle entry fee

MAPS: USGS *White Tank Mountains;* maps at entrance and maricopacountyparks.net/maps

FACILITIES: Restrooms, water, picnic areas, visitor center, horse corral, competitive track

WHEELCHAIR ACCESS: None

CONTACT: 623-935-2505, maricopacountyparks .net/park-locator/white-tank-mountain -regional-park

COMMENTS: Dogs must be leashed at all times

access path as it crosses a dry creek north of the road and connects to Ford Canyon Trail. Turn west here and hike toward the mountains. Enjoy the unspoiled desert beauty, graced by tall saguaros, prickly chollas, and hardy creosote bushes. Pass signed junctions with Ironwood Trail and Waddell Trail at 0.4 and 0.6 mile, respectively. Continue hiking northwest to the mouth of Ford Canyon. At 1 mile, the trail climbs over a small saddle into a flat valley and heads west into Ford Canyon.

The trail begins to climb at 1.75 miles, crossing a series of dry washes along the way. The nicely packed dirt trail deteriorates into unsteady rocks and boulders. At 2.25 miles, the trail bends southwest and skirts some huge boulders. From here, catch your first view of the white granite that forms the dry riverbed. Continue climbing steep switchbacks for 0.25 mile, and come to the base of a large overhanging boulder, where obvious trail markers guide you up and around it. At 2.6 miles, you'll reach a rocky area atop the white granite boulders, and some small pools of water. The elevation here is about 2,100 feet—600 feet higher than at the trailhead.

At this point, the trail becomes somewhat hard to follow. Look carefully for cairns and footprints in the sand. When in doubt, go over any rock obstacles and head straight up the streambed. At 3.2 miles, a 5- to 6-foot rock wall obstructs your path. Climb this wall and look for an abandoned dam built of stones and mortar. Take a break here to enjoy the beautiful white rocks and pools of water.

Beyond the dam, Ford Canyon Trail continues to follow the sandy wash bottom and eventually turns south. Here, you can enjoy patches of shade created by small riparian trees and shrubs. Pass a side stream at 3.5 miles, and scale another 6-foot wall at 3.7 miles. The climb is easy, but watch your footing on the smooth, slippery rock.

The trail departs the sandy wash at 4 miles from the trailhead, gently ascending an open hillside replete with golden desert grasses that sway in the breeze like wheat in a Midwestern field. This part of the hike offers a completely different experience than going through Ford Canyon. The ascending trail takes you up to a ridgecrest where you

Ford Canyon Trail and Mesquite Canyon Trail

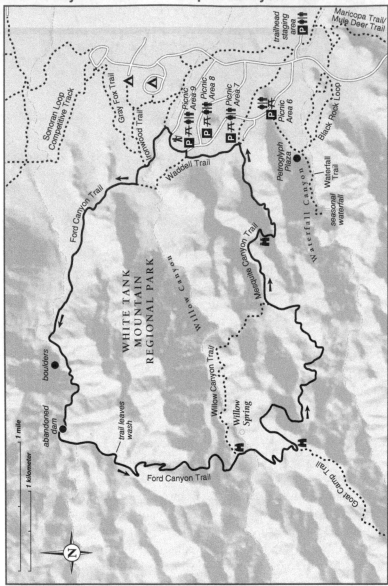

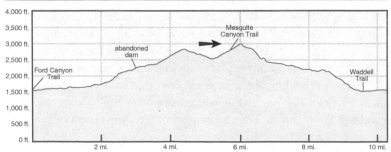

can see the radio towers atop Barry Goldwater Peak, the highest point in the White Tanks. At 5.5 miles, Ford Canyon Trail drops into a bowl where it intersects Willow Canyon Trail. The elevation here is 2,525 feet, and if you can't withstand another 400-foot gain in elevation, you should take Willow Canyon Trail east.

To finish Ford Canyon Trail, continue straight across the bowl and climb south. The remainder of Ford Canyon Trail ascends this slope via a series of long switchbacks to the highest point of the hike at 2,950 feet elevation. High on this ridge, 6.4 miles from the start, is the confluence of three major trails in the park: Ford Canyon, Mesquite Canyon, and Goat Camp. Turn east here onto Mesquite Canyon Trail.

Your return hike on Mesquite Canyon Trail begins with an impressive eastern view of the canyon below and the city in the distance. Next to the trail, shrubs such as Mormon tea and brittlebush paint the landscape in lively colors. A short but fairly steep descent on gravel-covered switchbacks at 6.75 miles requires careful stepping. Soon thereafter, hike across a small bowl full of jojoba, goldenrod, and prickly pear cacti. The trail can be somewhat faint here; be careful to follow it to the east.

Climb out of the small bowl and descend into a large drainage. The trail cuts to the south but makes a sharp bend north and intersects the lower end of Willow Canyon Trail at 7.9 miles. Had you taken Willow Canyon Trail earlier, you'd have emerged here next to a thicket of mesquite trees and a creekbed with the signature white granite and pools. Follow Mesquite Canyon Trail east along the creek. Half a mile on, you'll catch one last glimpse of the red rock–lined canyon ahead, then climb over a ridge to the southeast. At 8.6 miles you'll descend on long switchbacks into the next canyon and hike east for another mile to the Waddell Trail junction near Picnic Area 7.

Finish the hike by taking Waddell Trail north 0.5 mile to a sign that reads TRAIL-HEAD and points east. Turn east here and hike a short distance to the paved Ford Canyon Road. Follow the road northeast back to Picnic Area 9, completing the loop.

NEARBY ACTIVITIES

The park's **Waterfall Trail** is popular after heavy storms. **Wildlife World Zoo** (623-935-WILD, wildlifeworld.com) is 6 miles from the park entrance.

· ·

GPS TRAILHEAD COORDINATES N33° 36.010' W112° 30.606'

DIRECTIONS Drive west from Phoenix on I-10. At 9.5 miles west of Loop 101, exit onto Loop 303 north. Continue 7.5 miles on Loop 303 to Olive Avenue. Drive west (left) on Olive Avenue 4.5 miles to the entrance of White Tank Mountain Regional Park. Drive 3 more miles inside the park; then turn left onto Ford Canyon Road. Drive 0.5 mile to Picnic Area 9, where you'll see a sign for Ford Canyon Trail.

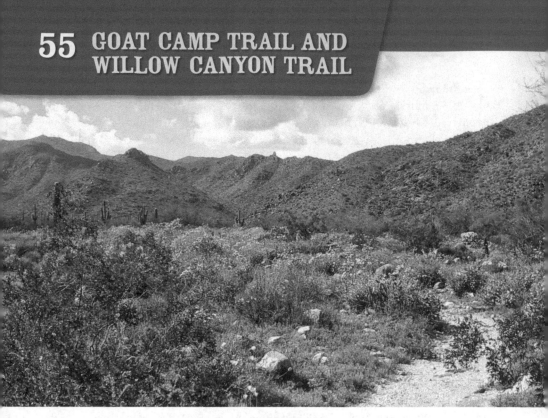

Goat Camp Trail passes through a field of wildflowers in White Tank Mountain Regional Park.

GOAT CAMP TRAIL is the most challenging hike in White Tank Mountain Regional Park, taking hikers on a long ascent through a canyon to the base of the antenna-studded Barry Goldwater Peak. Return on Willow Canyon Trail for another scenic tour.

DESCRIPTION

White Tank Mountain Regional Park encompasses nearly 30,000 acres of desert wilderness, making it the largest regional park in Maricopa County's park system. Within its boundaries many trails crisscross the eastern flank of the White Tank Mountains, which were named for the perennial pools of water that flash floods have carved from the white-granite canyons. This massive mountain range dominates Phoenix's western horizon and features excellent hiking trails. Hilltop views of the city are plentiful; plus, these trails take visitors through secluded wilderness areas.

From the park's many ramadas and trailheads, four main trails run deep into the hills: Ford Canyon, Goat Camp, Mesquite Canyon, and Willow Canyon. By taking this 11.5-mile one-way route, you touch them all. First, stash a shuttle vehicle at the Mesquite Canyon Trailhead in the Trailhead Staging Area, or save a mile of flat hiking by leaving your shuttle vehicle at Picnic Area 7.

DISTANCE & CONFIGURATION: 11.5-mile point-to-point

DIFFICULTY: Strenuous

SCENERY: Pristine desert, mountain vistas, rock formations, white-granite creekbed

EXPOSURE: Mostly exposed

TRAIL TRAFFIC: Light

TRAIL SURFACE: Packed dirt, sand, gravel, rocky creekbed

HIKING TIME: 5.5 hours

WATER REQUIREMENT: 3 quarts, 4 quarts during summer

DRIVING DISTANCE: 37 miles from Phoenix Sky Harbor Airport

ELEVATION GAIN: 1,495' at trailhead, 3,235' at highest point

ACCESS: Gates open 6 a.m.–8 p.m. (until 10 p.m. Friday–Saturday); $6/vehicle entry fee

MAPS: USGS *White Tank Mountains;* maps available at entrance and maricopacountyparks.net/maps

FACILITIES: Restrooms, drinking water, picnic areas, visitor center, horse corral, competitive track

WHEELCHAIR ACCESS: None

CONTACT: 623-935-2505, maricopacountyparks.net/park-locator/white-tank-mountain-regional-park

COMMENTS: Dogs must be leashed at all times

Begin the hike from the Goat Camp Trailhead, on Black Canyon Drive just inside the park's entrance. Head west toward the hills on Goat Camp Trail, which starts out fairly flat across the desert floor but eventually becomes the most challenging trail in the park. Pass intersections with Bajada and South Trails at 0.4 and 0.75 mile, respectively, as you approach Goat Canyon.

About 1 mile into the hike, you'll cross several dry washes as you continue west among creosote bushes and palo verde trees. A half mile on, the trail enters Goat Canyon and begins to climb up the white bedrock on the right side of the canyon below a chiseled summit. Cross the dry wash and ascend the left side of the canyon, hiking steep switchbacks. Turn around here and look through the end of the canyon. You can see Camelback Mountain through the V-shaped gap formed by the hillsides.

After the switchbacks the trail turns steeply uphill and gains roughly 600 feet in just 0.5 mile. Chug your way through this tough ascent on the southern side of the canyon. Look down into the canyon for "white tanks"—pools of water carved into white-granite bedrock along the dry wash. At 2.2 miles, you'll reach the head of the steep canyon, where a tattered saguaro seems to grow straight from the rock.

Beyond the saguaro, Goat Camp Trail enters a wide upper basin and flattens out considerably. Hike into the heart of the basin with the antenna-studded mountaintop directly ahead. The upper basin supports a wide variety of desert flora, including Mormon tea, ocotillos, agaves, various cacti, jojoba, and many desert grasses. At 2.5 miles, the trail begins to climb out of the upper basin, heading toward distant radio towers. Make a sharp turn north, and cross a dry wash. Begin ascending the right side of the basin toward a stand of tall saguaros. This section of trail, covered with broken rock, becomes rough and crumbly. An occasional blue paint spot marks the correct route. Reach a ridgetop at 3.1 miles, where another lone saguaro stands guard.

Goat Camp Trail and Willow Canyon Trail

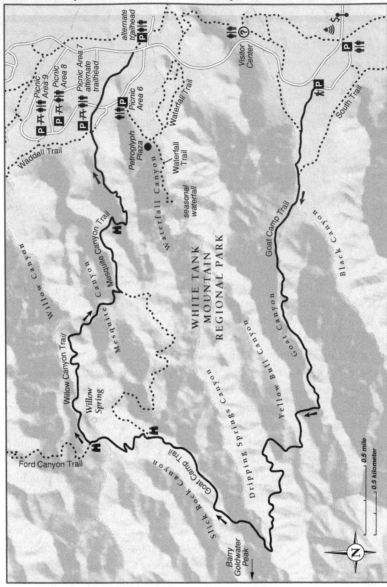

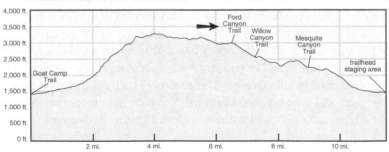

With most of the uphill struggle now behind you, you can enjoy the view as the trail begins to contour around the mountainside. First, traverse the drainage below the ridge, passing the highest point on the entire hike somewhere along the way. Then turn west in the direction of Barry Goldwater Peak (named after the legendary Arizona lawmaker), the tallest point in the White Tanks. Unfortunately, Goat Camp Trail doesn't reach its 4,083-foot summit. Instead, the trail crosses a drainage at 4.8 miles and makes a U-turn. As you skirt the next hill, look next to the trail for an intertwined pair of saguaros that appears to be frozen in a waltz. Hike atop a ridge with wide-open views of distant cities and the hills deep within the White Tank Mountains to reach a three-way junction with Ford Canyon, Goat Camp, and Mesquite Canyon Trails at 6.3 miles.

You could take Mesquite Canyon Trail (see previous hike) back, but I opted for the scenic but slightly longer Willow Canyon loop. From the three-way junction, follow Ford Canyon Trail down toward a wide basin below. The trail descends quickly via switchbacks, crosses a wide drainage at the basin's bottom, and intersects Willow Canyon Trail at 7.2 miles. Turn east onto the wide Willow Canyon Trail, lined by typical Sonoran Desert plants such as staghorn cholla, ocotillo, mesquite, and palo verde. A quarter mile on, the trail rounds a bend next to a fenced-off dike near Willow Spring before diving into a dry riverbed.

At 7.6 miles, you'll cut away from the wash and climb for a stretch, but the trail soon returns to the wash. Pass through a thicket of willows, and then emerge into a serene little valley framed by bleached granite and shining pools. Look for cairns to guide your egress. The trail eventually ascends the right bank, passing a rock outcropping at 8.1 miles. Take a quick break here to admire Willow Canyon, which is framed by chiseled hills and features many white tanks along the creekbed below.

Continue along Willow Canyon Trail to the top of a prominent saddle at 2,425 feet. Cross the saddle and descend into Mesquite Canyon, where the trail eventually meets Mesquite Canyon Trail near a stand of mesquite trees at 8.8 miles from the trailhead. Turn left onto Mesquite Canyon Trail, and follow it to the Waddell Trail junction and Picnic Area 7. Finish the hike by following Mesquite Canyon Trail east for another mile along flat desert, across Waterfall Canyon Road and White Tanks Mountain Road, and finally to the Mesquite Trailhead in the Trailhead Staging Area.

NEARBY ACTIVITIES

White Tank Mountain Regional Park contains many hiking trails, including the **Ford Canyon Trail** (see previous hike) and the **Waterfall Trail,** which is especially beautiful right after heavy storms. There is a multiuse competitive track inside the park. **Wildlife World Zoo** (623-935-WILD, wildlifeworld.com) is only 6 miles from the park entrance at Loop 303 and Northern Avenue.

GPS TRAILHEAD COORDINATES
N33° 35.246' W112° 29.991' (Trailhead Staging Area)
N33° 34.122' W112° 30.325' (Goat Camp Trailhead)

DIRECTIONS *Trailhead Staging Area:* Drive west from Phoenix on I-10. At 9.5 miles west of Loop 101, exit onto Loop 303 north. Continue 7.5 miles on Loop 303 to Olive Avenue. Take Olive Avenue west (left) 4.5 miles to the entrance of White Tank Mountain Regional Park. Inside the park, head north on White Tank Mountain Road; in 2.2 miles, turn right on Wildlife Way and make an immediate left into the Trailhead Staging Area to leave a shuttle.

Goat Camp Trailhead: From the Trailhead Staging Area, drive about 1.5 miles south on White Tank Mountain Road, take the first right, and park at the Goat Camp Trailhead on Black Canyon Drive.

Late-afternoon sunlight reflected by a small pool along Goat Camp Trail

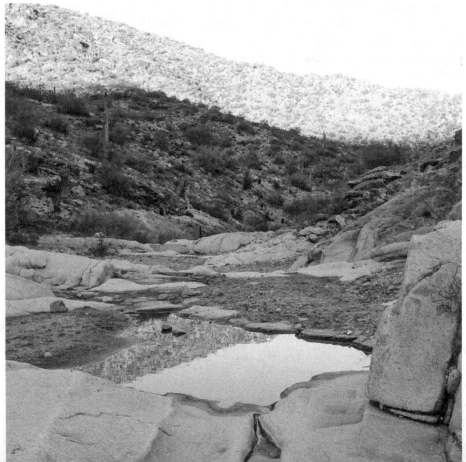

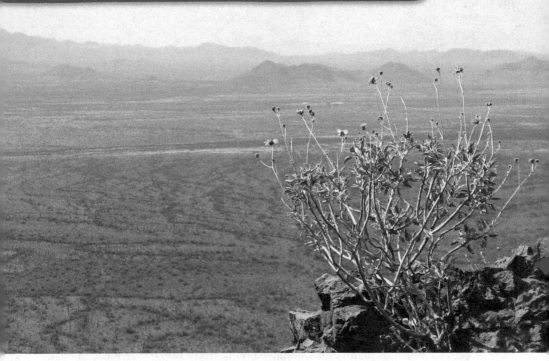

A lone brittlebush blooms on a rocky crag overlooking desert plains on Picacho Peak's Hunter Trail.

THIS SPECTACULAR CLIMB up Picacho Peak packs plenty of adventure into a short hike. The challenging Hunter Trail coils around sheer cliffs and rocky slopes. Cables assist in your scramble to a panoramic summit.

DESCRIPTION

As you drive along I-10 between Phoenix and Tucson, it's impossible to miss Picacho Peak, a prominent landmark resembling a tall volcanic cone rising 1,500 feet from the desert floor. From afar, its sheer cliffs appear insurmountable. As you approach Picacho Peak State Park on the eastern flank of the mountain, however, a kinder silhouette reveals itself. Challenging and steep, Hunter Trail is the most popular hike in the park, offering close-ups of rocky cliffs and fun cable-assisted scrambles.

The Picacho Peak area also boasts a storied past as the site of the only Civil War skirmish in Arizona. The Battle of Picacho Pass occurred on April 15, 1862, between Union forces led by Captain Calloway and Lieutenant Barrett and Confederate soldiers under the command of Captain Hunter. Calloway Trail, Hunter Trail, and Barrett Loop inside Picacho Peak State Park are all named after these Civil War soldiers.

This beautiful state park is also well known for its ostentatious displays of wildflowers after rainy winters. From February through April, folks flock to Picacho's

DISTANCE & CONFIGURATION: 3-mile out-and-back

DIFFICULTY: Strenuous

SCENERY: Picacho Peak, cliffs, desert, wildflowers, plains

EXPOSURE: Mostly exposed

TRAIL TRAFFIC: Moderate

TRAIL SURFACE: Gravel, rock, cable-assisted scrambling

HIKING TIME: 2.5 hours

WATER REQUIREMENT: 2 quarts

DRIVING DISTANCE: 70 miles from Phoenix Sky Harbor Airport

ELEVATION GAIN: 1,990' at trailhead, 3,374' at highest point

ACCESS: Park open 5 a.m.–10 p.m.; trails close at sunset; $7/vehicle entry fee

MAPS: USGS *Newman Peak;* maps available at entrance and azstateparks.com/picacho /explore/maps

FACILITIES: Restrooms, drinking water, picnic areas, visitor center, horse corral, competitive track

WHEELCHAIR ACCESS: None

CONTACT: 520-466-3183, azstateparks.com /picacho

COMMENTS: Consider bringing gloves for cable-assisted scrambles. Dogs are permitted on leash, but this hike is not recommended for them due to scrambling.

foothills hoping to see a blanket of golden poppies and blue lupines. Other colorful blossoms known to grace these mountainsides include purple filaree, white desert chicory, orange globemallow, yellow fiddleneck, and crimson ocotillo. The hotter climate of early summer brings a second wave of cactus flowers.

Begin your hike from the signed trailhead on Barrett Loop inside Picacho Peak State Park. Head south on a gravel trail and wooden steps toward the mountain and its imposing cliffs. When conditions are ripe, Mexican gold poppies and flower-laden racemes of blue lupine line the trail. At 0.25 mile, the trail becomes rockier and steeper and begins to ascend switchbacks toward the base of the cliffs. Use strategically placed steel cables for balance as you climb the volcanic rocks. Out of breath? Pause at a sharp bend in the trail beyond the cabled section to survey your ascent. You'll reach the base of the massive cliffs at 0.5 mile, where overhanging rock shelters you from the elements.

Turn left and climb 0.2 mile farther to an upper cliff, whose vertical walls shoot skyward. The eastern side of the cliff overhang affords splendid views of the valley below and the freeway running through it. Then turn west and climb a gentler slope along Hunter Trail until you reach a 2,960-foot saddle, where an inviting bench beckons. Admire open views to the south, and read the informative plaques next to the bench.

The trail crosses the saddle and takes a 250-foot plunge along the base of an incredibly steep, rocky, narrow precipice. Use the cables here to help you descend, and duck your head to avoid banging it against unforgiving rocks. At 1 mile from the trailhead, you'll reach the bottom of the cabled section, where the trail hooks left and begins to regain the lost 250 feet of elevation.

Warmer and drier, the southern slope of Picacho Peak hosts more cacti and appears sparsely vegetated. Shortly after resuming your ascent, you'll pass a rock

Picacho Peak: Hunter Trail

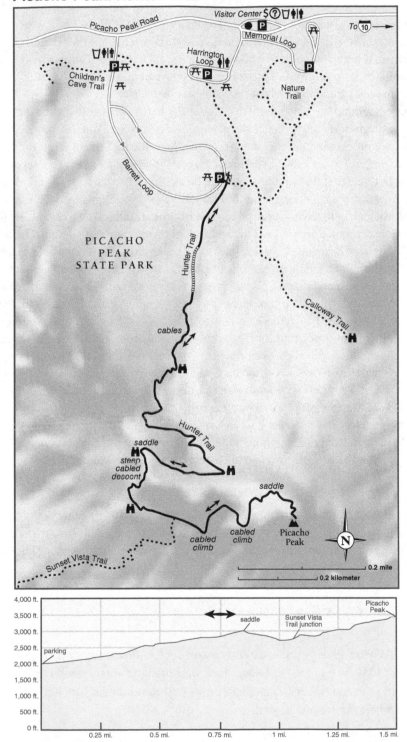

outcropping where you can enjoy a sensational view of the desert below. Hunter Trail intersects Sunset Vista Trail at 1.1 mile and soon reaches another cabled climb. Scramble up this narrow passage while hugging the rock wall, and enter a high basin full of saguaros, palo verdes, and creosotes. The overhanging cliffs from earlier in the hike are directly behind the walls of this semicircular bowl.

Contour around the upper basin to arrive at the base of yet another cabled climb. This is the toughest scramble, hence the presence of two cables. You'll clamber up the steep crevice only to find another scary section where the trail wraps around a large rock face. Rickety cables and a precariously placed wooden plank help you negotiate this part, but note that the wooden plank can be as slippery as ice when wet. I always wonder how much engineering went into the cables and metal posts driven into the rock, but they seem to have withstood the test of time. Hunter Trail was built by the Civilian Conservation Corps in 1932 to service a light beacon on the summit. The beacon has since been dismantled, leaving only a few rebar stubs as reminders of its past.

Reach the upper saddle at 1.3 miles from the trailhead and breathe a sigh of relief, because the remainder of this trail is easy and uneventful. Turn east and climb switchbacks to the wide summit of Picacho Peak, 1.5 miles from the trailhead. Park signs proclaim Hunter Trail to be 2.1 miles long, but my GPS usually doesn't lie.

From the 3,374-foot summit of Picacho Peak, you command a sweeping panorama of wide-open desert, broken only by I-10 and the Central Arizona Project canal. Newman Peak looms across the highway, and you can see the massive Catalina Mountains near Tucson on the southeastern horizon. Look for the nearly flat Table Top Mountain to the west, and the Sierra Estrellas to its right.

Return the way you came, or enjoy a longer hike around the mountain by taking Sunset Vista Trail from the junction on the southern side of the peak to Sunset Vista Point. Then hike back along the road to Barrett Loop and the Hunter Trailhead.

NEARBY ACTIVITIES

Sonoran Desert National Monument, 40 miles northwest of Picacho Peak, offers other excellent hikes, such as **Table Top Trail** (see Hike 59, page 298) and **Brittlebush Trail.** The **Catalina Mountains** north of Tucson are also a veritable haven for hikers.

• •

GPS TRAILHEAD COORDINATES N32° 38.560' W111° 24.148'

DIRECTIONS From Phoenix, take I-10 east toward Tucson. Drive southeast for 60 miles, and take Exit 219 for Picacho Peak Road. Turn west (right) to enter Picacho Peak State Park and pay the entrance fee. One-quarter mile past the entrance, turn left onto Barrett Loop, where Hunter Trail begins.

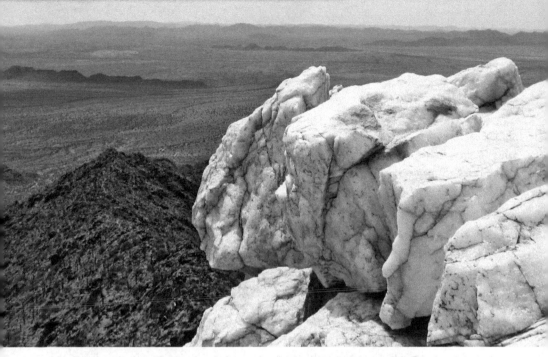

White quartz boulders adorn the summit of Quartz Peak high above Rainbow Valley.

THE PRISTINE WILDERNESS, a classic ridge walk, and expansive views from atop Quartz Peak provide plenty of rewards to those who tackle this challenging hike. This trail's remote location also ensures an absence of crowds.

DESCRIPTION

The Sierra Estrella, the broad, southwestern mountain range visible from nearly anywhere in Phoenix, captures the fancy of many hiking enthusiasts. Sierra Estrella means "mountain range of stars" in Spanish. From atop Quartz Peak, one prominent summit in the Estrellas, it certainly feels like you are gazing down from the stars. There is only one established trail in the entire mountain range—Quartz Peak Trail— but the Estrellas make up in quality what they lack in quantity.

Superbly managed by the Bureau of Land Management (BLM), Quartz Peak Trail is one of the finest desert hikes in the Phoenix area. This hike captures the rugged beauty of the 14,400-acre Sierra Estrella Wilderness and offers stunning views from high mountain ridges. Quartz Peak (4,052') provides even grander panoramas of the sprawling Phoenix metropolis.

Volcanic in nature, the Sierra Estrella range is rich in minerals. The remains of Crusher Mica Quarry lie in a small hill near the trailhead. Large white boulders cap

DISTANCE & CONFIGURATION: 6-mile out-and-back

DIFFICULTY: Strenuous

SCENERY: Pristine desert, Sierra Estrella, Butterfly Mountain, Quartz Peak, panoramic views

EXPOSURE: Mostly exposed

TRAIL TRAFFIC: Light

TRAIL SURFACE: Rock, gravel, packed dirt, some easy scrambling

HIKING TIME: 5 hours

WATER REQUIREMENT: 3–4 quarts

DRIVING DISTANCE: 52 miles from Phoenix Sky Harbor Airport

ELEVATION GAIN: 1,550' at trailhead, 4,052' on Quartz Peak summit

ACCESS: Sunrise–sunset; no permits or fees required

MAPS: USGS *Montezuma Peak;* Bureau of Land Management (BLM) *Arizona Sonoran Desert National Monument* (see avenzamaps.com /maps/488640)

FACILITIES: Toilet and picnic table, but no water

WHEELCHAIR ACCESS: None

CONTACT: BLM, 623-580-5500

COMMENTS: Very remote area; dogs permitted on leash but may not have the stamina to make it to the summit

the summit of the aptly named Quartz Peak, and one might find flaky mica crystals embedded in rocks along the trail, especially near the peak. If you happen to see a bright light near the summit as if someone's shining a mirror at you, it's likely sunlight reflecting off the shiny surface of a mica crystal.

Even though the Estrellas sit only 15 miles southwest of Phoenix, approaching Quartz Peak Trail can be an adventure that necessitates an extended drive through sandy desert terrain, since the only sanctioned access point to the trail is on the mountain's western slopes. Once there, though, hikers have the pristine desert all to themselves. The trail takes visitors up the spine of a long ridge to a quartz-covered summit 2,500 feet above the desert floor in just 3 short miles. Though very steep, Quartz Peak Trail is surprisingly manageable because it distributes the elevation gain fairly evenly over its entire length. Only the last half mile requires some scrambling and route-finding skills.

The BLM maintains Quartz Peak facilities very well, as it does most trailheads under its management. There is a large parking area and a clean toilet, but there's no water—always take plenty of extra water into a remote desert area like this. An informative plaque at the trailhead explains wilderness etiquette. Take note of the elevation profile and topographical map posted on the plaque to prepare mentally for the challenge ahead.

Begin by walking northeast, straight toward the twin peaks of Butterfly Mountain. Pass fields of teddy bear cholla, and admire stands of saguaros in the foothills. The trail initially follows an old mining road on the flat desert floor but soon turns left and begins to climb a straight, rocky path uphill. In the spring, colorful blossoms of brittlebush, phacelia, and filaree adorn the landscape, while tall saguaros stand like sentries on either side of the trail. Keep an even pace on the steep slope here because most of the hike requires the same level of effort.

Quartz Peak Trail

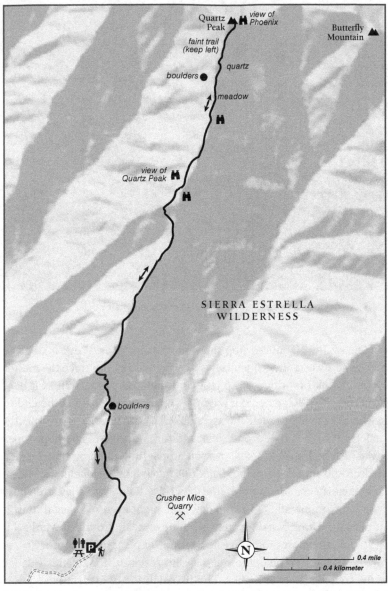

Quartz Peak
view of Phoenix

Butterfly Mountain

faint trail (keep left)

quartz

boulders

meadow

view of Quartz Peak

SIERRA ESTRELLA WILDERNESS

boulders

Crusher Mica Quarry

P

N

0.4 mile
0.4 kilometer

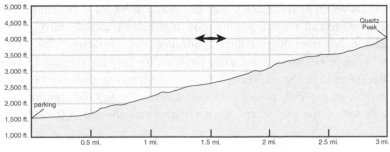

5,000 ft.
4,500 ft.
4,000 ft.
3,500 ft.
3,000 ft.
2,500 ft.
2,000 ft.
1,500 ft.
1,000 ft.

Quartz Peak

parking

0.5 mi.   1 mi.   1.5 mi.   2 mi.   2.5 mi.   3 mi.

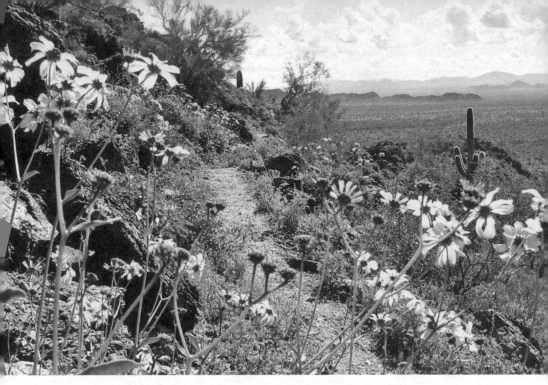

Springtime wildflowers line Quartz Peak Trail in the Sierra Estrella mountain range.

Most of Quartz Peak Trail lies atop sharp mountain ridges. Ridge hiking is especially rewarding because it offers open views to either side as you trace the mountain's spine. You'll attain the first ridge at 0.6 mile and then follow the trail as it heads to the left side of the hill. A large boulder outcropping blocks the path at the end of this short ridge where the trail turns left and ascends steep switchbacks to head north. Just beyond 1 mile, you'll reach the second ridge and turn northeast. The slope tapers off slightly for the next half mile or so, giving you ample time to enjoy this classic ridge walk. Steep drop-offs into deep ravines flank this much longer ridgeline, while jagged peaks loom in the distance. Behind you, the expansive Rainbow Valley stretches west from the base of the mountain. On a cold day, you might even see a giant mushroom cloud in the distance. Don't worry; it's only a plume of steam from Palo Verde Nuclear Generating Station, the most productive nuclear power plant in the country.

Near 1.7 miles into the hike, the steep ascent resumes. Ridge after ridge, crest after crest, the trail climbs ever higher. The first sighting of Quartz Peak pops into your peripheral vision as you reach a vista point at 2 miles from the trailhead. The unmistakable white cap on the mountaintop resembles unsightly bird droppings from a distance, but trust that it will be quite spectacular up close. The trail once again tapers in slope before reaching a tiny flat meadow atop the ridge at 2.5 miles.

The last 0.5 mile of Quartz Peak Trail is noticeably faint and may be rough in spots. However, strategically placed rock cairns mark the way. To complicate matters, there's a fork in the trail where one route heads for the top of the ridge while another skirts the hill to the left. When in doubt, just head for the ridgeline. The two paths converge later. At certain points, you'll need to scamper up the rocks, but no technical climbing skills are necessary. More and more white quartz and shiny mica crystals appear next to the trail as you near the summit.

The trail seems to end at a narrow saddle between two large boulder outcroppings just shy of 3 miles from the trailhead, and a sheer drop-off faces you. If you've been watching your feet on the rough trail over the last 0.2 mile, you might not realize that Quartz Peak is just above your head to the left. Head back down the trail about 15 feet, turn left up a rocky slope, and then scramble 20 feet to the top.

Seemingly chiseled out of blocks of snow-white stone, Quartz Peak is unique among summits near Phoenix. At an elevation of 4,052 feet, it also provides an impressive panorama. From the summit, a sweeping view opens toward Phoenix, its urban sprawl stretching as far as the eye can see beyond the Gila River Indian Reservation. From this vantage point, South Mountain appears diminutive in the distance. The twin peaks of Butterfly Mountain lie directly to the east, while Montezuma Peak, the highest point in the Estrellas, lies to the southeast. After soaking in the scenery, retrace your steps to return to the trailhead.

NEARBY ACTIVITIES

Estrella Mountain Regional Park, about 7 miles south of I-10 on Estrella Parkway, offers many hiking trails, including **Rainbow Valley** and **Butterfield** (see next hike). Farther north, **White Tank Mountain Regional Park** also provides excellent trails, such as **Ford Canyon** (see Hike 54, page 276) and **Goat Camp** (see Hike 55, page 280).

• •

GPS TRAILHEAD COORDINATES N33° 11.940' W112° 14.402'

DIRECTIONS Drive west from Phoenix on I-10, and exit onto Estrella Parkway. Drive south on Estrella Parkway 8.3 miles, and then turn west (right) onto Elliot Road. Take Elliot Road west 2.6 miles. Turn south (left) onto Rainbow Valley Road, and follow it 9.3 miles to Riggs Road. Turn east (left) onto Riggs Road; then drive 4 miles to the intersection with Bullard Avenue. Turn right and then make an immediate left onto a dirt road under the telephone poles. Follow the dirt road east 5.3 miles until it ends. Note that the last section of this road past Rainbow Rancho is narrow and sandy. At the end of the road, under large power lines, look for a small TRAIL sign, and turn right. Continue under the power lines 1.9 miles. Turn left at another TRAIL sign, and drive 1.9 miles to the trailhead.

Note: Sections of these dirt roads are rough and sandy, crossing several eroded washes. High-clearance vehicles are required.

A rare cristate saguaro cactus found along Rainbow Valley Trail in Estrella Mountain Regional Park

ESTRELLA MOUNTAIN REGIONAL PARK sits at the northern tip of the Sierra Estrella range. Many trails crisscross foothills and plains in the park, and Rainbow Valley Trail and Butterfield Trail touch nearly all of them, forming countless loops. You can customize the hike distance by choosing different return routes.

DESCRIPTION

West Phoenix hikers have several excellent mountain parks to choose from. Encompassing nearly 20,000 acres, Estrella Mountain Regional Park, on the northern tip of the Sierra Estrella range, offers everything from picnics to rodeos, from camping to fishing, and from baseball to golf. Visitors sometimes overlook the park as a hiking destination, though. There are, in fact, more than 33 miles of trails inside the park, most of them lying in the foothills and desert plains at the base of the Estrellas. These trails offer abundant views of the distant city and the rugged Sonoran Desert.

Rainbow Valley Trail, named for a huge plain west of the Sierra Estrellas, leads you on an enjoyable loop that touches several other trails. Rainbow Valley Trail, along with a combination of Toothaker, Pedersen, Gadsden, and Butterfield Trails, creates an excellent route through the park. The western half of the loop is hilly, whereas the eastern portion runs through an expansive desert valley. Although the highest peaks in the Estrellas appear jagged and rough, the foothills trails make for a moderate hike.

DISTANCE & CONFIGURATION: 8.8-mile loop

DIFFICULTY: Moderate

SCENERY: Desert, Sierra Estrella views, Rainbow Valley, Gila River access, wildlife

EXPOSURE: Completely exposed

TRAIL TRAFFIC: Light

TRAIL SURFACE: Gravel, packed dirt, sand

HIKING TIME: 5 hours

WATER REQUIREMENT: 4 quarts

DRIVING DISTANCE: 28 miles from Phoenix Sky Harbor Airport

ELEVATION GAIN: 1,020' at trailhead, 1,360' at highest point

ACCESS: Gates open 6 a.m.–8 p.m. (until 10 p.m. Friday–Saturday); trails close at sunset; $6/vehicle entry fee

MAPS: USGS *Avondale SE*; park map available at entrance and maricopacountyparks.net/maps

FACILITIES: Restrooms, water, picnic areas, youth camp, rodeo grounds

WHEELCHAIR ACCESS: Near trailhead

CONTACT: 623-932-3811, maricopacountyparks.net/park-locator/estrella-mountain-regional-park

COMMENTS: Hike may be shortened by taking alternate loops; dogs must be leashed. You're likely to encounter a few mountain bikers and equestrians on this hike.

Begin at a small trailhead on the rodeo arena's western side. The trail heads west and soon reaches a fork where Toothaker Trail veers left. Trail markers use two-letter abbreviations that match those found on the park map; the designation for Rainbow Valley Trail is RB. Keep right at the fork and continue west on Rainbow Valley Trail, which begins a gradual ascent at 0.25 mile. Typical desert plants such as creosote and palo verde line the trail and cover the slopes. Buzzing grasshoppers and darting lizards remind you that the desert is full of fauna as well as flora. At the head of the basin, the trail breaks left and climbs to a saddle a half mile from the trailhead.

As you hike up the ridge, enjoy views of the White Tank Mountains to the northwest and the peaks of the Sierra Estrellas to the southeast. The park's lush golf course resembles a desert oasis below. The Phoenix skyline lies in the distance, flanked by the familiar silhouettes of Camelback Mountain, Piestewa Peak, and Four Peaks. Winding around the north-facing hillside, this section of Rainbow Valley Trail truly earns its name in the spring when colorful wildflowers brighten the slopes. Blue lupine, azure delphinium, golden poppy, yellow brittlebush, fuchsia hedgehog cactus, white Fremont's pincushion, and purple owl clover all thrive here, often blooming concurrently.

At 1.5 miles, the trail climbs to a 1,300-foot hillcrest graced with a stunning panoramic view of the wide valley west of Phoenix. Crossing over to the drier southern slopes, you'll see the flora changes abruptly, as if you've passed through a door into the Sonoran Desert, entering the domain of cacti and creosote bushes. The trail descends a steep hill covered with loose rocks—be careful with your footing here.

In the valley below, a DS sign marks Dysart Trail at 2.1 miles from the trailhead. If you're already tired, Dysart Trail can take you back to the trailhead in 1.7 miles via Toothaker Trail. For a longer outing, continue south on Rainbow Valley Trail.

Rainbow Valley Trail begins to climb again at 2.3 miles, heading toward a gap in the hills. Reaching a high basin a half mile farther, you leave the western plains behind.

Rainbow Valley Trail and Butterfield Trail

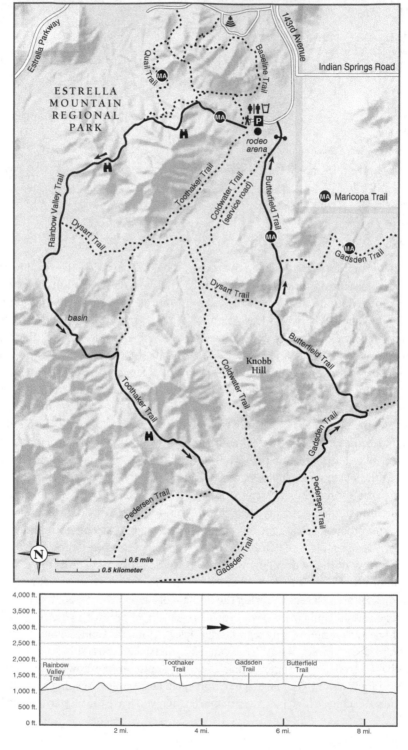

Thick grasses encroach on the trail, as this section is sometimes overgrown. Forge ahead toward the 1,350-foot saddle due east of the basin; then descend into a deep valley where you find a junction with Toothaker Trail at 3.5 miles. Again, you can turn left and head back early on Toothaker, which returns you to the trailhead in 2 miles.

To continue, turn right onto Toothaker Trail and head south across a deep wash. The trail slowly climbs again and bends southeast. At 4.1 miles, reach a flat mound with what is arguably the best view of the Sierra Estrellas' summits from anywhere on the loop. And at 1,360 feet elevation, this is also the highest point on the entire circuit. Begin a gradual descent into Rainbow Valley, where stands of saguaros dominate the landscape. Near 4.9 miles, look for an extremely rare saguaro, whose down-bent arm displays a cristate formation in its midsection. A cristate, or crested, saguaro is one that develops an abnormal growth pattern resulting in the formation of a crown on the tip of the cactus. It's rare, and rarer still to find a cristate formation in the middle of an arm.

Soon after the cristate cactus, reach the Gadsden Trail junction in a wide, sandy wash. Keep left here and hike Gadsden Trail northeast in and out of more washes. Pass Coldwater Trail at 5.4 miles from the trailhead. Then, at 5.6 miles, find the marked junction of Pedersen and Gadsden Trails. Pedersen Trail turns right—continue straight on Gadsden Trail. Hike another 0.7 mile and cross a major wash to reach Butterfield Trail.

Turn left onto Butterfield Trail, which heads back toward the rodeo arena. There are a few strenuous hills on this segment, but most of the work is now behind you. Pass the other end of Gadsden Trail at 7.8 miles from the trailhead. The remainder of the hike traces a portion of Maricopa Trail. Continue north another 0.7 mile to the end of Butterfield Trail on a wide dirt road. Follow the road north to a large parking area on the east side of the rodeo arena; then hike around the arena to return to your starting point.

NEARBY ACTIVITIES

Before you leave, consider visiting the **Gila River,** north of the park. Find a hidden passage near the park boundary fence next to the Navy Area, a signed picnic area located roughly at the northeastern corner of the park. Take the small hidden trail out of the park and across the street where a wider trail leads to the riverbanks. Gila River nourishes a wide variety of riparian plants and wildlife. You'll likely see some herons or ducks frolicking in the water—an unlikely scene in the middle of a desert.

• •

GPS TRAILHEAD COORDINATES N33° 22.222' W112° 22.358'

DIRECTIONS Drive west from Phoenix on I-10; exit onto Estrella Parkway, and follow it south 5 miles. After crossing the Gila River bridge, turn east (left) onto Vineyard and continue 0.6 mile to Estrella Mountain Regional Park. Follow the main park road about 2 miles to the rodeo grounds. Park near the trailhead, on the western side of the arena.

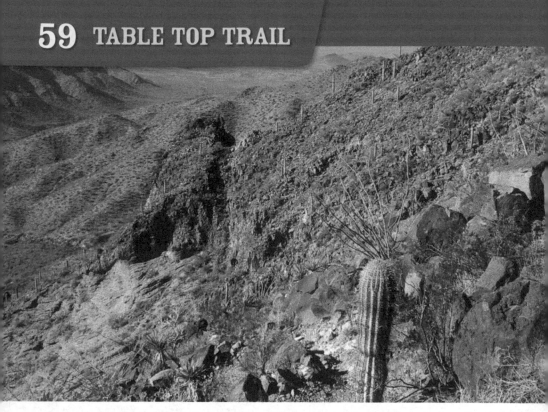

The pristine Sonoran Desert stretches for miles around Table Top Mountain.

HIKERS WHO ENJOY solitude will love this trail in Sonoran Desert National Monument. Table Top Trail offers pristine desert scenery, unobstructed panoramas, and a challenging 2,000-foot climb to the top of Table Top Mountain.

DESCRIPTION

Occupying nearly half a million acres, Sonoran Desert National Monument contains three mountain ranges, encompasses wide expanses of open desert, and hosts a large variety of indigenous flora and fauna. Table Top Mountain is the tallest point inside the preserve, and its distinctively flat peak can be seen for many miles.

The Bureau of Land Management manages all trails in the area, including Table Top Trail. This rugged and remote hike to the top of Table Top Mountain celebrates the pristine Sonoran Desert, untainted by development or overuse. It showcases forests of saguaros and ocotillos, the volcanic landscape, a historic trail with signs of ancient cultures, panoramic views, and the strange and unique grassland on Table Top's wide summit. Getting to the trailhead requires a long haul from town and considerable off-road driving in a high-clearance vehicle, but the time and effort pay off handsomely with a challenging yet rewarding hike.

As you approach Table Top Wilderness from Vekol Valley, an odd sense of complete isolation overwhelms you. When you reach the trailhead, however, civilization

DISTANCE & CONFIGURATION: 7.8-mile out-and-back

DIFFICULTY: Strenuous

SCENERY: Pristine desert, Table Top Wilderness, panoramic views

EXPOSURE: Completely exposed

TRAIL TRAFFIC: Very light

TRAIL SURFACE: Packed dirt, gravel, rock, loose rock

HIKING TIME: 4.5 hours

WATER REQUIREMENT: 3 quarts

DRIVING DISTANCE: 69 miles from Phoenix Sky Harbor Airport

ELEVATION GAIN: 2,360' at trailhead, 4,350' at Table Top Mountain

ACCESS: Sunrise–sunset; no permits or fees required

MAPS: USGS *Little Table Top;* BLM *Arizona Sonoran Desert National Monument* (see avenzamaps.com/maps/488640)

FACILITIES: Toilet, campground, picnic area, but no water

WHEELCHAIR ACCESS: None

CONTACT: BLM, 623-580-5500

COMMENTS: Very remote area; dogs must be leashed at all times

returns in the form of a surprisingly clean toilet, a small campground, and picnic facilities. Water is not available here, so bring a few extra gallons just in case.

Pick up a brochure from the trail register near the toilet, and begin hiking northeast on a wide, level dirt road. Table Top Mountain looms large ahead, and the surrounding desert offers little sound to drown out the shuffling of your feet along the trail. It's so quiet that you can almost hear your own heartbeat. Follow the flat trail as you admire forests of giant saguaros on nearby hills and dodge "land mines" left by wandering wildlife. A wooden plaque marks the official trailhead at 0.7 mile into the hike. Sign in at the trail register, and continue along the prominent trail as it bends north.

A rich variety of desert plants adorns your route. Saguaros, chollas, creosotes, prickly pears, and ocotillos. Fallen ocotillos often litter the trail, while live ones bloom with brilliant crimson flowers in spring. Cross a wide, dry wash at 0.9 mile, and follow the trail directly toward Table Top Mountain as you begin a gradual climb.

At 1.5 miles, pass a mound of twisted and layered rock. The next half mile of Table Top Trail snakes around the base of the mountain, crossing another dry wash as it approaches the foothills. Beyond 2 miles, the trail begins to climb in earnest. Smooth trail gives way to crushed rock as the vegetation becomes denser and brushier. The terrain changes abruptly at 2.3 miles as the trail merges with a dry creekbed laden with ancient river rock. Pink puffs of fairy duster blossoms can often be seen nearby.

Cross the dry wash again at 2.9 miles, and climb a bunch of loose boulders; look for a small cairn to guide you in case you lose the trail here. A quarter mile farther, the trail begins a punishing ascent up a series of switchbacks next to a large talus of volcanic rock. When negotiating the north-facing legs of the switchbacks, you'll see a large rock outcropping with a vertical cliff face directly ahead jutting out from the side of the mountain. Continue laboring up this seemingly endless climb.

At 3.7 miles, as you near the top of the mountain on loose, pale gravel, you'll notice a series of low walls constructed from stacked rocks. Similar features can be

Table Top Trail

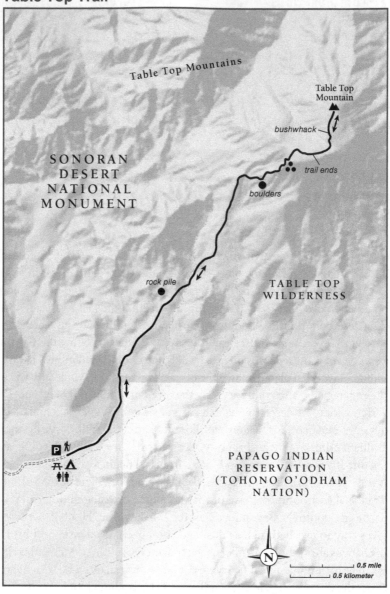

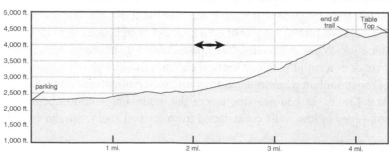

found on Elephant Mountain Trail (see Hike 45, page 232), north of Phoenix. Did the Hohokam, who inhabited central Arizona hundreds of years ago, build them? Are they wind shelters or protective walls? No one knows for sure. Hike a bit farther to reach a ridgecrest where you can see the summit. From this vantage point, it's evident that there are really two flat summits separated by a large dip in the connecting ridge.

When the trail reaches the top of Table Top Mountain, the landscape changes dramatically again. An eerie field of desert grasses, yuccas, ocotillos, and sickly-looking yellowish cacti blankets the entire plateau. Unlike the mountainsides below, the peak is entirely devoid of saguaros. Continue to Table Top Trail's terminus at an unceremonious post 3.9 miles from the trailhead. The elevation here is 4,350 feet, more than 2,000 feet higher than the parking area.

The top of the mountain yields expansive views in all directions. I-8 is just to the north, while Casa Grande and Picacho Peak lie toward the east and southeast. Looking northeast, you'll notice that the other Table Top summit is actually slightly higher than the peak at the end of the trail. If you simply must stand atop the true peak, you'll have to bushwhack through a half mile of cactus minefield toward some metal poles planted on the far summit. Given the effort required and the fact that the only sight of note on the true summit is a USGS marker, I recommend forgoing the aggravation. Return the way you came, and don't forget to sign out in the trail register.

NEARBY ACTIVITIES

The park's other remote and secluded hikes include **Brittlebush, Margie's Cove,** and **Lava Flow Trails. Picacho Peak** (see Hike 56, page 285), about 40 miles due east, is another excellent hike. A collection of rock mosaics rests near a wide turnaround about 1,000 feet west of a cairned turnoff on Vekol Valley Road, 4.7 miles south of I-8.

• •

GPS TRAILHEAD COORDINATES N32° 42.990' W112° 9.557'

DIRECTIONS Leave Phoenix on I-10 and head toward Tucson. Exit onto AZ 347, Queen Creek Road/Maricopa Road, and follow it south for 29 miles until it reaches a T-junction with AZ 84. Take AZ 84 west (right) 6 miles to I-8. Continue 7 miles west on I-8, and take Exit 144 onto Vekol Valley Road. Turn left as if to get on eastbound I-8, but take the turnoff to Vekol Valley Road before you reach the on-ramp. Reset your odometer here and continue south on Vekol Valley Road, which soon becomes a dirt road. At 2.1 miles, stay right at the Vekol Ranch turnoff, and follow the TRAIL signs. At 11.3 miles, turn east (left) across a large cattle guard onto a smaller dirt road. Follow this rough road another 4.3 miles to the trailhead parking, staying to the right at any forks in the road. *Note:* A high-clearance vehicle is necessary to reach the trailhead.

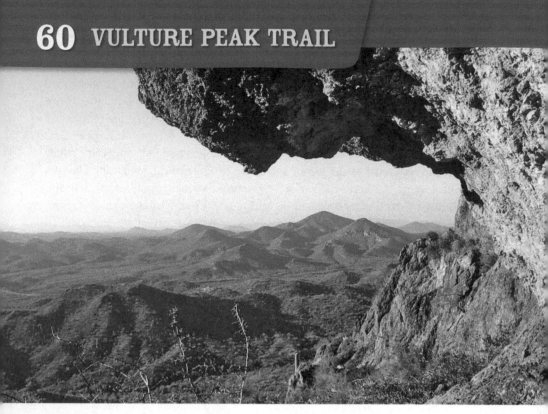

A rocky overhang on Vulture Peak Trail frames the distant desert foothills.

THOUGH LOCATED IN a remote area, iconic Vulture Peak attracts plenty of visitors. This challenging trail takes hikers to a prominent saddle point overlooking expansive desert wilderness. Experienced hikers can scramble up another 240 feet to the summit for an even more impressive panoramic view.

DESCRIPTION

When you arrive at the Vulture Peak Trailhead in the middle of the desert, it's difficult to believe that this remote mountain and the nearby Vulture Mine played key roles in the births of Wickenburg and Phoenix. Back in 1863, a German immigrant and prospector named Henry Wickenburg struck gold and founded Vulture Mine, which became one of the most successful gold mines in Arizona history. One of the financiers for the stamp-mill operation that processed ore from Vulture Mine was Michael Goldwater, the grandfather of the legendary Arizona lawmaker Barry Goldwater. Henry Wickenburg also provided financing for a young entrepreneur named Jack Swilling, who used the funds to excavate and improve irrigation canals left by the ancient Hohokam people along the Salt River.

The resulting community spawned by Swilling's canals was named Phoenix because it allegorically arose from the ashes of the ancient civilization it supplanted. Wickenburg worked Vulture Mine for a few years but then sold it to a man named

DISTANCE & CONFIGURATION: 4.2-mile out-and-back

DIFFICULTY: Moderate

SCENERY: Pristine desert wilderness, Vulture Peak, mountain vistas

EXPOSURE: Limited shade near summit; otherwise exposed

TRAIL TRAFFIC: Moderate

TRAIL SURFACE: Packed dirt, gravel, optional scrambling near summit

HIKING TIME: 3 hours

WATER REQUIREMENT: 2 quarts

DRIVING DISTANCE: 75 miles from Phoenix Sky Harbor Airport

ELEVATION GAIN: 2,490' at trailhead, 3,658' on Vulture Peak summit

ACCESS: Sunrise–sunset; no permits or fees required

MAPS: USGS *Vulture Peak;* BLM *Arizona Sonoran Desert National Monument* (see avenzamaps.com /maps/488640)

FACILITIES: Shaded ramada, restrooms, and picnic area, but no water

WHEELCHAIR ACCESS: None

CONTACT: 602-506-2930, maricopacountyparks .net/vulture-mountains-recreation-area

COMMENTS: Beautiful desert hike away from it all, yet popular among Wickenburg locals; dogs must be leashed at all times

Phelps and retired near a settlement that eventually became the town of Wickenburg. Phelps's name is still one of the most recognizable in the Arizona mining industry.

From the town of Wickenburg, Vulture Peak resembles a giant thimble protruding high above the desert floor. This distinctive profile appears imposing and unconquerable, but it is merely an illusion caused by the foreshortening of the summit's true form. When viewed from the trailhead west of the mountain, one can see that Vulture Peak actually sits on a long ridge, challenging but definitely attainable.

Maricopa County Parks is working with the Bureau of Land Management to develop a recreation area here. As it stands, there are two departure points for this hike: the main trailhead near Vulture Mine Road and an upper trailhead accessible only by high-clearance off-road vehicles. Should you choose to drive the 1.25 miles to the upper trailhead, make sure that you bring a capable off-road vehicle and some steady nerves: the primitive dirt road is very rough in spots, and there are plenty of places where protruding rocks aim to puncture the floor pans and damage the underbody components of unworthy vehicles. Climbing over a 50-foot dirt berm and traversing sandy Syndicate Wash will also challenge your vehicle's all-terrain capabilities. Four-wheeling enthusiasts may enjoy this drive even more than the hike!

In stark contrast to the nerve-wracking off-road adventure, hiking to the upper trailhead is an exercise in tranquility. A pleasant stroll in the pristine desert, this trek measures 1.4 miles and gains only 150 feet. Enjoy up-close views of the hardy flora that thrives in this arid climate. Desert plants adapt to the environment well and respond quickly to the limited amount of rainfall. After seasonal storms, the desert seemingly changes overnight into a lush green landscape full of new life. In the spring, golden flowers—from Mexican poppies, brittlebushes, and palo verdes—blanket the foothills.

The trail begins from a gap in the fence near the picnic tables and enters a desert wonderland of saguaros and teddy bear cholla. A pair of benches near 0.2 mile

Vulture Peak Trail

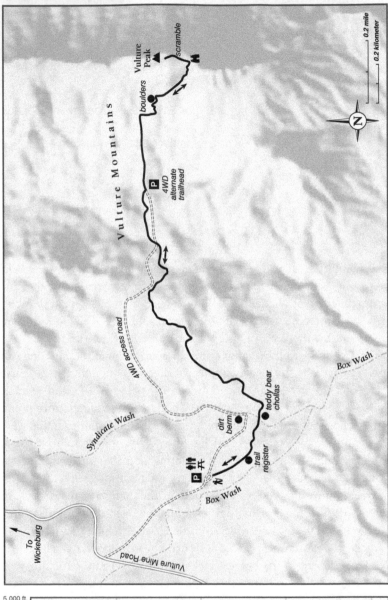

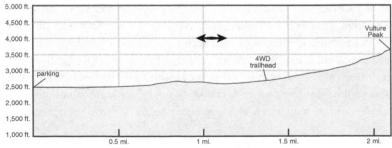

provide a scenic rest area to gaze at Vulture Peak. From here, descend into and cross Syndicate Wash. Continue hiking through unspoiled desert foothills and climb a moderate hill at 0.7 mile. The trail snakes around gentle slopes and once again enters a dry wash at 1.1 miles. This time, stay in the wash and follow the trail signs until you eventually cross the dirt road leading to the upper trailhead. At 1.4 miles, the trail converges with the road at the upper trailhead.

The remainder of the hike to Vulture Peak is notably steeper and considerably more challenging than the stretch along the desert floor. Begin by crossing an equestrian barrier and head east straight toward the mountain. The trail initially remains flat among classic Sonoran Desert brush but soon begins to increase its slope as it nears the base of the mountain. At 1.7 miles from the main trailhead, the trail bends south and starts to climb in earnest as it ascends some zigzagging switchbacks.

As you climb higher, turn around occasionally to admire the valley below and the unbroken expanse of desert hills to the west. It's easy to understand why this hike is a favorite among Wickenburg residents. Near 1.8 miles the trail ducks around the base of a large rock outcropping at 3,070 feet elevation to mount a steep climbing traverse toward a gulley at the base of the summit saddle. Pick your way through some bushes as the trail enters the ravine, which provides some cool shade during hot summer months. Forge ahead up the final section of tight switchbacks to a saddle at 2 miles from the main trailhead.

The view improves dramatically when you reach the 3,420-foot saddle because you can now see toward the east as well as the west. Casual hikers should stop here and make this spot their turnaround point. More experienced adventure seekers can continue climbing north to the 3,663-foot summit of Vulture Peak. The final stretch is short but requires scrambling up a steep, rocky crevice. From the wide summit of Vulture Peak, sweeping panoramic vistas will take your breath away. Break out the snacks, and soak in unobstructed views of the surrounding desert and the town of Wickenburg. Don't forget to sign the summit log before returning the way you came.

NEARBY ACTIVITIES

Hassayampa River Preserve (nature.org), a Nature Conservancy preserve near Wickenburg, offers guided nature walks and the opportunity to see unique plants and wildlife. Historic and rustic **Vulture Mine** (vultureminetours.com), 5 miles south of Vulture Peak Trail, offers self-guided tours of the remaining buildings and the mine site.

(Continued on next page)

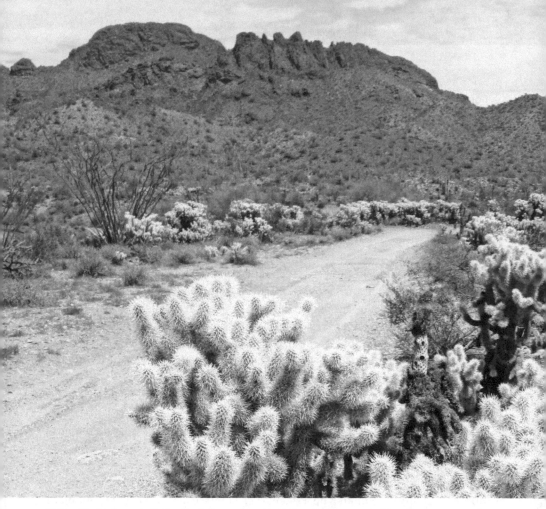

Fields of teddy bear cholla line the 4x4 access road to Vulture Peak's upper trailhead.

· ·

GPS TRAILHEAD COORDINATES N33° 52.628' W112° 49.045'

DIRECTIONS Drive to the town of Wickenburg, 50 miles northwest of Phoenix via US 60, or take I-17 north, AZ 74 west, and then US 60 west. From the junction of US 60 and US 93 in Wickenburg, continue west 2.5 miles on US 60; then turn south (left) onto Vulture Mine Road. Proceed 7 miles—do *not* take the Vulture Peak Road turnoff—and then turn east (left) into Vulture Peak Trailhead between mile markers 19 and 20. Continue 0.4 mile to the main trailhead. High-clearance four-wheel-drive vehicles can follow a very rough dirt road 1.25 miles to the upper trailhead.

APPENDIX A: Hiking Stores

ARIZONA HIKING SHACK
hikingshack.com

- 3244 E. Thomas Road
  Phoenix, AZ 85018 • **602-944-7723**

BIG 5 SPORTING GOODS
big5sportinggoods.com

- 10745 E. Main St.
  Apache Junction, AZ 85220 • **480-357-0162**

- 1623 N. Dysart Road
  Avondale, AZ 85323 • **623-535-0384**

- 2050 N. Arizona Ave.
  Chandler, AZ 85225 • **480-821-9226**

- 4180 S. Arizona Ave., Ste. 3
  Chandler, AZ 85248 • **480-812-8926**

- 965 S. Val Vista Drive
  Gilbert, AZ 85296 • **480-892-2043**

- 5490 W. Bell Road, Ste. A
  Glendale, AZ 85308 • **602-548-5794**

- 41800 W. Maricopa–Casa Grande Highway
  Maricopa, AZ 85138 • **520-217-3231**

- 1244 S. Gilbert Road, Ste. 101
  Mesa, AZ 85204 • **480-507-0137**

- 2930 N. Power Road
  Mesa, AZ 85215 • **480-854-1889**

- 10030 N. 91st Ave.
  Peoria, AZ 85345 • **623-878-0399**

- 1717 W. Bethany Home Road
  Phoenix, AZ 85015 • **602-242-1806**

- 3560 E. Thomas Road
  Phoenix, AZ 85018 • **602-955-9601**

- 1919 W. Bell Road
  Phoenix, AZ 85023 • **602-863-1309**

- 4623 E. Cactus Road
  Phoenix, AZ 85032 • **602-953-0305**

- 7710 W. Thomas Road
  Phoenix, AZ 85033 • **623-848-4800**

- 3610 W. Baseline Road, Ste. B2
  Phoenix, AZ 85041 • **602-237-9080**

- 4722 E. Ray Road
  Phoenix, AZ 85044 • **480-783-4800**

- 10202 Metro Parkway W.
  Phoenix, AZ 85051 • **602-674-3189**

- 34648 N. Valley Parkway, Ste. 130
  Phoenix, AZ 85086 • **623-581-0402**

- 3330 Hayden Road
  Scottsdale, AZ 85251 • **480-941-4387**

- 14987 N. Northsight Blvd.
  Scottsdale, AZ 85260 • **480-948-9277**

- 12801 W. Bell Road, Ste. 125
  Surprise, AZ 85374 • **623-974-3043**

- 921 E. Southern Ave.
  Tempe, AZ 85282 • **480-491-4511**

BLUE PLANET OUTDOORS
blueplanetoutdoors.com

- 44 S. San Marcos Place
  Chandler, AZ 85225 • **480-525-6189**

COLUMBIA SPORTSWEAR OUTLET STORE
columbia.com

- 4976 Premium Outlets Way
  Chandler, AZ 85226 • **480-426-7232**

CABELA'S
cabelas.com

- 9380 W. Glendale Ave.
  Glendale, AZ 85305 • **623-872-6700**

DICK'S SPORTING GOODS
dickssportinggoods.com

- 2269 San Tan Village Parkway
  Gilbert, AZ 85295 • **480-899-3993**

- 7680 W. Arrowhead Towne Center
  Glendale, AZ 85308 • **623-334-8366**

- 7000 E. Mayo Blvd.
  Phoenix, AZ 85054 • **480-212-0260**

DICK'S SPORTING GOODS *(continued)*

- 2350 W. HAPPY VALLEY ROAD
  Phoenix, AZ 85085 • 623-434-3388

- 7014 E. Camelback Road, Ste. Anc 03
  Scottsdale, AZ 85251 • 480-240-4409

- 8550 S. Emerald Drive
  Tempe, AZ 85284 • 480-592-0938

iRUN
irunshop.com

- 4730 E. Indian School Road
  Phoenix, AZ 85018 • 602-368-5330

**LOWERGEAR OUTDOOR
RENTALS AND SALES**
lowergear.com

- 2155 E. University Drive, Ste. 107
  Tempe, AZ 85281 • 480-348-8917

MERRELL
merrell.com

- 4976 Premium Outlets Way
  Chandler, AZ 85226 • 480-639-1779

REI
rei.com

- 870 N. 54th St.
  Chandler, AZ 85226 • 480-940-4006

- 12634 N. Paradise Village Parkway
  Phoenix, AZ 85032 • 602-996-5400

ORVIS
orvis.com

- 2011 E. Camelback Road, Ste. C10
  Phoenix, AZ 85016 • 602-626-7558

SPORTSMAN'S WAREHOUSE
sportsmanswarehouse.com

- 10145 W. McDowell Road
  Avondale, AZ 85392 • 623-745-0700

- 19205 N. 27th Ave.
  Phoenix, AZ 85027 • 623-516-1400

- 1750 S. Greenfield Road
  Mesa, AZ 85206 • 480-558-1111

APPENDIX B: Sources for Trail Maps

MAPS & FACTS UNLIMITED
powermaps.com

- 2525 E. Arizona Biltmore Circle, Ste. c131
  Phoenix, AZ 85016 • 602-381-6883

HOLMAN'S, INC.
holmans.com

- 1403 W. 10th Place
  Tempe, AZ 85281 • 480-967-0032

NAVTEQ
navteq.com

- 4700 S. McClintock Drive, Ste. 190
  Tempe, AZ 85282 • 480-615-7787

REI
rei.com

- 870 N. 54th St.
  Chandler, AZ 85226 • 480-940-4006

- 12634 N. Paradise Village Parkway
  Phoenix, AZ 85032 • 602-996-5400

U.S. FOREST SERVICE
www.fs.usda.gov

PRESCOTT NATIONAL FOREST
www.fs.usda.gov/prescott

- Bradshaw Ranger District
  344 S. Cortez St.
  Prescott, AZ 86303 • 928-443-8000

TONTO NATIONAL FOREST
www.fs.usda.gov/tonto

- Cave Creek Ranger District
  40202 N. Cave Creek Road
  Scottsdale, AZ 85262 • 480-595-3300

- Mesa Ranger District
  5140 E. Ingram St.
  Mesa, AZ 85205 • 480-610-3300

U.S. GEOLOGICAL SURVEY
nationalmap.gov/ustopo,
store.usgs.gov

WIDE WORLD OF MAPS
maps4u.com

- 2133 E. Indian School Road
  Phoenix, AZ 85016 • 602-279-2323, ext. 1

- 17232 N. Cave Creek Road
  Phoenix, AZ 85032 • 602-279-2323, ext. 3

- 2155 E. University Drive
  Tempe, AZ 85281 • 602-279-2323, ext. 4

APPENDIX C: Hiking Clubs and Organizations

ARIZONA BACKPACKING CLUB
meetup.com/arizona-backpacking

ARIZONA DESERT HIKERS
meetup.com/arizona-desert-hikers

**ARIZONA HIKING & OUTDOOR
TRAIL EXPLORERS**
meetup.com/ahote-hiking

ARIZONA MOUNTAINEERING CLUB
arizonamountaineeringclub.org
meetup.com/arizona-mountaineering-club

ARIZONA HIKING AND TRAVEL CLUB
azotc.com

ARIZONA TRAIL ASSOCIATION
aztrail.org

ARIZONA TRAIL BLAZERS
azhikers.org

**BACKPACKING, CANYONEERING,
& HIKING CLUB**
meetup.com/bchclub

EARLY RISE HIKERS
meetup.com/early-rise-hikers

FRIENDS HIKING CLUB
friendshiking.com

GLENDALE HIKING CLUB
glendaleazhikingclub.org

HIKING HIKERS HIKING GROUP
meetup.com/threeh

PHOENIX (2-HOUR) BEGINNER HIKERS
meetup.com/phoenix-beginner-hikers

**SIERRA CLUB, ARIZONA
GRAND CANYON CHAPTER**
arizona.sierraclub.org

SOUTHWEST OUTDOOR CLUB
groups.yahoo.com/group/soctempe

TAKE-A-HIKE ARIZONA
meetup.com/take-a-hike

TLC HIKING GROUP
meetup.com/tlc-hiking-group

TRAIL MIX HIKING
meetup.com/trail-mix-hiking

WANDERING SOLES HIKING CLUB
meetup.com/wandering-soles-hiking

GLOSSARY

ARROYO A deep gulley cut by an intermittent stream; a dry gulch.

BALLOON A hike configuration composed of a loop and an out-and-back section.

BELAY To secure a rope to a rock or other projection, or to a partner, during climbing.

BERM A natural or man-made raised bank of earth that forms a low ridge.

BOULDERING Basic or intermediate climbing, practiced, usually without rope, on relatively small rocks that can be traversed without great risk of bodily harm in case of a fall.

BUSHWHACKING General term for traveling off-trail, though such travel doesn't necessarily involve going through bushes.

CAIRN A stack of rocks created as trail markers or as a memorial. Hikers often construct cairns to mark the way on faint trails.

CANYONEERING A sport in which participants travel within a canyon, involving a combination of hiking, swimming, scrambling, climbing, and rappelling. Also known as *canyoning*.

CLASS + NUMBER A reference to the Yosemite Decimal System (see entry on next page) for ranking the difficulty of climbs, i.e., Classes 1–5.

DEADFALL Downed trees or brush obstructing a trail.

DESERT VARNISH A thin layer of clay minerals and manganese oxides, activated by bacteria over thousands of years, that imparts a bronze or dark-brown color on exposed surfaces of rocks and boulders in the desert. Also known as *rock varnish* or *patina*.

EXPOSURE The potential for physical harm in the event of a fall.

FOURTEENER Popular nickname for a mountain whose summit elevation exceeds 14,000 feet. Within the 48 contiguous US states, there are 54 such peaks in Colorado, 15 in California, and 1 in Washington State.

HOODOO A strangely eroded rock column, usually found in clusters.

JAVELINA A small wild hog (*Tayassu tajacu*) with a range from the Southwest United States to northern Argentina, having a gray and black coat with a white band from the back to the chest. Also known as a *collared peccary*.

MOUNTAINEERING The sport of climbing mountains. Often refers to technical ascents involving roped climbs or glacier traversal.

ORIENTEERING A cross-country race in which competitors use a map and compass to navigate between checkpoints along an unfamiliar course.

PATINA See Desert Varnish, above.

PETROGLYPH A carving or line drawing on rock, especially one made by prehistoric people.

RAMADA An open or semienclosed permanent shelter designed to provide shade, often covering benches, picnic tables, and grills.

RIPARIAN ZONE Vegetation corridors adjacent to streams or rivers.

SCREE Loose rock debris.

SHALE A fissile rock composed of layers of claylike, fine-grained sediments.

TALUS A sloping mass of rock debris at the base of a cliff.

USE TRAIL An unofficial trail that develops from frequent foot traffic.

YOSEMITE DECIMAL SYSTEM A popular rating system used to rank the difficulty of climbs. Classes 1–4 do not require ropes, while Class 5 has subdivisions between 5.0 and 5.13 for increasing difficulty of technical climbing. For purposes of this book, Class 1 means hiking on a trail, and Class 2 means some route-finding is necessary and the hiker may need to use hands for balance. Class 3 requires scrambling over rocks or obstacles, and Class 4 indicates a very steep, exposed, and potentially hazardous scramble requiring climbing skills. Ropes and belays may be used for safety on Class 4 routes. (There are no Class 5 routes in this book.)

INDEX

ABOUT THE AUTHOR

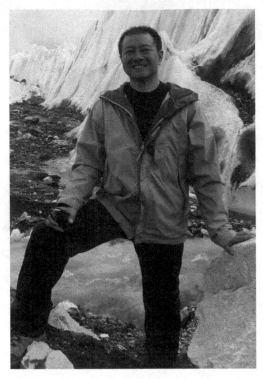

Charles at Mount Everest base camp

CHARLES LIU immigrated to the United States from China in 1980 and settled in a suburb of Phoenix with his extended family. During his formative years at Arizona State University, Charles grew increasingly fond of the Grand Canyon State's diverse outdoor offerings. Hiking quickly became his passion; in particular, he adopted a keen preference for challenging day hikes and alpine mountaineering. An avid outdoorsman and active member of several hiking clubs and creator of his own hiking group, Charles has led countless hikes over the years, including annual treks to the depths of the Grand Canyon and to the 12,633-foot summit of Humphreys Peak, Arizona's highest point.

An engineer by trade, Charles spends much of his spare time hiking, photographing, and writing about trails in and around Phoenix. He can often be found racing up Camelback Mountain after work, relieving stress from a high-tech career, or traipsing through the Superstition Wilderness on weekends.

Aptly nicknamed "Mad Hiker," Charles finds fulfillment in tough hiking challenges. He has recently conquered Mount Whitney in California, Mount Rainier in Washington, and all of Colorado's 58 "fourteeners." He has also climbed challenging peaks worldwide, including Kilimanjaro, Aconcagua, and Elbrus. Charles's extensive hiking experience, attention to detail, and passion for hiking make him an ideal trail guide for the 60 Hikes Within 60 Miles series.

To contact Charles with comments or suggestions, email him at madhiker @gmail.com or visit his website, madhiker.org/6060.

CPSIA information can be obtained
at www.ICGtesting.com
Printed in the USA
LVHW020507301220
675362LV00001B/1

9 781634 040747